Therapeutic Communities

Therapeutic Communities:
reflections and progress

Edited by
R. D. Hinshelwood and Nick Manning

ROUTLEDGE & KEGAN PAUL
London, Boston and Henley

First published in 1979
by Routledge & Kegan Paul Ltd
39 Store Street, London WC1E 7DD,
Broadway House, Newtown Road,
Henley-on-Thames, Oxon RG9 1EN and
9 Park Street, Boston, Mass. 02108, USA
Set in 10/11 Press Roman by
Hope Services, Abingdon
and printed in Great Britain by
Lowe & Brydone Ltd
Thetford, Norfolk

British Library Cataloguing in Publication Data

Therapeutic communities.

1. Therapeutic community – Great Britain
– Addresses, essays, lectures
I. Hinshelwood, R D II. Manning, Nick
362.2'0425   RC489.T67   78-40987

ISBN 0 7100 0109 6
ISBN 0 7100 0108 8 Pbk

Contents

Contents

Biographies

Colin Archer   A former Administrative Officer with the London County Council Children's Department, later trained in community work at the National Institute for Social Work. Since 1971 he has been Assistant Director (Community Services) with the Social Services Department of the Royal Borough of Kensington and Chelsea.

Joel Badaines, PhD   A clinical psychologist trained in the USA. Before coming to London in 1972, he worked for two years in a half-way house for people (adults and adolescents) coming out of mental hospital in Texas. He came to London to direct the training house of the Richmond Fellowship (an organization which runs a variety of therapeutic communities). In 1975 he became a groupwork adviser to a London Borough Social Services Department and worked freelance as a groupwork consultant. Since 1977 he has done that on a full-time basis and leads groups for Growth Centres in Britain and Europe, specializing in sensitivity and relationship groups as well as psychodrama. He has run training groups and published several articles on psychodrama. He also maintains a private practice in individual and group psychotherapy.

Jeff Bishop   Qualified as an architect and worked in private practice. During this time was architect to the Friends of a psychiatric unit. Moved to Kingston Polytechnic to teach and research, working on a study of a day unit, perception and environmental education. Now at the School for Advanced Urban Studies, Bristol.

Raymond Blake   Following a training in and short practice of individual psychotherapy, including working with R.D. Laing, he moved to the therapeutic community model, supervising a range of residential communities. He then applied the therapeutic community model to psychiatric day care in the social services of Kensington and Chelsea, with the accent on co-ordinating Health and Social Services.

Anna Christian Trained at the London School of Occupational Therapy. Head occupational therapist, Marlborough Hospital therapeutic community for eight and a half years. At present occupational therapy consultant and project officer for the Mental Health Association (MIND) for Kensington and Chelsea. Interested in the development of realistic work groups (creative, administrative, etc.) for therapeutic as well as preventive purposes.

Richard Crocket, MD, FRCP (Edinburgh and Glasgow), FRCPsych, DPM Scottish psychiatrist, trained in Glasgow and Edinburgh before and after 1939-45 war. Five years in the RAF. Psychiatrist at Leeds University for four years, specializing in psychosomatic medicine and psychotherapy. Since 1954 in charge of the Ingrebourne Centre, Hornchurch, Essex, where he has been facilitating therapeutic community procedures in a district general hospital, and contributed latterly to structuralist theory as a basis for integrating sociology and psychotherapy.

Anne Crozier Formerly a patient at Marlborough Hospital for eighteen months.

Angela Foster Has a Master's degree in social work from the London School of Economics. She was Assistant Director of Phoenix House, and has been working at the Marlborough Hospital for four years. She also teaches on the social work course at North London Polytechnic and is staff consultant for LINK, a residential project for young adults.

Marta Ginzburg, MA A clinical psychologist who trained and worked in Argentina. She lived in Israel, where she worked with immigrant adolescents and their families. She has been living in London since 1972 and has worked in drug rehabilitation and as an advisor in groupwork for a social services department. At present, Ms Ginzburg leads workshops for various Growth Centres in Britain and Europe, and is involved in leading a psychodrama training programme. She also is a staff consultant to a number of helping and counselling organizations as well as to various university programmes; Ms Ginzburg is also a psychotherapist.

Sheena Grunberg Graduated in psychology in 1964 at Edinburgh University. Trained as Educational Psychologist in Leicester, 1964-8. Began groupwork in 1968, first in Social Psychiatry with Joshua Bierer, 1968-70. Subsequently studied at the Institute of Group Analysis (London) and qualified as Group Analyst in 1975. Studied Rorschach, psychotherapeutic skills at Tavistock Clinic from 1968 to 1971. Member of the Association of Therapeutic Communities. At present working at

Marlborough Day Hospital as Senior Clinical Psychologist. Member of British Psychological Society.

Brian Haddon Born 1940. 1966, general nurse, then postgraduate psychiatric nurse training. 1968, staff nurse for one year at Roffey Park Hospital, then charge nurse for three years at Paddington Day Hospital, and nursing officer for one and a half years at Shrodells psychiatric unit, Watford. 1973, resigned from the Health Service. After three months as temporary charge nurse at Henderson Hospital, joined Surrey Community Development Trust Ltd as a community worker and company secretary–book keeper. 1972-3, treasurer of the Association of Therapeutic Communities, and editor of the *ATC Bulletin*. In 1977 he worked for a diploma in advanced studies in community education.

Peter Hawkins Director of St Charles House, Kensington, which is the training house for the Richmond Fellowship (an international organization for running half-way-house therapeutic communities and for mental health education). Works also in freelance teaching of group work and drama-therapy, and is researching the ways in which various communities facilitate self-learning.

R.D. Hinshelwood Psychoanalyst, Consultant Psychotherapist at St Bernard's Hospital, Consultant Psychiatrist to Royal Borough of Kensington and Chelsea, with seven years' experience in orientating a day community along therapeutic community lines at the Marlborough Hospital. Currently with a finger in various therapeutic community pies (St Luke's Project, Denbigh Project, Connolly Unit). Editor of the *ATC Bulletin*.

Bob Hobson, BA, MD, FRCPsych, DPM Consultant Psychotherapist, Manchester Royal Infirmary and University Hospital of South Manchester. Honorary Reader in Psychotherapy, University of Manchester. Regional Adviser on Training in Psychotherapy. Training Analyst, Society of Analytical Psychology. Founder member of Association of Therapeutic Communities.

Maxwell Jones One of the pioneers of the therapeutic community, he developed his early ideas running an effort-syndrome unit during the war. With backing from the Ministry of Labour he opened a unit for rehabilitating the unemployed at Belmont Hospital in 1947. This developed subsequently into a specialist facility for treating 'psychopaths' with group and community methods; it became Henderson Hospital in 1960. At this time Maxwell Jones left for a short spell in the

USA, returning to Dingleton Hospital, Melrose, Scotland, in 1962. Here he facilitated the decentralization of the hospital and its extension out into the community, through crisis intervention. Returning to the USA in 1969, he has recently devoted himself to applying his experience of social change in psychiatric hospitals in wider fields, especially education. Maxwell Jones has not only accomplished a great deal in his long career, but also committed many of his ideas to paper; a selection of his writings appears in the bibliography.

David Kennard   Studied psychology at Manchester University, trained in clinical psychology, and since 1970 has worked at Littlemore Hospital, Oxford. He has carried out research into aspects of patient change in therapeutic communities, and is at present training to become a group analyst. For the past two years he has been convenor of the Training Group of the Association of Therapeutic Communities.

Janine D. Kirk   Gained an MA in Modern History at St Hilda's College, Oxford, in 1970. Trainee mental health social worker for the London Borough of Greenwich, 1970-1. Unqualified social worker, Bedfordshire, 1971-3. Gained MSc in Applied Social Studies /CQSW, Department of Applied Social Studies, Oxford University, 1975. Worked as a social worker for the London Borough of Wandsworth, 1975-7. Interested in working with adolescents and residential work.

Nick Mahony   Meet me in Chapter 9.

Nick Manning   MA in Economics, and Social and Political Sciences at Emmanuel College, Cambridge, 1971. MPhil, University of York, 1975. 1972-3, research assistant, Health Services Unit, department of Social Administration, University of York. 1973-4, research sociologist, Henderson Hospital. Since 1974 lecturer, Faculty of Social Sciences, University of Kent at Canterbury. Has written several articles on the therapeutic community, and is preparing a book on the sociology of the therapeutic community movement. He is interested too in comparative social policy studies, and is preparing a book on the Soviet social welfare system.

Alan Mawson   Consultant Psychiatrist to the therapeutic community at the Marlborough Hospital. He also has Consultant Psychotherapist sessions at the Tavistock Clinic. He was previously at the Maudsley Hospital for six years, and is a Psychoanalyst. He has written on a variety of topics from behaviour therapy and research methodology to psychoanalysis and creativity.

Isabel Menzies   Gained an MA in Economics and Psychology at St Andrews University. She practised psychoanalysis with adults and children, and is a Fellow of the British Psychological Society. After lecturing in Economics at St Andrews and working as a psychologist with the army during the war, she joined the Tavistock Clinic in 1946, retiring in 1976. Since 1954 she has practised psychoanalysis privately. She rejoined the Tavistock in 1977. Her work at the Tavistock has been mainly on institutions for children of various ages.

David W. Millard   A lecturer in Applied Social Studies, University of Oxford, and Honorary Consultant Psychiatrist, the Warneford Hospital.

J.K.W. Morrice   Consultant Psychiatrist and Clinical Senior Lecturer, Aberdeen, for the past ten years. Runs day hospital, Ross Clinic, as a therapeutic community. Also interested in rehabilitation of long-stay patients. Previously at Dingleton Hospital and Fort Logan, Denver. One time Visiting Psychiatrist, Edinburgh Prison. Author of *Crisis Intervention: Studies in Community Care.*

Ken Myers, BSc, MB, BCh, MRCPsych, DPM   Born in London, 1929. School and Medical School in South Wales. Following army service in the Far East, started psychiatric training at Whitchurch Hospital, Cardiff, and subsequently Fulbourn Hospital, Cambridge. After three years of research into the effects of therapeutic community treatment at Fulbourn, appointed Consultant Psychiatrist at Middlewood Hospital, Sheffield, in 1969. Publications on drug addiction and therapeutic communities.

Malcolm Pines, FRCP, FRCPsych, DPM   Consultant Psychotherapist, Maudsley Hospital; President of Group Analytic Society, London; Member, Institute of Psychoanalysis, London; Member, Institute of Group Analysis, London. Formerly Senior Lecturer in Psychotherapy, St George's Hospital. Consultant Psychotherapist, Cassel Hospital. Founder member of the Association of Therapeutic Communities.

Stuart Whiteley   The Medical Director of Henderson Hospital, where his twin interests of group treatments in psychiatry and the exploration of psychopathic disorder came together. He is a member of the Group Analytic Society and a founder member of the Association of Therapeutic Communities, of which he was Secretary from 1971 to 1978.

Stephen Wilson   Qualified in medicine from the Royal Free Hospital in 1968. He specialized in psychiatry at Fulbourn Hospital, Cambridge, and studied medical sociology in London. Since 1973 he has worked at Littlemore Hospital, Oxford, researching into aspects of the therapeutic community and practising psychotherapy.

Preface

This book explores a major difficulty in therapeutic community work
− that of the tension between innovation and routine, between discovery
and management. This, of course, is a classic sociological problem discussed by Max Weber, and to this extent therapeutic communities illustrate quite clearly many of the processes surrounding other social innovations which have developed into social movements (Manning,
1976a).

Many therapeutic community innovators pushed their ideas and
communities into new, and little-explored, social psychiatric territory
in the 1960s. Since then progress within the therapeutic community
movement has not been innovatory so much as extending geographically and numerically. Inevitably this has brought about issues of standardization and conformity − the antithesis of innovation. As the nature
of therapeutic communities is to explore and to give freedom to the
individual to innovate within his own life and circumstances, the direction of the movement as a whole (towards standardization) conflicts
with the aims of the therapeutic community method. This dilemma
characterizes the state of the therapeutic community movement in the
1970s.

In this book the tension between innovation and routine is explored
as an important dilemma for the movement as a whole; as a difficulty
that appears in the life of the communities themselves; as a sociological
phenomenon in the development and change in organizations; and as an
example of the relationship between new medical and psychiatric
treatments and older, standardized ones.

This collection contains many articles previously published in the
Bulletin of the Association of Therapeutic Communities, or presented
at the Association Conferences. The establishment of the Association in
1972 (there are now over 300 members) marked a step forward in the
struggle to develop new forms of care for mental patients and other
dependent groups. Through its meetings, steady progress has been made

in thinking about institutional dynamics. This concern is particularly timely in view of the White Paper *Better Services for the Mentally Ill* (DHSS, 1975), in which it is recognized that community care services are minimal and likely to remain so in the near future. As a result institutional care will not disappear, as was expected back in the early 1960s, and hence problems of institutional life remain with us to be tackled directly (Bransby, 1973; Maynard and Tingle, 1975).

The book is organized into seven sections, but underlying this categorization is a basic dimension running between theory and practice. The former, as developed by various writers in the last twenty-five years, is a multi-disciplinary exploration of problems surrounding personal change in social group situations. The latter is concerned with the implementation of these ideas in the real world of the British National Health Service and Personal Social Services, and particularly the traditions of the mental health services.

We have aimed to bridge an important gap in the available literature in the field of psychiatry, group work, institutional life, and health service policy. This gap has opened up partly because other publications tend to report either theory or practice, but not both; but also because the issues which must be faced in institutional life have tended to be swept under the carpet since the 'Community Care bandwagon' of the 1960s and early 1970s. The failure of this movement to materialize actually in terms of resources has meant a return to the institutional scene. We are therefore, presenting the issues that the present generation of therapeutic community workers are preoccupied with. They have reworked the traditional principles of therapeutic communities in relation to present-day political issues, recent developments in psychotherapy and group therapy, and developments in general scientific outlook (e.g., systems theory).

We hope that this collection, the most extensive ever to appear on this topic in Britain (and the most extensive in the USA since the 1950s), will stimulate and co-ordinate a greater interest in the social environment and its impact on mental health and illness. We cannot afford to waste this valuable resource in a new era of economic constraint.

Acknowledgments

As editors we have been midwives to a book which has really been spawned by the Association of Therapeutic Communities. This collection is entirely due to the ATC as a medium of communication and contact, which has enabled us to draw on a very wide field of experience for the contributions. In turn we must also acknowledge the enormous debt to the even wider field of patients and colleagues amongst whom we and the contributors have gained the necessary experience and enthusiasm. Finally we must recognize the endless task of typing up the final copy which was so willingly shouldered by Miss Maureen Humphries and Mrs Joan Denning.

For permission to reproduce extracts from T. S. Eliot's 'Easter Coker' in his *Four Quartets*, the editors and publishers wish to thank Faber & Faber Ltd, London and Harcourt Brace Jovanovich, Inc., New York.

R. D. Hinshelwood and Nick Manning

1

The therapeutic community, social learning and social change

Maxwell Jones

How did my colleagues and I develop our early concept of a therapeutic community? How did we come to deviate from the strict orthodoxy of the Maudsley Hospital in London? The Second World War acted as a stimulus, and in 1940 I was put in charge of a 100-bed unit to study and treat effort syndrome. Working with cardiac neurosis in armed forces personnel we started out on a 'scientific' study of the physiology of exercise fatigue, but circumstances almost forced my colleagues and myself to depart from traditional psychiatric practice. To have a unit of 100 soldiers all with a similar syndrome seemed to demand that we discuss their problems with all 100 men at the same time. Was this innovative or merely common sense? There was a common theme: heart disease. We gave them feedback from our physiological researches, in which they were intensely interested. The nursing staff comprised many assistant nurses from all walks of life who were conscripted to help in the war effort. They did not think like most nurses, but reflected their training in art, ballet, or acting. We were in London, where the bombing contributed to a high morale and a feeling of closeness and interdependence. Traditional hospital barriers slowly gave way to an intimacy and democratization which might well have been impossible in peacetime. The creativity of this group of 100 'patients' and staff was remarkable, epitomized by a Christmas season when our unit was transformed into a medieval village (Maxwellton) replete with a banqueting hall (the 'patients' conned antique dealers into lending whole suits of armour), the artists painted appropriate scenes (the Yuletide log) and the staff acted as waiters and waitresses. We had a realistic post office, pub and antique store.

In retrospect, this was the beginning of the notion of a therapeutic community (Jones, 1953). The 'patients' took over many of the staff functions as they grasped the physiological mechanism of their symptoms (Jones, 1948), and the staff were largely resource personnel (facilitators).

In an interesting study of innovation, Manning (1976a), a sociologist, states, 'Most writers list three (developmental) stages: an early stage of unrest, perhaps with certain surrounding social strains or tensions; an enthusiastic mobilization or popular appeal when the movement takes off; and a final stage of institutionalization when there is often goal displacement and stagnation.' He points out that this describes only internal development.

> External development depends crucially on the role of advocacy of a movement amongst the wider society, and whether it is consciously encouraged or repressed by the prevailing power structure. And at a less conscious level, the movement's growth will be enhanced to the extent that it can attract general support by resonating with other emergent social groups or values in the wider society.

This sums up many aspects of our struggle to introduce a therapeutic community approach in psychiatry. The war years heightened the dissatisfaction that many of us felt with traditional psychiatry and gave birth to a new ideological approach (therapeutic communities). Because the social climate was ripe for changes in many directions, parallel developments were occurring elsewhere, notably among the ex-Tavistock Clinic army psychiatrists at Northfield Military Hospital, where they were inspired by Kurt Lewin's concept of life space. To me, the final stage of stagnation and institutionalization of the therapeutic community movement has not occurred. I like Manning's concept of resonance. After twelve years of helping to develop the original therapeutic community in London (1947-59), I found, as expected, little resonance at Stanford University Department of Psychiatry. An approach to 'treatment' based on social organization and using the social environment of the 'patient' to effect change, had little appeal for academic psychiatry. Moreover, my image was tied to the treatment of 'psychopaths' and so my relevance to psychiatry was limited to this particular area. After a year, I gladly accepted an offer to go to Oregon State Hospital, determined to prove that therapeutic community concepts had relevance for the whole field of psychiatry.

Four years in Oregon more than met my goal. Not only were my ideas positively supported by the power structure, but three other effects were apparent:

(a) Many hospitals, mainly in California, sought consultations with a view to establishing therapeutic communities of their own. A new facility in Denver, Colorado, was still in the planning stages when Dr Alan Kraft visited us, and Fort Logan Mental Health Center was opened as a therapeutic community. It has served as a model for this

2

approach in the American scene for the past seventeen years, and I worked there myself for five years (1969-74).

(b) The California Corrections Agency asked me to consult with them and, in four years, some eleven therapeutic community projects were established (Jones, 1962). The prisoners (usually in units of sixty men) again demonstrated the power of the peer group and the possibilities of social learning in such a setting.

(c) At Oregon State Hospital, we began to infiltrate into the surrounding community, setting up clinics in the counties which we served. These units antedated by three years the Community Mental Health Act of 1963, which led to the establishment of Community Mental Health Centers throughout the USA.

This trend towards a total mental health service from the home to the hospital was further developed when I became physician superintendent of Dingleton Hospital in Scotland (1962-9). Here, diffusion of therapeutic community principles extended into the school system and into behavioural science departments at Edinburgh University. We also had an important part to play as a model of complementarity between local authorities and mental health care systems. This, in turn, affected the nature of the new mental health plan for Scotland.

On returning to the USA in 1969, I became very much aware of the similarity between Organizational Development (a process applied by social psychologists to industry), systems theory, and therapeutic community principles. In fact, with my increasing contact with industry, the church, and education (mainly elementary schools), it seemed more appropriate to talk about social systems for a change and to drop the term 'therapeutic community'. As a consultant at Fort Logan Mental Center, I began to realize that the therapeutic community as I had known it was an early model of an open system, before systems theory was a recognized entity. I have become increasingly convinced that the social organization of a hospital, or a church, or a classroom (Jones, 1974) will influence the behaviour of the subjects in ways as yet not well understood. In other words, the social movement which, for me, started as a therapeutic community in 1940 has an increasing relevance to everyday life and would appear to be 'resonating with other emergent social groups or values in the wider society' (Manning, 1976a). In other words, it has not become institutionalized or stagnant.

Another common belief is that a movement ceases to be innovative when the leader moves elsewhere. I know that when I left Henderson Hospital after working there for twelve years and having been the innovator of the movement many people predicted that the hospital would not survive. This was eighteen years ago and Henderson is still an excellent example of a therapeutic community. The same argument applies to Dingleton Hospital which I left eight years ago, after being the physician superintendent for seven years. My explanation of this viability, if not vitality, is that the very nature of a therapeutic community, with its delegation of responsibility and authority to the system, implies that, through time, the formal leader will become largely redundant. This was certainly the case at Dingleton, where, for my last three months, I had little to do. In fact, we convinced the National Health Service that I should not be replaced, and they agreed to a leadership of six people from four different disciplines as the responsible body for the running of the hospital.

When movements die following the loss of the leader, it seems to imply that the social organization was hierarchical, and multiple leadership in a multidisciplinary setting had not evolved. This may well apply to Summerhill, where A. S. Neill, the charismatic leader, did not create an open system, and his death may have left an irreplaceable gap.

To me, an open system such as Dingleton Hospital came to be is in a constant state of flux, and responds sensitively to changing circumstances, e.g., the arrival of a new staff member. Such a system has its own dynamic and cannot stand still. It has a built-in system of checks and balances expedited by the open communication system, e.g., frequent meetings of all staff and patients where tendencies to become smug or to become too staff-centred, etc. can be recognized and countered.

The literature on therapeutic communities or milieu therapy invariably assumes that we are 'treating' some form of 'illness'. Starting with this medical frame of reference puts severe restrictions on the scope of a social environmental approach to change. If we talk of art therapy, we imply that a 'sick' person is participating in some form of art with a view to ameliorating his/her symptoms. But at what point does art cease to be 'therapy' and become an education in the expression of abstract feelings or whatever it achieves for the subject?

The fact is that medicine cornered the market on deviancy when, at the beginning of this century, the early psychoanalysts began talking about psychopathology. In a manner typical of the arrogance which characterizes the modern mental health movement, the term 'psychopathology' was coined so that certain forms of deviancy, later to be elaborated into ever more diagnostic categories, were created as types of 'illness', and so 'treated' by doctors.

The tendency of powerful elements in society to establish norms of behaviour, and to label the values of other groups as deviant, is a sinister aspect of the abuse of power, and is as old as history; e.g., the witch hunts of the Middle Ages, followed by the incarceration in mental institutions in the seventeenth century.

But medicine claims to be scientific and should be proof against such abuses of power.

Had deviancy been looked at as a manifestation of environmental

stress, and separated from those relatively few cases of true pathology
and illness, what a different picture we would have today. It is impossible to guess what form the mental health movement might have taken,
but certain deductions can be risked. Presumably, mental hospitals,
modelled in part on general hospitals, and so retaining the term 'hospital', would not have emerged. Instead, we might have had supportive
'asylums' or 'retreats' which characterized the moral treatment era of
150 years ago. But, even though these 'retreats', such as the York
Retreat in England, were run by doctors, humanistic values prevailed
and useful roles like productive work were made available to the
residents. Stripped of medical labelling, deviancy might have escaped
the insulation and isolation which inevitably followed its image of
'sickness'. Like lepers, these unfortunates were seen as dangerous and
unpredictable, to be put out of sight and, it was hoped, out of mind.
Even Szasz (1974), who describes so eloquently the myth of mental
illness, does not provide an alternative approach to psychiatric 'illness'.
In another book (Szasz, 1970), he says:

> I do not here propose to offer a new conception of 'psychiatric
> illness' or a new 'therapy'. My aim is more modest and yet also more
> ambitious. It is to suggest that the phenomena now called mental
> illness be looked at afresh and more simply, that they be removed
> from the category of illnesses, and that they be regarded as the
> expression of man's struggle with the problem of how he should live.

One admirable attempt to involve society in more responsible roles
in conjunction with mental health professionals has been attempted by
Mansell Pattison (1976). He describes the evolution of what he calls
psycho-social systems therapy. Starting with individual psychotherapy
at the turn of the century, he describes how, around 1920, the child
guidance involvement emerged, then group psychotherapy in the 1930s,
family therapy in the 1940s, multiple family therapy in the early 1960s,
and how finally, in recent years, the social network of relationships has
been made the focus of psychotherapy. He sees this evolution from
the point of view of the psychiatrist, and defines therapy as a healing
intervention on behalf of a specific individual who has identifiable
dysfunctional behaviour – this includes internal behaviour (thoughts,
feelings), or external behaviour (words, actions). He distinguishes
psycho-social treatment systems from psycho-social care systems. He
says, 'We gain social sanction to define and treat to the extent we can
demonstrate appropriate skills and knowledge that justify a social
mandate to treat' (Pattison, 1976). If we reverse this, and ask how
willing psychiatrists are to treat those cases which society sees as being
in greatest need, the social casualties in the lower socio-economic range,

5

the aged, the 'psychopath', the criminal, we see how the psychiatrist keeps a firm grip in deciding who gets 'treatment'. We are back to labelling and the control the medical profession has in deciding who is 'sick' and who requires 'treatment'. This hierarchy of values determines the distinction Mansell Pattison makes between psycho-social treatment systems and psycho-social care systems (social clubs, church groups, etc.). A care system stops short of 'treatment' and makes relatively less demand on mental health professionals.

I find it hard to accept this distinction between what is treatment and what is care, linked to the degree of involvement of the mental health professional. It implies a hierarchy of values, with the medical man at the top. After all, the whole field of medicine (perhaps more strikingly in the USA than in the UK) is on trial (Illich, 1975), and there is an increasing demand for accountability by the consumer. This applies equally to psychiatry. In fairness to my own profession, many psychiatrists have rebelled against the rigid conformity of the medical schools, and the whole evolution of social psychiatry can be seen as an attempt to become more involved with the patient and his social world, and complement the original model of psychotherapy with many forms of group interaction. My objection to the use of the word 'treatment' in relation to what is 'done' for the patients in therapeutic communities is that it implies a relatively subservient role for the 'patient'. This cuts across what to me is the most important lesson that therapeutic communities have shown, i.e. the importance of the 'patient's' own peer group. But, to make this a reality, we have to go to the other end of the spectrum compared with the typical hospital or even community treatment environment — from a closed to an open system. In my latest book (Jones, 1976), I have defined a system as an organized whole unit that includes the interactions of its interdependent component parts, and its relationship to the environment.

Virtually everyone in the mental health field knows that the latent potential of 'patients' to help themselves is not a high priority; and this applies in hospitals and in the community mental health programmes. It is quite sickening to see the administration, both medical and non-medical, deciding what is 'best' for 'patients' — often not even consulting the staff who are in daily contact with 'patients', far less the 'patients' themselves.

Perhaps the most important lesson of my life was the twelve years (1947-59) spent with 'sociopaths' at Belmont Hospital, later renamed Henderson Hospital, near London. We knew of no effective 'treatment' for this condition and had to turn to the 'patients' for help. Thus started the chain reaction of daily community meetings with all 'patients' and staff present (approximately 100 people), information-sharing, identification of problems, setting priorities, and shared decision-making, if possible reaching consensus.

One could say that this experiment was forced on us by the very fact of our ignorance, but might one not extrapolate and suggest that all 'treatment' units might follow this pattern and attempt a fresh start, questioning all their preconceptions and prejudices, and involving the 'patients' as people from the start?

Such a re-examination of what we mean by the term 'treatment' would, hopefully, raise the issue of the traditional treatment modalities based on the idea of psychotherapy (both individual and group) and the physical therapies (drugs, ECT, etc.), but would also examine the importance of social forces in the environment in preventing mental illness, as well as in effecting change once illness patterns had emerged.

It seems to me that this is the area where the application and development of therapeutic community principles can be most innovative and potentially useful.

If we dispense with diagnostic labels, except for mental 'illnesses' which are organically determined (e.g. brain damage), or genetically determined (e.g. Huntington's Chorea), we are left with conditions which are the result of adverse social forces in the individual, family, group, neighbourhood, city, or national environment. Admittedly, the etiology of many conditions, especially schizophrenia, is highly controversial, but even schizophrenia may eventually be understood in terms of a psychotic defence against an unbearable reality. If we adopt this position, then most cases of mental 'illness' would appear to call for a reversal, or at least an adjustment, of the social forces which resulted in the aberrant behaviour in the first place. This would include individual psychotherapy, but would usually involve the social matrix of the individual. We have already discussed what Mansell Pattison calls psycho-social systems therapy and how I see the term 'therapy' as limiting us to psychopathology and the medical model. I would like to suggest that, as all 'therapy' is clearly part of a process of learning, we should use a term such as 'social learning', which would include what is at present called psychotherapy, or extended to include the social matrix, psycho-social systems therapy, and now add learning techniques extended to problems of living and prevention. By social learning, I mean two-way communication in a group, interaction motivated by some inner need or stress, leading to overt or covert expression of feeling, and involving cognitive processes and change. The term implies a change in the individual's attitude and/or beliefs as a result of the experience. These changes are incorporated and modify his personality and self-image.

In this context, social learning can be seen to apply to any form of psychotherapy, to psycho-social systems therapy, and to problems of living in general. It has particular significance in the field of prevention.

My own experience working as a facilitator in a classroom setting has convinced me that social learning could, with advantage, be added to the formal curriculum from elementary school onwards. Briefly, we needed a headmaster who was favourable to such an approach, and who asked the teachers to volunteer for weekly training seminars. These were much like encounter groups and involved three months of weekly two-hour groups of approximately ten teachers. They began to examine their feelings for each other and become aware of interpersonal problems and their resolution. Even such a brief exposure to problem-solving techniques seemed to give them the confidence to tackle problems in the classroom or the playground, etc. In company with a mental health professional trained in group dynamics, they now confided to the class that, for an hour a week, there would be no formal instruction and asked the children to leave their desks, sit in a circle and talk about their experiences at school and in the classroom.

Given the opportunity, children can become interested in human behaviour and learn skills in problem-solving. In this process of social learning, they begin to sense their own need for close ties with other people and the power of the peer group. At present, in most schools, this power is manifest in patterns of conformity. Physical size is equated with an individual pupil's power, which can express itself negatively in bullying, or, more acceptably, in athletic success. In either case, a stereotype exists that largely precludes the questioning of group (classroom) values. The nonconformist in dress, social attitudes, activities, or interests is a 'deviant' and may face rejection from his peers. Here lie the seeds of later mental health difficulties. The artistic, creative, sensitive, withdrawn or independent child, the physically handicapped, small of stature or obese, may fail to find acceptance by his peers and drift into isolation, 'illness', drugs, or delinquency. Why wait until an alien environment identifies him as 'ill' and refers him for treatment, whereupon he is identified as a patient, which further estranges him from his peers (and maybe his family) and reinforces his own negative self-image?

This switch from a passive teaching situation, with one-way communication from teacher to pupil, to social interaction and, through time, expression of feeling, runs a course familiar to all group workers. The exposure to an open system may shock many, and it may be months before the level of trust is such that it is 'safe' to express feelings with and about one's peers.

Moreover, as word leaks out, and rumours and distortions about the 'group' get to the school at large, there will be many negative reactions based on fear and misunderstanding. The same applies to the parents, who may see this process as a threat to their authority and moral values.

It is here that an understanding headmaster is essential to lead the process of social learning.

Looking back over my thirty-seven years' experience with therapeutic communities, I find a remarkable similarity between the struggle to evolve a therapeutic community for the treatment of psychopaths in London at Henderson Hospital, and the difficulties in establishing a social system for change and social learning in a classroom. Both require sanctions from above in order to succeed, both require psychodynamic skills, commitment, and courage to face the inevitable resistances to change. By and large, everyone grows up in a relatively closed hierarchical system, and an attempt to develop an open system strikes at the very roots of our culture. Nevertheless, therapeutic communities continue to symbolize one such approach.

In conclusion, I see relatively little difference between residential therapeutic communities in the USA, the UK, and Europe. I refer only to those establishments which have seriously pursued such a goal. In the USA practically every hospital claims to be a therapeutic community but, more often than not, this is a meaningless figure of speech. Where serious attempts to develop an open system in either country have been made, remarkably similar general principles seem to hold true. In both countries, decision-making by consensus is more an ideal than a practice. The power of veto is usually retained by the top authority, an attitude which I deprecate.

This book brings together many experiences in the establishment of therapeutic communities in Britain and raises questions about the future of the movement. The establishment of a Therapeutic Community Association with regular conferences may look like an institutionalization process. But the important question is: Does this movement have a positive influence in psychiatry and counter many of the abuses of authority and devaluation of the 'patient' so familiar in traditional psychiatry? I am hopeful that therapeutic communities, or open systems, will act as a springboard and will revitalize many of our social organizations.

9

Part I

The therapeutic community

The whole of Part I is designed to provide the reader with a brief guide to the history and basic ideas of the therapeutic community movement in Britain. There are classic texts already published which have set out some of these ideas in the making (Rapoport, 1960). Here we wish to explore the current position to which those earlier developments have brought us, rather than to restate the original model. These first chapters are intelligible to the newcomer to this area, but they also contain fresh insights and modern reflections on some well-known issues for the more experienced to ponder.

Section A
History and current status

The four chapters in Section A review the development of the therapeutic community in Britain over a considerable period of time (Chapter 2). The breadth to which this aspect of social psychiatry has spread is affected by government policies. When money is short such communities may be seen as a luxury, yet they offer an opportunity to use a freely available source of therapeutic power (the social environment). Again, the current popularity of planning tends to drive out the less demonstrably effective methods, as does the traditional medical dominance of research in a more sociologically appropriate area. However, the fortunes of the therapeutic community have in fact been more significantly dominated by the fashions of psychiatry and social work than by government policy.

Thus, in Chapter 3 Malcolm Pines explores the extent and limit of the influence which the therapeutic community has exercised in academic psychiatry; while in Chapter 4 Colin Archer welcomes and supports the expansion of therapeutic community work within the non-medical arena of the personal social services. These two chapters highlight the limited opportunities for therapeutic communities to develop in conventional psychiatry on the one hand; on the other hand, the social services have a greater 'resonance' with the basic approach of this kind of work, which can only lead to its much wider acceptance in a field short of good workable models of group and community functioning.

In Chapter 5, Brian Haddon sets the therapeutic community movement of the 1970s in an explicitly political context. Not only does he favour the replacement of a medical by a social approach in the mental health services, but he also challenges the notion of professionally defined (and therefore rigid) goals and structures. He favours a more flexible and responsive leadership of community mental health which aims at meeting needs as imaginatively as possible. Strict professional education closes options rather than opens them.

2
Progress and reflection

Stuart Whiteley

Since the Second World War the therapeutic community has had a fluctuating popularity both in psychiatry and in the more general social setting. In the first decade there was a period of enthusiastic application of therapeutic community ideas. Civilian mental hospitals were influenced by psychiatrists returning from the war and rightly proud of the part that this approach had played in the treatment of war neuroses (Jones, 1956; Clark *et al.*, 1962). Psychiatrists had little else of value to offer at this time. There were no psychiatric equivalents of penicillin or sulphonamide nor of the advanced surgical techniques that the war had encouraged.

In the 1960s, however, physical and particularly pharmacological methods of treatment were developed and rapidly absorbed by the psychiatric profession. This period became one of troubled implementation of the therapeutic community. Papers appeared describing the failure of the method (Wilensky and Hertz, 1966), the break-up of therapeutic community hospitals (Crabtree and Cox, 1972; Stotland and Kobler, 1965), and the conflict between therapeutic community aspirants and those who favoured physical or psychoanalytic methods (Kosin and Sharaf, 1967; Talbot and Miller, 1966). Gradually the therapeutic community faded from prominence except in a few isolated centres. Clark (1965) signalled the surrender when he wrote of the therapeutic community approach in those hospitals which had largely returned to medical care although not entirely dismissing the lessons learned about the social situation. The term 'therapeutic community proper' he reserved for a few units which still adhered to the original philosophy and practice. Of these, he later wrote (1977), there were but six in existence in England in 1966.

A later tour of selected hospitals and other establishments using large group meetings was conducted by Crocket from 1970 to 1972. His terminology was slightly different from Clark's but, although he was surprised to find wide interest in social psychiatry methods and partial practice of therapeutic community ideas, he found an even smaller number of hospital units employing the full therapeutic community method. These he calls psychotherapeutic communities. A few schools for maladjusted children, drug-addiction, alcoholic and adolescent units also came within the category. The strongholds of the movement, whether in the more general application of the ideas or in therapeutic communities proper, seem all to have been either led by a committed, charismatic figure (Clark at Fulbourn, Martin at Claybury, Crocket at Ingrebourne), or had a long-standing association with the philosophy (Henderson), or both (Main at the Cassel). Lesser-known therapeutic community wards or units waxed and waned as younger psychiatrists visited or read about the therapeutic community and attempted to implement the ideas back home. The therapeutic community smouldered on into the 1970s, occasionally sparking into life but becoming neither fully extinguished nor widely established.

New beginnings

A meeting at the Henderson in 1970 initiated a new era, one of thoughtful evaluation. Because of the situation outlined above, a round table conference invited a dozen or so psychiatrists, psychologists, nurses or social workers who had researched into, written about or contributed to therapeutic communities. The meeting fanned into flame the smouldering embers. Links were established between isolated workers in the field, problems were shared and mutual support was given. Exchange of ideas and experience revived interest. Even as the first meeting was being held a secondary meeting of those who had not been invited to the round table was hastily assembled to debate similar issues at a less expert but perhaps more grass-roots level! For eighteen months or so the curious situation prevailed. Members of host communities (Fulbourn, Dingleton, etc.) clamoured to join in and expressed considerable anger and envy at being excluded from what seemed to be the 'secret conclave'.

At last, in 1972, it was decided to form an Association of Therapeutic Communities (ATC) open to all who worked in therapeutic communities or were interested in the method. The regular meetings and the publication of the ATC *Bulletin* have set up a strong network of support and a communicational link. It has drawn attention to the continued existence of therapeutic communities. Research has been stimulated, and papers published in the 1970s have been increasingly analytical. Sociological exploration of the therapeutic community process has complemented outcome studies more typical of medical research. In this way, there has been a return to the approach taken by Rapoport and his team in the 1950s (Rapoport, 1960; Manning, 1976a, 1976b, 1976c; Kennard and Clemmey, 1976).

This resurgence is not due solely to the stimulus of the ATC. We have learned of similar research in Holland. A thoughtful re-appraisal of the therapeutic community has also occurred in the USA where Zeigenfuss (1976) in an unpublished thesis has reviewed the world-wide literature on therapeutic communities from 1970 to 1975. He studied 270 papers published in this period from the widest variety of countries, and concluded that the term therapeutic community is ill-defined and covers a wide range of methods and applications, but that interest in a social approach to psychiatric treatment is universal.

More definitive research is needed now, to respond to the demand from general psychiatrists and from administrators to 'prove it works'. What explorations have been made into therapeutic communities have neither satisfactorily proved it works nor proved it doesn't work. Rather, it works in some cases but not in others: interaction between subject and method is crucial (Clark and Yeomans, 1969; Clarke and Cornish, 1972; Whiteley *et al.*, 1972). Moreover, encompassing this basic interaction is the prevailing social climate which either facilitates or mitigates against a successful outcome. Thus, a 'living-and-learning' situation for neurotic young adults was most effective at a time when social pressures and political and economic expediency encouraged a successful outcome. In the thirty or so years following this wartime experience, neither the subjects nor the method have changed much but the social environment has changed considerably. To look at the current status of the therapeutic community we therefore need to appraise it from all three perspectives: the subjects, the method and the social climate.

The subjects

The pioneers of the therapeutic community optimistically believed that the approach could be universally applied across the field of psychiatric treatment. Bitter experience and careful research demonstrated that this was not the case. Rapoport (1960) showed that subjects with weak ego-strength could be damaged by exposure to the harsh confrontative techniques. Other studies in their turn discarded various diagnostic categories as unsuited — depressives, paranoids, psychopaths — until it might have seemed that no clinical group was suitable for the treatment. Letemendia and others (1967) in a comparative study of schizophrenics in a country mental hospital showed that there was no difference in outcome at follow-up between those treated in a therapeutic community and those treated by more traditional methods.

However, in a more selective appraisal of the results of treatment, Myers and Clark (1972) showed that it was the disturbed, often hallucinated and deluded schizophrenic who could respond to the therapeutic community, whereas the withdrawn and apathetic could not. The patients who were still 'struggling with their fate and reacting against their institutional environment' could interact meaningfully with the dynamic life of the therapeutic community. Again, whereas Craft (1965) had demonstrated in a controlled study that psychopaths of low intelligence actually did worse in a therapeutic community than those treated by a benignly authoritarian regime, studies at Henderson Hospital found that the psychopaths who respond to the challenge of the therapeutic community are those with some personality resources on which to build. The very inadequate psychopath is often more disturbed by the responsibilities put upon him in a therapeutic community, whilst the primitive, aggressive psychopath of low maturity also finds it difficult to cope with the stresses aroused (Whiteley, 1970). Indeed, it has become possible to predict from past life experience just who will be able to respond positively (Copas and Whiteley, 1976).

The question of what facets of personality the therapeutic community can affect is illustrated by the studies of Miles (1969, 1972) on psychopaths of low intelligence and schizophrenics in long-term hospital workshops. Her findings were that the therapeutic community produced a change for the better in the attitudes to authority in the former, whilst in the latter there was a significant increase in the social awareness and social networks of the patients treated in the therapeutic community-style workshop when compared with a traditional workshop. Not long ago Caine and Wijesinghe (1976) have investigated the personality attributes of patients entering group treatments, their pre-treatment expectations and the outcome. Those most likely to respond to group psychotherapy are the ones who are open-minded, having an 'inward' direction of interest and a generalized 'liberal' attitude to life as opposed to the more rigid, closed-minded, patients who are more likely to prefer and show a response to a medical or behaviourist type of approach. Psychiatric staff were studied by Caine and Smail (1966). The therapeutic community doctor is someone who is less likely to distinguish sharply between neurosis and psychosis, and he believes more in communication made on the basis of individual personality than in communication determined by professional roles or authority. The movement is thus away from the concept of disease and its cure towards the understanding and resolution of behavioural conflicts that arise between the individual and society. These manifest themselves in a variety of ways according to the means available to that individual and depend upon his personality maturity, resources and background experience.

The method

From the first dogmatic beginnings when slogans such as 'opening up the communications', 'flattening of the staff hierarchy' and 'blurring of the roles' set a rather rigid and ritualistic pattern, the therapeutic community has developed into a more subtle appreciation of its basic tenets and a more flexible application of the ideology. In the early days a religious zeal was probably required to convert rigid custodial mental hospitals into more open therapeutic communities, but experience has led to variations on the basic theme. In different situations, different modalities are practised. Maxwell Jones (1968a) has commented that there is probably no one model for a therapeutic community; and Moos (1974) cites four different examples, commenting that each programme offered a different type of milieu but each accepted the basic notion that the treatment milieu has important influences on treatment outcome. Maxwell Jones, working with the Belmont group of neurotic and personality disorders, stressed involvement, peer-group support, autonomy and the expression of feeling. Fairweather (1964), working with chronic mental patients, also encouraged involvement and peer support but stressed a practical task organization. Sanders (Sanders *et al.*, 1967) working on chronic schizophrenics showed that a maximally structured situation led to involvement and support without the need for stressing personal feelings. Coleman (1971) also found that a programme with a strong task-orientation was superior to a non-directive therapeutic milieu, for delinquent young males.

Sociological exploration of mental hospital life continues to be the tradition of therapeutic community research and as such is a far cry from the customary 'spot-the-winner' type of medical research into disease and its cure. Clark (1967) showed how patient participation was related to patient improvement. Wilensky and Hertz (1966) showed that when authority was consciously decreased it might well be replaced by a paternalism that was just as stifling for the patient. Bierenbroodspot (1972) distinguished power-sharing in which the staff retain considerable influence, from delegation of power in which total resources must come from the patient group. Authority and democracy have been more clearly interpreted (Crocket, 1966b) and the role and function of leadership in a therapeutic community have been explored (Furedi *et al.*, 1974). Maxwell Jones (1976) writes of charismatic leadership at the outset moving into a phase of multiple leadership and then on to self-sufficiency of the organization with leaders acting as facilitators or even from the outside as occasional interventionists. There are problems in multiple leadership, not least of which are envy, rivalry and the avoidance of responsibility on occasion. In another form of leadership, focal leadership (Whiteley, 1978), the designated leader of the community responds to the transferential demands and forces of the close-knit community and does not deny the identifications that are thus invested in him. Schiff and Glassman (1969) ascribed to the leader of a large group the functions of gate-keeping (bringing in or excluding individuals), reality maintaining, the selection of topics for exploration and modelling. The latter is much bound up with the strong transference relationship that develops in the therapeutic community.

Doctors and nurses usually lack experience and expertise in sociodynamics. Their basic training is directed toward the medical model of treatment of the disease in the passive patient. Perhaps this is one of the reasons why the therapeutic community has made few inroads into the general psychiatric hospital and has remained in isolated enclaves of enthusiasts who are often regarded as eccentric or even deviant by their colleagues. Teaching hospitals make some acknowledgment of the therapeutic community as a treatment modality and most have or have had a small ward or unit designated as a therapeutic community. But the other demands on the teaching hospital (such as the education of students and the selection of patients for their teaching and research potential) weigh against the all-out application of full therapeutic community methods.

Outside the psychiatric hospitals, however, the therapeutic community has not suffered from the same internal or external constraints. Membership of the ATC reveals a wider allegiance to the therapeutic community method outside the strictly therapeutic areas. Approved schools, after-care hostels, day centres and even prisons have proclaimed themselves as therapeutic communities.

The problem is whether they are really therapeutic communities, or rather communities for therapy? In how many are the social dynamics and interpersonal interactions of the members fully utilized in the pursuit of growth toward personality and emotional maturity? Zeitlyn (1967), in a critical examination of therapeutic community practice, suggests, for instance, that in many hospitals when all other treatments have failed or been abandoned, the final back ward is designated a therapeutic community as if to instil hope in both patients and staff. Chaos reigns behind the locked door, while staff discuss the ward's problems endlessly and without insights in the ward office. Similar processes have developed in a Borstal recall wing for the failures amongst the failed. In hostels the aims and objectives of staff and clients can be quite different from each other. These aspiring therapeutic communities lend support to the movement when it is flourishing; but when the movement is under attack they are the weak spots that crumble or are crushed out of existence. Such a place is the experimental wing at Barlinnie Prison which had considerable praise from the media and from the establishment a few years ago, until it became the object of attack and repudiation when the general social climate changed from liberalism to one of authority and control.

In many peripheral or fringe therapeutic communities there may well be a hidden authoritarian dependency structure beneath the apparent democratic model put forward by the staff. This is not necessarily a deliberate deception, for many of the clients may not share the therapeutic community ideals and aspirations of the staff. Even in the authentic therapeutic community the aims of the staff and of the patients may not altogether coincide (Manning, 1976b; see also Chapter 14). White (1967) in an interesting and provocative paper suggests that a community democracy model is not really appropriate in a hospital situation, and what should be used is a labour-relations model where staff and patients bargain and compromise with each other to get the best deal for each side.

One of the most significant and far-reaching developments at Henderson Hospital in the post-Maxwell Jones era was the institution of a selection group for prospective patients wherein present patients and present staff (the latter slightly fewer in number) in a group setting select on the principle of one man one vote irrespective of status. It cannot be denied that staff carry a considerable influence in this power-sharing task but this is one of the most endurable, satisfying and least avoided groups at the unit. It is a co-operative working group in which it is spelled out to the candidate how we work, what expectations we would have of him, and what expectations he must have of all of us. He makes a verbal contract with us and we with him. So if it becomes necessary to remind him of the treatment contract as time passes there is no problem of divided aims or different expectations arising to obscure the issues. Other units have gone further than this in actually drawing up a written and signed contract of treatment.

The social climate

During the Second World War it was both politically and economically expedient to foster the development of the therapeutic community to preserve manpower for the war effort. In the years of austerity and restrictive control that followed the objectives and aims of the therapeutic community remained attractive and were in keeping with the new democracy and social aspirations of the post-war era. The general principles of open communications, power-sharing and the relaxation of authoritarian controls were absorbed into our general social setting as well as into the world of the mental hospital. The therapeutic community offered no new message in the 1960s, indeed the pedantic-seeming insistence on 'putting it to the community' and 'no unilateral decision-making' took on something of a dogma and ritual in a society

21

which was accepting these values. This was the era of the therapeutic community approach. But when the pharmaceutical companies broke into the field of mental health many mental hospitals quickly slipped back into the medical treatment of psychiatric disorder and the abandonment of the social approach. Not only did hospitals and hospital staff quickly revert but the general attitudes of the patient group also seemed to favour the resumption of the passive patient-role and a surrender to medical omnipotence. To entrench further this medicalization of mental illness and its treatment, the poor living and working conditions in the mental hospitals has resulted in native-born doctors and nurses leaving psychiatry, and the mental hospital in particular, to be replaced by staff less able to grasp British social and group problems.

A therapeutic community in such a society with obvious communicational barriers is difficult to establish or maintain. The role of the doctor and the nurse has become to administer physical treatment in the best physical environment that the Department of Health can afford. Emphasis is on the physical environment, rather than the treatment milieu, to avoid further public scandals and outcry. A new mental health profession — that of social therapist — should be encouraged for native-born young graduates with the necessary sociological and psychological skills and with the all-important language and cultural background.

As the 1960s came to an end the freedom of expression and the increased tolerance for deviant behaviour, disinhibition and the general throwing-off of authoritarian controls resulted in a near anarchy in some European countries, and instituted a generalized threat to the stability of many societies. The therapeutic community, with its well-known goals of freedom of expression and replacement of authoritarian direction by democratic process, has come to be seen as a similar threat to the established order of the health services as perhaps never before. The myths of anarchy and loss of control have been resurrected, and there have been instances in both Germany and Holland where links between therapeutic communities and anarchist groups have been alleged and dealt with by police intervention. In our own society we have recently seen the tightening up of prison security and of the regulations for the treatment of mentally abnormal offenders, recommendations for secure units in mental hospitals, and the revision of the Mental Health Act to exclude 'psychopathic personality' as a mental disorder 'requiring or susceptible to medical treatment'.

The therapeutic community today finds itself the victim of its own success. The general ideas have been taken up in hospitals and in society at large but the means have become separated from the meaning. In many cases what has purported to be a community democracy model is no more than a superficial gesture toward open communication and power-sharing, without real understanding of the principles involved.

3
Therapeutic communities in teaching hospitals

Malcolm Pines

In this chapter I shall describe the evidence for the influence of the therapeutic community concept on the practice of teaching hospital psychiatry in the United Kingdom. The teaching hospital is normally understood to be a component of a university department granting degrees in medicine. Historically, departments of psychiatry are relatively recent additions to the basic clinical disciplines of medicine, surgery, obstetrics, gynaecology and the minor specialities. Many undergraduate teaching hospital departments of psychiatry are relatively new, and quite small in numbers of staff and in their influence on the teaching curriculum. Their work is mostly concerned with out-patients and liaison within the hospital; in-patients are usually few in number and are housed in sub-sections of the main general hospital. Few teaching hospital departments of psychiatry have separate units for in-patients of any substantial size (say, of over fifty beds). Teaching hospitals may often have connections with nearby large mental hospitals, but these are usually more for the purpose of teaching and research than for direct clinical and administrative responsibility.

We need to grasp this historical development in order to view the context for the practice of in-patient psychiatry in teaching hospitals against which the influence of a therapeutic community concept can be assessed. As this concept arose from the experience of the psychiatrists working with quite large numbers of patients, as at Northfield Hospital and at Henderson Hospital, it can readily be appreciated that there has been little scope for applying therapeutic community concepts and practice within the teaching hospitals. Even if there had been a more suitable environment, whether the concept would have taken further root and been established in practice is a moot point, for a number of reasons which I shall try to discuss.

The argument will begin at the level of the doctor–patient relationship and will move on from the individual to the social frame of reference, and finally to a view of the hospital culture as a whole.

23

Doctor–patient relationship models

In the models offered by Szasz and Hollander (1956) there are three basic types of doctor–patient relationship, based upon the degree of helplessness of the patient and the attitude and response of the doctor to this:

(1) A high degree of helplessness is characteristic of patients with acute medical or surgical emergencies where the appropriate response is for the staff to take more or less complete responsibility for the survival of the patient. The model of the unconscious patient and the highly skilled and fully conscious medical and nursing staff pertains here; these features lead to the creation of a stable social system where the highly active doctor or nurse can dis-identify with the helpless patient and thereby is enabled to act upon the patient calmly and relatively objectively.

(2) When the patient is less helpless a social system is developed between a patient who is seeking help and who is willing to co-operate with a doctor who is seen as a parent figure. This gratifies the doctor's need to feel superior and to give help to the weaker. This model is the traditional one for the doctor–patient relationship in our society, and appears appropriate to conditions of chronic illness where the patient seems to need continued guidance in a prolonged dependent relationship.

(3) The model of mutual participation, of relative equality of roles, between two adults interacting fairly completely is unusual in medical models; but this is characteristic of the psychoanalytical or psycho-therapeutic doctor–patient relationship. The psychotherapeutic model of adult-to-adult relationships is evidently out of step with the models that operate in most other hospital-based relationships, where the patient is seen as relatively childlike or infantile.

From these differences in levels of relationships and types of social systems it follows that both patients and staff have to make a considerable readjustment of role relationships when they enter the field of psychiatry. However, even within the province of psychiatry this level of adult relationship does not have to be applied. Evidently, this does not have to be the case where a department of psychiatry treats a patient as ill in much the same way as any other patient with a physical illness. Such departments are more easily integrated with other parts of the hospital (medical, surgical and so on) and are less likely to arouse the quite considerable boundary problems which inevitably arise when two spheres of influence overlap with each other. The more the socio-cultural attitudes within these two separate spheres contrast with each other the more likely there is to be a realm of anxiety, mistrust, ambiguity and confusion where they overlap (Pines, 1976).

Staff and patient training

It follows from this that the training of both staff and patients for their roles in the social encounter of clinical psychiatry is radically different in the therapeutic community setting from that in other branches of medicine. Attitude surveys have shown that both staff and patients (Caine and Smail, 1969) who feel comfortable in the therapeutic community situation are those with divergent rather than convergent personality styles, with democratic rather than authoritarian attitudes. Convergent and authoritarian attitudes are in many ways appropriate to persons dealing with acute medicine and surgery where a rapid assumption of responsibility is often required of staff. Thus difficult decisions involving dis-identification with the patient, who is temporarily disregarded as a person, can be made about physical welfare.

Nurses and occupational therapists find the transition from the ordinary ward to the psychiatric unit quite difficult in itself, and when to this is added the usual therapeutic community ideology that staff–patient role distinctions should not be made too sharply there is often considerable difficulty in adjustment. The self-definition of the trainee nurse, for instance, has to a considerable degree incorporated both the uniform and relatively uniform patterns of interactions with medical and surgical patients. Doing without both uniform and previously learned patterns of behaviour is a considerable test of psychological flexibility and produces a considerable degree of stress for which the person requires much support.

Senior nursing and ancillary staff have even greater problems of adjustment if a unit changes from a more orthodox psychiatric stance to that of a therapeutic community, and resignations and stress reactions are not at all uncommon when this takes place.

Models of social organization

The same factors apply to the models of social organization that are often evolved in teaching hospital departments other than those of psychiatry. These models tend to be pyramidal with a great deal of authority vested in the most senior members of the hierachy; and information passing up the social structure is quite extensively controlled and censored. Hence it follows that free exchange of information between those at the bottom of the hierarchy, that is the most junior staff and the patients, and those at the top of the hierarchy, that is the most senior staff, is considerably restricted and curtailed. This model applies to both the clinical management of patients and to the teaching of medical students and nurses. Information is handed out by those

25

with authority and knowledge often in such a manner as to demonstrate that discussion and questioning of this information is unwelcome.

As the model of the therapeutic community usually implies the flattening of this social structure and the free exchange of information between all members of the social organization, there are very considerable and powerful social obstacles that have to be overcome before the social structure can be altered. The therapeutic community approach is basically the application of social, psychological and psychotherapeutic principles to the organization of a treatment unit and its transactions with the consumers, that is, the patients. As most university departments of psychiatry have a rather cool attitude towards psychodynamic and socio-cultural theories it is not surprising that so radical a step as the adoption of the therapeutic community concept and principle has not often been taken.

I shall in the remainder of this chapter describe some personal experiences of the introduction of therapeutic community principles to the in-patient unit of a teaching hospital, and also describe those few departments where the therapeutic community concept has to some extent been practised and can be said to be established.

Some examples

University of London

My own experience at St George's Hospital has already been partly described (Pines, 1975). My training in therapeutic community methods was largely under Dr T. F. Main at the Cassel Hospital, where we worked with a neurotic population in a highly sophisticated setting. Individual psychoanalytic-orientated psychotherapy was provided in the setting of a carefully monitored psycho-social environment. The nursing staff received a special and intensive training in group dynamics from their own specialized senior nursing staff and were largely responsible for the running of the community (Barnes, 1968).

One notable nursing gradutate of the Cassel Hospital, Eileen Skellern, received her training both at Henderson and at the Cassel and went on to become the Chief Nursing Officer of the Maudsley and Bethlem Royal Hospitals. There she helped to design a special unit for in-patient psychotherapy, the Hood Unit, in collaboration with the consultant psychotherapist, Dr Robert Hobson (see below). Though the Cassel Hospital taught many psychotherapists their trade in conjunction with a training at the Institute of Psychoanalysis, the hospital was not part of a teaching hospital unit. The reasons for this being so are complex, but it is a matter of considerable regret that the great expertise to be found in the hospital, where many innovations of in-patient treatment on psychotherapeutic lines were created, was never part of an academic unit either for the purposes of teaching or for research.

Part of my brief when I was appointed senior lecturer in psychotherapy at St George's Hospital under Professor Arthur Crisp was to introduce therapeutic community methods into the in-patient unit at Atkinson Morley Hospital. The setting for this challenging work was an in-patient unit of some forty beds under three consultants, each of whom had special research interests ranging from metabolic aspects of psychiatric disturbances to a specialized research programme in psycho-surgery. The unit admitted a very wide range of psychiatric disorders: acute and chronic psychosis, organic disorders, patients for psycho-surgery, neurotic and personality disorders, alcoholism and drug dependency problems.

A regime was gradually introduced which allowed both small and large group meetings, but it was clear that it would never be possible to bring together all the members of staff regularly at these meetings. The multiplicity of roles which is essential for the treatment and maintenance of both the therapeutic community situation, and senior academic and clinical staff in a teaching hospital, not only makes it difficult for staff to attend but also actively to participate in the activities of the large community group.

An academic department has many functions. There is responsibility for introducing medical students to the basis of psychiatry in a two-month period, and for training junior medical and nursing staff for research and clinical work with the patients. These functions compete for priority, and clear lines of demarcation are needed for them to be carried out simultaneously. For instance, research may require the vigorous discipline of data collection by medical and nursing staff, and may well clash with what they feel is an appropriate clinical response to their patients' needs and behaviour. The responsibility for teaching students and junior staff again imposes conditions on the in-patient regime that often clash with the therapeutic community method and ideology.

Despite these and many other problems it was possible to introduce a significant degree of re-organization within the in-patient unit, though I categorize this more as the creation of a milieu therapeutic approach than a therapeutic community proper (Clark, 1965). Indeed, a joint Senior Registrar training post in psychotherapy has recently been created that links St George's Hospital with Henderson Hospital. This confirms both the acceptance of the therapeutic community in an academic department, and the academic status of Henderson Hospital.

The therapeutic community

Maudsley and Bethlem Royal Hospitals

A very interesting attempt was made to organize an in-patient psycho-therapeutic unit at the Bethlem, the Hood Unit. An intensive day regime of group interaction with the medical, nursing and occupational therapy staff was linked to a night hostel scheme where patients looked after themselves without the aid of nursing staff. Since the hostel was situated in the hospital grounds, night-nursing staff were available in emergencies. For a variety of reasons, amongst them being a lack of internal support from the rest of the hospital, the expense of running a small unit with a relatively high staff ratio, and the competition of other items in the hospital budget for priority, the unit closed after a few years (see Chapter 22). The major problem in the running of this unit was that of selection of patients, who had both to warrant the offer of in-patient treatment for a considerable length of time (up to and sometimes over a year), and yet who were thought to be able to maintain a considerable degree of autonomy within that setting with its inevitable and powerful inducement to ego regression.

The other unit within the joint hospitals that uses therapeutic milieu methods, Ward One, Maudsley Hospital (consultant Dr Murray Jackson), is a unit that accepts more severely disturbed patients, psychotic and borderline states. Treatment is firmly based on therapeutic milieu methods and on individual psychoanalytically-based psychotherapy.

University of Edinburgh

Professor Henry Walton, a trainee of Dr S. F. Foulkes of the Maudsley Hospital, has introduced therapeutic milieu methods into in-patient wards of the Royal Edinburgh Hospital, and some interesting research has been initiated there (Walton, 1970, 1971; Johnstone *et al.*, 1969). Therapeutic community and group analytic methods have been applied to the functioning of general psychiatric units and to the treatment of alcoholism. A particularly interesting and important application of therapeutic community methods has been to the work with in-patient adolescents. A series of papers by the staff of the Young People's Unit (Evans, 1970, 1976; Clark, 1970; Canizares, 1976) clearly outlines the history of its development, the treatment methods applied, and the means by which the medical and nursing staff are helped to acquire the necessary skills.

University of Oxford, Littlemore Hospital

This medium-size mental hospital is part of the Oxford teaching hospital group. Therapeutic community methods were introduced by Dr Bertram

Mandelbrote in 1956 (Mandelbrote, 1965; Mandelbrote and Gelder, 1972; Mandelbrote and Trick, 1970; Sugarman, 1968; Kennard and Clemmey, 1976, Kennard, Clemmey and Mandelbrote, 1977; Letemendia *et al.*, 1967). Later Dr Mandelbrote was joined by Dr Pomryn, who had worked at Henderson Hospital with Maxwell Jones. Though the hospital was part of a teaching hospital group and therefore included the teaching of medical students in its work, the staff of Littlemore Hospital were allowed to carry out large-scale reorganizations without interference. The hospital is notable for several innovations. These include a highly regarded alcoholism treatment unit where group therapy methods have been adapted to the needs of this special population, and the counselling centre (ISIS) for students and young people situated in the town centre (research). Mandelbrote (personal communications) was greatly stimulated by the innovations used by Dr T. P. Rees at Warlingham Park Hospital, which in the 1950s provided a vigorous example of hospital reorganization along therapeutic community lines, adapted however to the needs of a large mental hospital.

University of Cambridge, Fulbourn Hospital
(Clark, 1964, 1965, 1974, 1977)

The outstanding work of Dr David Clark at Fulbourn can only be mentioned in passing, as this hospital has only recently become part of the Cambridge teaching hospital organization. Until the opening of the Cambridge Clinical Medical School in 1976 there was no medical student teaching in the Cambridge district.

University of Birmingham

Uffculme Clinic   This clinic was founded in 1956 and provides both in- and out-patient psychotherapy services in the Birmingham area. About fifty patients are in treatment daily, up to thirty-five as in-patients; the others attend as day-patients. The Director, Dr John Harrington, a Maudsley-trained psychiatrist, had also been introduced to group therapy by Dr S. H. Foulkes, and the treatment has retained a strong group-analytic orientation. The clinic is a major psychotherapeutic resource for the treatment of neurotic patients in the Midlands.

John Connolly Hospital   There is a direct link between the organization of this early treatment centre on therapeutic community lines and the work of Henderson Hospital, since Dr Hayden Taylor, who succeeded Maxwell Jones as Director of Henderson Hospital, was closely involved in the formation and organization of the John Connolly.

29

University of Aberdeen (Morrice, 1973, 1974)

This university has for many years been noted for its support of the psychotherapeutic aspect of psychiatry. Through the work of Dr J. K. W. Morrice (see Chapter 6), who was a colleague of Maxwell Jones at Dingleton, there is a definite therapeutic community approach to the university department. A day hospital, a regional out-patient centre (Ross Clinic) and several wards in the mental hospital (Royal Cornhill) are all run on therapeutic community lines. Dr Morrice also ran a unit on therapeutic community lines in Edinburgh Prison between 1960 and 1966, and this may have influenced the practice at Grendon Underwood Prison in England, an institution which is notable for the extent to which offenders are treated in therapeutic groups (personal communications).

Conclusion

It seems clear that the most successful applications so far of the therapeutic community approach to treatment in the teaching hospital setting depend on two factors. First, the decision to introduce the therapeutic community approach is made by a person who is in a position to implement and to develop this approach by virtue of his position of authority in the hospital organization. Second, the unit is sufficiently clearly defined and separate from other units, so that its development does not impinge upon them to such an extent that boundary problems ensue.

This is the case when the unit is large but separate, as at Littlemore Hospital, Oxford, or small but separate, as at the Young People's Unit, Edinburgh. In such situations the boundary problems that arise from the clash of treatment methods and their underlying ideologies are relatively small and can be coped with. A consistent model of staff–patient relationships in the therapeutic milieu can be maintained, especially at times of stress and crisis. Where the unit is less autonomous and the therapeutic community approach competes with other models for the allegiance and support of staff and of patients, the methods are less consistently applied and are apt to be discarded at times of stress and crisis (see Chapter 15).

The further development of the therapeutic community approach in the teaching hospital setting will continue to depend on the initiative and encouragement of the heads of departments. Relatively few of these are trained in and sympathetic to the therapeutic community and psycho-dynamic approach, and the organization of in-patient units and further progress in this area will remain slow.

4

The therapeutic community in a local authority day care programme

Colin Archer

This chapter draws on the experience of a service-organizer within one local authority Social Services Department of using therapeutic community concepts within a day-care programme; and suggests that an opportunity which may now exist for wider national developments on these lines will be missed unless appropriate support systems for staff can be developed, and practitioners become better able to share the overall task in ways which place value on a wide variety of provision.

More day centres

It has been said that 'development and change, not stability and equilibrium, are the dominant features of the social services' (Donnison and Chapman, 1965). In the social services, it is particularly important that management should be concerned with both maintenance (by which I mean the holding, supporting, and sustaining) and development in terms of improvement in provision, practice, and performance, even if, with current restrictions on public expenditure, the scope for expansion is limited. Yet looking around one, what development does one see in the provision of psychiatric day centres by local authorities?

Fifteen years ago, Richard Titmuss wrote that:

> Beyond a few brave ventures, scattered up and down the country . . . pioneered by statutory and voluntary bodies, one cannot find much evidence of attempts to hammer out the practice, as distinct from the theory, of community care for the mentally ill (Titmuss, 1968).

It does not seem to me that the situation has changed very much in a decade and a half. The situation in Kensington and Chelsea has until recently been typical: a token provision comprising just one small centre largely 'silted up' with long-term highly dependent clients. Then in

31

1974, assisted by funds under the Urban Aid Programme, we set up St Luke's — again small, but committed to a totally different philosophy, that of the therapeutic community proper.

The question now is whether St Luke's is just another rare 'brave venture', a flash in the pan. Or does it signal something more, in one community at least?

Certainly one sees little evidence that, even in theoretical consider-ations of 'community care', day centres are yet generally seen as a crucial element. In one substantial and classic guidebook to the social services I find much written about the role of social workers in com-munity care for the mentally ill, and about hostel provision, both of which are admittedly very important. But the only reference to psychi-atric day centres which I find is: 'ancilliary services, such as social clubs and day centres, are also provided under this legislation' (Forder, 1969). To quote Titmuss again: 'It may be said, and no doubt the Minister said it yesterday, that the future looks more promising for community care than the past' (Titmuss, 1968).

While sharing Titmuss's obvious distrust of ministerial statements about a rosier future, I think there are now a number of government statements about community care for the mentally ill which are fairly specific, which seem to me to be very significant, and which we, who work in varying capacities in the community, might really make some-thing of. The first was the 1975 White Paper *Better Services for the Mentally Ill*. This did at least concede that 'day care services are at present perhaps the least developed of all mental health services', and it envisaged considerable expansion (DHSS, 1975).

Then in 1976 came the consultative document *Priorities for Health and Personal Social Services in England*. This was in my view even more important, because it dealt with hard cash, and it placed the needs for development in this field against the claims of all other health and social service work. In this contest of priorities, day care for the mentally ill came out particularly well, better even than residential provision, and better in fact than any other aspect of the health and social services. An additional 1,200 day places were envisaged each year between then and 1980. This document specifically stated that the availability of day care 'may be a critical factor in determining the success with which a person recovering from mental illness is able to readjust to life in the Com-munity' (DHSS, 1976).

The latest government statement (September 1977) hints at some backsliding, a recurring feature of national planning in this field, by stating that 'the latest statistics have shown a need to change the base and projections in the consultative document for local authority day care places for mentally ill people' (DHSS, 1977). Nevertheless, I am confident that we can still anticipate a significant increase in local authority psychiatric day centres, especially if we can avoid expensive purpose-built structures and share premises with others, as does St Luke's (playing Box and Cox with a youth club) and indeed our latest centre, opened in 1977, in church premises.

The relevance of a therapeutic community approach

I am sure that ministers and top civil servants, surveying the national scene from such heights, do not have any very clear ideas about the types of practice which might emerge from the implementation of their grand strategic plans. I do not expect most of them even to have heard of 'therapeutic communities'.

The task of exploring the scope and possibilities of psychiatric day centres is one for local Social Services Departments. Some centres – maybe many – will be based on therapeutic community principles. A local authority Social Services Department provides in many ways a natural home for therapeutic communities, whether these are expressed in a residential or a day-care setting. I will advance four reasons why.

First, the traditional principles upon which most social casework is based (Biestek, 1961) are reflected in a day centre run on therapeutic community lines: belief in the purposeful expression of feeling; controlled emotional involvement by staff; acceptance and non-judgmental attitude towards people; confidentiality of the relationship – here within the group; belief that each person must make his own choices and decisions about his own life. Even the 'individualization' on which social casework places such store is reflected in a therapeutic community: individual need has not been lost in the needs of the group.

Second, social work has a growing interest and involvement in group work, and within therapeutic communities there is a reservoir of knowledge and experience which can, over time, irrigate a Social Services Department.

Third, social work is also entering, however uncertainly, the ill-defined field of community work, and St Luke's is not just in the community, it is of the community. It is having some effect upon community attitudes. It is linking its members not just with each other, but also with the wider community, recognizing the truth of the statement that 'to feel completely alone and isolated leads to mental disintegration just as physical starvation leads to death' (Fromm, 1960).

Fourth, St Luke's is really doing what the Seebohm Report (Home Office, 1968), which founded Social Services Departments, urged, which is to 'reduce the rigid distinction between the givers and the takers of social services'.

The therapeutic community approach is closer to a social work model than to a traditional medical model. With this closeness of interest between social work and the therapeutic community, and with the possibilities of expansion which now exist, all might seem sweetness and light, and we can walk together, social services and therapeutic communities, hand in hand, towards the promised land waiting for us somewhere on the horizon. Alas, it is not like that! Although we may be natural bedfellows, it will be, at times, a stormy marriage. But because it has a solid basis, we must see that it does not end in separation or divorce.

Issues and problems

There are a number of minor issues. How, for example, would you explain to a Borough Treasurer an overspending of the food budget, if this were due to making the members responsible for buying; or inaccuracies in certain returns, which you have delegated to a member because his experience of paperwork is greater than yours, but still not great enough? Bureaucracies do like things right, for perfectly understandable and indeed good reasons. Unfortunately, they sometimes, quite inappropriately, ask for them to be not only right but tidy. Life is never tidy.

But beyond the sometimes deadly, sometimes merely hilarious, administrative expectations by bureaucracies, lie more important issues about this kind of work: where one recruits the staff with the very special experience, knowledge, and skills to work on therepeutic community lines; whether, within the rigidities of local authority salary scales, one can offer adequate salaries; how one defines the boundaries between the role of the social worker and that of the project staff. How do we ensure skilled and appropriate psychiatric support – of the kind which has proved so valuable at St Luke's – now that central government regulations will not allow Social Services to retain the services of a psychiatrist, insisting instead that they must rely on whoever – if anyone – the Area Health Authority can make available?

These are all important issues, but I want to draw special attention to two particular management issues, selected because I think that they are of fundamental importance in the relationship of the therapeutic community to its departmental environment, and because I think that we can, though with difficulty, do something about them ourselves. They are staff support and the need to share. If we do not attend to these issues, we will undoubtedly lose the real chance that now presents itself to us.

Support systems for staff

Work in therapeutic communities is difficult, mentally exhausting, emotionally draining. Those engaged in it need skilled support. Traditional local authority organizational structures are not guaranteed to provide this. These structures, basically bureaucratic and hierarchical, may be very appropriate to much of the work of a local authority, and indeed to many of the service-giving activities of a Social Services Department. But the more personal the work, the greater its depth, the less suitable these simple structures become. This has been recognized — though I think only partially — in the social work element of Social Services Departments. It has not been recognized at all adequately in relation to other provision, particularly in day centres.

Hierarchies are not, of course, the only way of organizing things, and Jimmy Algie (1970) of the National Institute for Social Work, has developed ideas of what he calls 'polyarchic' structures. It was these ideas, maybe in a bastard form, which led me to set up the St Luke's 'support group'. Now, this does not consist of hand-picked 'nice guys'. It consists of people whose roles within the department inevitably impinge upon St Luke's. Thus, in addition to the staff of the project, and the staff (like me) who are managerially responsible for all day centres (and whose managerial accountability remains), we have the Consultant Psychiatrist, the Department's Social Work Advisor on Mental Health, the local Area Officer, the Training Officer (whose interest includes placements of social work students at St Luke's), and at times the Research Officer.

The therapeutic community approach is a relatively new one, at least in the local authority psychiatric day centre field, and all the people I have referred to are likely to respond to it differently. A support group enables these differences to be hammered out. But it goes deeper than this. The work of a therapeutic community does in fact arouse very strong feelings — both positive and negative — among service providers. These cannot be explained simply by different intellectual stances towards this particular way of working. A therapeutic community is handling very strong and often primitive feelings among its members. I am sure that these spill out in all kinds of ways into those who have contact with it, touching something within themselves. The support group works on these feelings, though not always openly. The support group is also an appropriate reflection that group work is central to the project itself; it is symbolically right.

It may sound from all this that the last thing that the support group actually does is to provide support! In fact I think that it does. But this is not the key point. It is the experience of the group which enables the members to exercise their individual roles within the department in a

way which is supportive of St Luke's. I think that this is so important
that any psychiatric day project based on therapeutic community principles would find it very difficult to survive for long in a Social Services
Department without some such system of group support. It would
either — to develop an earlier analogy — fall out of bed, or be kicked
out of bed, or tip the whole bed over.

The need for sharing

I have recently extended this kind of support group to other centres in
the borough: the one long-established centre (which has now undergone
radical change), and a new centre which has just opened. And this brings
me to the second issue, which is about how different centres can between them meet a wider range of need.

Therapeutic communities certainly have a very valid and effective
way of working. They contain much truth, and they shed much light.
I sometimes wonder, though, whether they see themselves as possessing
the way, the truth, and the light. I need not make out a detailed case
why this is not so, as I am sure even the most committed therapeutic
community zealot would agree with me that human need is infinitely
varied. The same person has different needs at different times, and it
would be quite wrong if every psychiatric day centre the length and
breadth of the land were based on the purest of therapeutic community
principles.

Yet I suspect that our zealot's agreement would sometimes merely
be an intellectual one, and that some of his actions, as opposed to his
words, would spring from very different and maybe not fully conscious
feelings. He may act as if in his heart of hearts he wished the therapeutic community were a cure-all. Does he see a therapeutic community
as an 'absolute'? I do not. I see it as based on a collection of valuable
ideas, which in various combinations can inform the work of many
different centres. Does he think that the only alternative to a therapeutic
community is a non-therapeutic institution? I do not. Does he think
that all staff at psychiatric day centres who are involved, by whatever
means, in meaningful work, need similar support? I do, and I set up the
St Luke's support group before the decision that it should be based on
therapeutic community lines.

I hear of people going to other places because they are not 'ready'
for a therapeutic community. What does this imply? That the job of
any other centre is merely to 'contain' people until they are somehow
ripe for the Real Thing? Is our zealot colleague simply 'doing his own
thing'? He must beware of becoming old-fashioned. Doing 'one's thing'
was a feature of the 1960s. The 1980s will be all about sharing one's
thing, and sharing other people's things.

All those involved in the therapeutic community movement could have a head start in this sharing process if they could adapt and use their knowledge of how people and groups work to a wider context, including that of how organizations work. Yet I fear that some of those who have this opportunity, and have this to offer, simply live within and defend their own boundaries, suspicious of everyone outside them. To these I would commend a new slogan: 'All those who are not against us are for us.' It is at least worth trying.

I make this point about fitting into, and influencing, the wider scene, and I make it very strongly here and now because it seems to me that all those involved in therapeutic communities have some work to do in considering their stance towards other kinds of community provision. Also because — to return to an earlier analogy — I fear that the white heat of enthusiasm for therapeutic community ideas might inadvertently start a fire which would burn us all in our bed!

These two central issues about the structural relationship of a therapeutic community day centre to its environment, and the issue of its functional relationship to other centres, can be resolved. But they do need to be worked on speedily and hard. John Wesley wrote that 'he who is not free is not an Agent but a Patient'. Day centres should and can offer chances for some who, in other places or at other times, are called 'patients', to become agents — not only free agents in control of their own individual destinies, but agents for change in others and in the society in which they live.

5
Political implications of therapeutic communities

Brian Haddon

The leader of the first reported therapeutic community proper (Bion and Rickman, 1943) was removed from post for his trouble. This event has its parallels in mental hospitals and therapeutic communities today. My aim in this chapter is to expose some of those influences for study, and to offer some interpretations. I do not draw on an academic background, but write from personal experiences.

Political issues surrounding psychiatric units

I left general nursing for psychiatric nursing in 1966, mainly because I felt that the concentration on a person's sick part to the exclusion of healthy attributes was in itself unhealthy. To insist on an adult reverting to the status of a child was often a humiliation that was totally unjustified except, of course, in making the management of a ward easier. Someone's personality is often a factor in physical illness, and physical illness always affects a person's state of mind. This relationship between mind and body is usually ignored in the interests of management. It came as a shock to find that labelling and management were even more dominant in psychiatry. The process of helping patients was influenced by factors other than therapeutic techniques.

Horton Hospital (large mental hospital)

I had assumed that doctors were the best people to be responsible for the treatment of people with problems, but I found that, in large psychiatric hospitals, it is the nurses who do the work and often make the decisions too. Since these actions often included brutality toward, and humiliation of, helpless patients, I felt that the doctors were often betrayed by my nursing colleagues. Although they acknowledged the hypocrisy of pretending to treat a patient who had not responded to similar treatment for many years, the nurses also pointed out that a large population of patients kept them in employment. When I suggested a change from 'treatment' to caring, of changing the hospital into a community home with no pretence of most residents leaving, the senior nurses agreed with the logic, but pointed out that the power was with the doctors, and that their salaries depended upon people being labelled 'patients'. This situation has not changed.

Shrodells Psychiatric Unit

When Shrodells Psychiatric Unit opened in March 1973, I had already made clear the therapeutic community ethic for the treatment area on the ground floor.

At first, the General Hospital and the Hospital Adminstration did not know what to make of us. As we had our own physically separate unit, this wariness did not matter too much. Some of us made a considerable effort to involve the Assistant Administration Officer in the unit processes. When this was unsuccessful, my efforts to get him replaced were the cause of friction with other unit leaders, as they suggested a policy of appeasement. I should have been better prepared for this style of hospital administration, which I now know to be common.

The most extreme example of hospital process opposing my attempts to resist bureaucracy overcoming common sense, happened in 1973. When representing the unit at a hospital group catering meeting, I pointed out that the unit patients doing quite active physical work required more food than patients recovering from surgery. During the discussion someone said the needs of the unit were not fully understood by many in the hospital group. This was relayed to the Chief Nursing Officer as a statement that she didn't know what she was talking about. She, without attempting to speak to me at all, instructed my senior to reprimand me. He merely told me to be careful about what I said to some people, while seeming in no way to disagree with what I had said. He then left the unit to go on sick leave, but had issued a written notice to all, except me, that I had been demoted in his absence and could not act with my previous authority.

Further examples

At least three therapeutic communities came under attack from hospital management authorities in 1971–2: Paddington Day Hospital, Marlborough Day Hospital and Halliwick Hospital were 'looked at' with a view to 'modification of arrangements' which would effectively have ended their therapeutic community style. During negotiations one source of threat to the administration became clear. Sheena Rankin

Grunberg (1973) has written of the need to prepare for negotiations with outside groups with care, if the statutory authorities are not to be provoked, through discomfort, to hostile actions. The group process itself threatens people who are used to meetings controlled rigidly by agendas, minutes and chairman. This is one reason why many medical leaders of therapeutic communities go alone to their meetings with management.

A clear example of reaction to group penetration into a controlled atmosphere was an experience at Pentonville Prison. Whilst working at Paddington Day Hospital, I took 'classes' at the Prison. These sessions were really introductions to psychotherapy. I tried to interest the prison authorities in the possibility of organized change, while I continued to strengthen the group identity, including the few prison officers occasionally involved. With the co-operation of other staff, I offered an out-patient group in Paddington Day Hospital with a psychiatrist and one prison officer in training. I would continue to hold a group inside the prison and 'feed' the outside group with people as they were released from prison. The prison officers, after their training, would do more groups inside the prison. This arrangement was well received by an Assistant Governor who supported the project, but when the prison psychiatrist heard about it he stopped the plan. He would meet neither the psychiatrist from Paddington Day Hospital nor myself with the Assistant Governor.

Political issues within the therapeutic community

Even those units which consciously avoid bureaucratic control and try to respond flexibly to the needs of the patient and his social environment, can be merely playing at democracy. Esoteric theory, or dominant leadership, may be a barrier to real patient participation. A sure sign of such a situation is resistance to self-examination, for this might expose the anxiety which is being hidden by pseudo-participation.

Roffey Park Hospital (forty-bed neurosis unit)

Roffey practised the middle-class notion of therapeutic community. The patients were certainly treated with a great deal of courtesy and respect, but their realistic ability to take part in decisions affecting the hospital was strictly limited. Rules were quite clearly made by the staff team. This changed during the year that I was there, especially in recognition of non-medical practitioners of group techniques. Difficulties started when I involved patients in practical work within the hospital and its grounds. The work load of this project was sometimes quite heavy, and also required planning and responsible execution. The patients responded positively, as they usually do, and quickly began to take part in the overall management of the group. This was encouraged by me as a logical extension of the group's function. This intrusion into decision-making by patients and a lowly staff nurse assaulted the sensitivities of some heads of departments. The group was then judged, not on its merits, but by stereotypes.

Paddington Day Hospital

I joined Paddington Day Hospital as a charge nurse in 1968. Virtually everything in the community took place in groups. There were two kinds: those that sought to make decisions, and those that tried to find out why things happened the way they did. In both types of group, some of the techniques imported from the Henderson Hospital were used though interpretation was used more than confrontation. The main departure from common practice in therapeutic communities was the increasing emphasis on collective interpretations of the group rather than the individual. By 1970, I was aware of working as a member of a dynamic team with some of the staff, and occasionally patients, especially in large groups, sometimes as large as forty-five members.

The larger groups came to interest me more, whilst my confidence in small-group analytical psychotherapy diminished. By this time Basil Gregory had left, and Julian Goodburn was the senior doctor. By this time also, I was regularly fulfilling the requirements of the authorities for paperwork, statistics, etc. In summer 1971 a conflict began to develop between my argument for a degree of structure and Julian's preoccupation with analysis of situations from an observer stance. This involved a class issue that disturbed me. Julian analysed in the small group the need for medical certificates, rather than signed them. The group barricaded the door until he had promised to deal with the administrative aspect that would allow them to pay rents and survive. I argued that the experimental therapeutic community which Julian wanted must be seen within boundaries mutually agreed if it was to be valid, and perhaps even survive.

Henderson Hospital

The Henderson is famous for the clarity of its techniques of social organization. It controls behaviour by social pressure exerted by the whole community rather than just staff. These well-known processes have become a little clouded by the increasing introduction of small-group psychotherapy (see Chapter 14) but it still seems to me to be the most potent therapy practised. However, the hierarchy still caused great

41

problems. Stuart Whiteley is the statutory head of Henderson. He is also accepted as the 'spiritual' leader. I find the acceptance of an ongoing leader inconsistent with the Henderson community's regular criticism of statutory authority outside the unit. I was also irritated by everybody's insistence that all staff were psycho-social therapists, and also that the Henderson was not really a hospital. This attitude always changed dramatically every time there was any blood around. What was most depressing to me was to find that doubts were seen as negative, and that such discussion was not common in the community.

It is always exciting to feel part of a cohesive team activity, and the Henderson provides more consistency in this than most other therapeutic communities. Even more exciting is the feeling that the whole community is working together and in this, too, the Henderson is often the best example. However, excitement is not a valid indicator without measuring techniques that will demonstrate the effective processes.

Medical politics

It seems to me that medical leadership, while initially commanding a 'breathing-space' for the development of democratic psychiatry, eventually determines the limits of that democracy (see Chapter 1). Professional status, while losing its more formal and divisive trappings, is not ultimately relinquished: after all it provides a good salary and often 'instant leadership'. But, perhaps more correctly, doctors are functionally important for social control in our society, and hence serve political ends dimly perceived in the detail of therapeutic work.

Association of Therapeutic Communities

In March 1972, a few of us went to a conference at Halliwick Hospital determined to push the concept of a working Association of Therapeutic Communities. A steering committee was set up, most of whom were not doctors; and in fact, all of the people who undertook the practical organizational chores were either nurses, occupational therapists, or social workers of some sort. The steering committee for the association hoped for an exchange of ideas through group meetings and educative newsletters. There was no consensus about the degree of organization or whether patients should be welcome to join, though only a doctor argued against patient representation.

The association was officially started at the Littlemore Conference in July 1972. The working aim was 'for the prime task of furthering our particular work by the exchange of ideas in meetings, large and small, in publications for the promotion of research into the method and installation of a training programme into therapeutic community techniques' (ATC *Newsletter*, 1972). The three people who undertook to do the necessary work were nurses.

By October, there were 111 members of the association, none of them patients, though there had been no stated policy of exclusion. No therapeutic community was encouraging its resident population of patients to join the association. The work load was still being carried by non-medical staff. By May 1973, there were 148 individual and eight group memberships. Almost all members were from the Health Service hospitals. The speakers at conferences were mainly senior doctors, but the people doing the work or organizing the association and newsletter were non-medical staff. Arguments about the disadvantages of bureaucracy diminished, as did the attendance of those who advocated more radical alternatives to medically-dominated therapeutic communities.

I regret now the urgency with which I pursued an organizational framework for the association. It was to be undoubtedly another bandwagon which the medical profession would use for consolidating their position as leaders of the therapeutic community movement. Many of us at the beginning wanted the ATC to examine objectively the therapeutic community role in helping individuals and providing examples of healthy organization. This examination should have included the possibility that problem people should be seen not as a medical concern, but rather as a social problem to be dealt with outside the Health Service altogether. Medical control of therapeutic communities does discourage the examination of this possibility.

A person's environment is a major factor in determining his mental health. It has a positive or negative influence in helping him to overcome his problems. All therapeutic communities insist to a greater or lesser extent that their members are part of a social system. Some therapeutic communities consider that social pressure is one of the major therapeutic forces. The Henderson is one of those. Others, like the Ingrebourne Centre, insist that in psychotherapeutic communities social pressures should not be allowed to infringe on the therapeutic sessions too much. Neither type of community can avoid being a political entity; both acknowledge that social pressures are at work. Politics is the science, or art, of government, no matter how small the organization.

Therapeutic communities tend toward the environmental school of psychiatry, though many use drugs. Multi-disciplinary decision-making and role blurring are common, but doctors continue to be seen as the prime authority. Many therapeutic communities outside the Health Services use a psychiatrist for direction.

The politics of psychiatry

Ivan Illich (1975) questions the assumption that doctors are the best guardians of society's physical health. Though the activities of the medical profession have some scientific support, political attitudes are naive. Slogans like 'patients before politics' can perhaps be tolerated but never condoned in doctors dealing with physical disorders. Physical medicine developed in response to illness and injury; it was not a political decision to create the profession. Psychiatry can have no such claims to a natural scientific birth. The decision that the medical profession should be the guardians of the society's mental as well as physical health was made by Parliament with a powerful medical component. It was a decision of political expediency.

People did go mad before the twentieth century, but were catered for by families and small communities. Some people started businesses to cater for unwanted 'lunatics' (and others): the private madhouses. One of the first charitable institutions in Britain was the poor-house, where many people, now called schizophrenic or inadequate, were housed. Large lunatic asylums soon followed. There was little notion of calling such problem people ill until the medical profession redefined their problems. Doctors invariably came to treat those unfortunates because of the physical state that was caused by neglect and abuse.

With shocking revelations made about the conditions in these institutions, Parliament was obliged to investigate and prevent excessive abuses. An inspectorate was set up. The political decision in favour of the medical interests provided politicians with a willing custodian for those who did not accept society as organized by politicians. Millions of pounds have been spent on trying to give some scientific support to the original political decision. After 150 years or so, the scientific basis for organic psychiatry is still a subject for argument on its most basic tenets.

The driving force behind the Henderson Hospital, Paddington Day Hospital, Dingleton Hospital, Shrodells Psychiatric Unit, and other therapeutic communities comes from young staff, enthused with the prospect of challenging the bastions of corrupt psychiatry. The movement away from physical and chemical control techniques is a challenge to traditional forms of psychiatry. The motivation for most people involved in therapeutic communities is not to effect more humane control, but to liberate.

How do we explain the fact that, whilst expertise in the therapeutic processes practised in therapeutic communities is not a feature of the training of a doctor, it is doctors who are seen as the leaders of the community? Many doctors openly court popularity by acknowledging other staff and sometimes patients as their peers, but carefully retain their medical status. Further progress must lie in social action or community development organizations, where the leadership is determined by the current social needs, rather than one profession's interpretation of those needs.

Therapeutic communities have served a great purpose in insisting that individuals can be understood and helped (and can understand and help) much better if seen as part of a social entity. The real community, however, must comprise a range of interdependent factors. If some people insist unilaterally that they have special importance, and if they have the power to maintain that importance, then that organization cannot really call itself a community. So long as it is politically expedient for the medical profession to be the guardians of society's mental health, then doctors will be propped up in their artificial leadership role. The development of a community will be limited by the needs of its leader, and not by the needs of its members.

Conclusion

Although Britain is supposed to be a democracy, the status of the citizen is low. Citizenship is not featured in school curricula despite being embodied in the 1944 Education Act. A substitute status is that given to membership of the middle class. This equates with the range of welfare institutions in Britain being based on the old, emasculating charity systems, and not on social institutions responding to democratically agreed needs.

The middle class controls all powerful social institutions from Parliament to primary schools. Therapeutic communities that use group methods as techniques devised by middle-class professionals are useful only if middle-class norms are those to aspire to. Only therapeutic communities and community development projects that do a realistic situation analysis of their target population, respond to the needs demonstrated and then evolve an ongoing dynamic process, can be said to be truly working in the best interest of the people.

Section B
The basic idea

This section gives an outline to some of the basic ideas in therapeutic community theory and practice. It is not comprehensive, but rather deals with the more important aspects. The staying power of the original concepts is explored by Morrice in Chapter 6. He reflects critically on permissiveness, democracy, confrontation and communalism, arguing that experience has elevated some concepts to a more central position than others. He is acutely aware of the mystification that can result from the use of such concepts as slogans.

The use of groups is fundamental to the therapeutic community, but these are constrained by physical space. That space may be used in ways which reveal some of the hidden structures of a community. Bishop explores these issues in Chapter 7, pointing out that the use of groups can be enhanced by a suitable architecture.

Finally, the more spontaneous and emotional side of therapeutic community life is explored in Chapters 8 and 9. Marta Ginzberg and Joel Badaines point out the connections with the 'new' therapies, while Nick Mahony has written an insightful and evocative account of his own deepening involvement and change as a community resident. These two written accounts obviously cannot be spontaneous themselves, yet they have successfully captured some of the fleeting and ever-changing emotional landscape. Indeed, this tension between what is changing and what is stationary, highlighted by the occasional conflicts between 'new' therapists and more traditional therapeutic community staff, is a small example of the fundamental problem for social psychiatry: the institutionalizing of a spontaneous and critical therapeutic method.

6

Basic concepts: a critical review

J. K. W. Morrice

The four fundamental themes originally suggested by Rapoport (1960) as characterizing the therapeutic community are still worthy of general acceptance. They are: democratization, permissiveness, reality confrontation, and communalism. The words themselves lack euphony, but they represent important concepts and so may be forgiven their polysyllables. The implementation of these principles involves certain practices which over the years, have become identified with the therapeutic community, are now hallmarks of its authenticity, and may even be somewhat hallowed with time. It may be that these principles and practices are not so much hallowed as cliché-ridden and ritualistic. But, without doubt, there are theories at the bottom of the jargon and reason behind the ritual.

Familiar practices include freeing of communications, flattening of the authority pyramid, sharing of responsibility, decision-making by consensus, analysis of events, provision of living-learning opportunities, and examination of roles and role-relationships. This list, which might be considerably extended, indicates how deeply the therapeutic community has been preoccupied with social structure and function, the nature of leadership, the exercise of authority, and the working relationships of staff and patients. Behind all this again, in an attempt to inform the whole atmosphere of the community, is the requirement that each individual experience his own feelings and help others to experience theirs in an open, concerned and hopeful fashion. In such an atmosphere, the expectation is that each person will feel free to make mistakes, discover himself, grow and learn. How valid are such concepts and practices? How have they proved themselves? What is their place now and in the future?

Democratization

This term, like the word 'therapeutic' itself, tends to disarm any disagreement. It is not only a principle, but also possesses the characteristic of a humane and liberal attitude which all 'right-thinking' people must surely accept and strive to implement. Over the past twenty-five years, within most institutions as in society at large, there has been a considerable movement away from rigid and authoritarian control towards more flexible and participative administration. But, how democratic must an organization be before it is said to embody the principle of democratization? When we use terms like 'democratization' or talk about 'freeing communications', how far are we engaging in the fashioning of ideological slogans and how closely are we examining what is desirable and attainable in a particular set of circumstances? If there are many kinds of therapeutic community, as Maxwell Jones has affirmed, there may be many different levels of the democratization process appropriate to different situations. So, the distinction drawn by Clark (1965) between 'the therapeutic community approach' and 'the therapeutic community proper' — which is an important, valid, and useful division in many ways — may be too neat in actual practice. This sort of labelling may also lead to the easy but mistaken assumption that some of the highly valued elements of the therapeutic community (like open communications and the promotion of criticism) are specific to it, rather than representing sound administrative practice in any situation, including those not seeking to be therapeutic.

The facts of life, as they exist for most of us, set obvious limits to the democratic process. For example, patients in hospital do not elect the medical staff who, in turn, are responsible to a medical director or a board appointed to that position. Within such limits, however, a democratic structure can be either encouraged or blocked. It is facilitated by opening channels of communication vertically and horizontally, encouraging face-to-face encounters, and by sharing in a relevant way the responsibility for decisions. But what is possible and realistic in a small psychiatric unit may be foolhardy in a large hospital, a school, or a prison. And even within the same unit, because of fluctuations in the number and quality of staff or the nature of patients under care, techniques and expectations have to be suitably modified. All too often, failure and even disaster attend unskilled attempts to translate appropriate ideals into inappropriate action.

In essence, democracy in a bureaucratic organization like a psychiatric hospital is concerned with where and with whom decisions are made. If a democratic social structure exists, staff and patients have a say in the conduct of their work and treatment. But democracy has become confused with equality, and it often seems that people believe that everyone has a right to have something to say about everything. This ensures messy management, delayed decisions, and general inefficiency; and such difficulties arise from the fallacy of supposing that all administrative problems are soluble by better communications. Often, what we need is not simply better communication, but rather, something better to communicate. In the name of democracy we have seen in recent times the urgent work of hospitals, schools, and factories disrupted or halted, as it seemed quite capriciously and without any sense of priority or responsibility.

As the Cummings (1962) have pointed out, 'in any social structure, decisions should be made at the places in which they can most effectively forward the goals of the structure, once the major values *about* decision-making itself have been taken into account'. So, if a therapeutic milieu has a clear appreciation of its goals and values, the location of decision-making follows logically. This certainly failed to happen in traditional mental hospitals, where aims and methods were obviously mismatched, where decision-making was jealously guarded and centralized, and nursing staff and patients had next to no say in their own affairs. Now, with the establishment of the multidisciplinary team, with formation widely disseminated in ever-multiplying meetings amid snowstorms of directives, and with the enfranchisement of those low in the hierarchy, how effectively do we make our decisions, fulfil our values, and reach our goals? Not too well, perhaps. We seem to have ignored Schumacher's advice that 'small is beautiful'.

It is true that even in therapeutic communities there exist difficulties in communicating, sharing, and taking responsibility; that values and norms are not clearly established or agreed; and that goals may be vague. Indeed, examination of certain ideas and assumptions about therapeutic communities proves in practice that they may be inaccurate or misleading. The present writer has previously suggested (Morrice, 1972) that, since there is always a difference between what we do and what we say we do, and since there is an even greater discrepancy between our actual practice and our stated ideals, it is inevitable that myth becomes part of all behavioural codes and methodologies. Moreover, the therapeutic community entails an understanding of inexact concepts that are put into practice in what are often difficult and demanding circumstances. Myth — it is easy to see — grows up as a defence against anxiety. But it needs to be recognized and examined, the kernel of truth preserved, and the empty shell discarded. But he who wields the nutcracker invites accusations of disaffection or even heresy. This may have something to do with the beleaguered position of social psychiatrists in their early days and the missionary quality that may still invest some advocates of the method. There is also the charismatic type of leadership which is clearly present in many therapeutic communities and which may encourage a closely guarded set of relationships. Such a group resents criticism from without and distrusts it from within. While it is true that the diffusion of innovation is less like the sharing of good tidings and more like civil war, one must try to practise what one preaches. Self-evaluation and open communication are undoubtedly risky, but there is little hope of progress without them.

Disparate notions of authority and leadership bedevil the process of democratization in therapeutic communities as in the outside society. It is understandable that, disillusioned by the failure of self-styled experts and in a flight from authoritarianism, from medical dominance, and oppressive bureaucracy, many have called the whole idea of leadership into question. But it is a paradox worth remembering that a democracy needs good leadership and can be efficiently maintained only from a position of power. The task of leadership in a therapeutic community is burdensome and exposed. But abdication or the 'killing off of father' solves nothing. More useful and satisfactory is the acknowledgment that different situations need different leaders, and this is ensured by what Jones (1968a) has termed multiple leadership. The role is then not the prerogative of one individual, but instead is shared appropriately and according to ability. But, and sometimes it is a big but, this assumes the group's cohesiveness is repeatedly destroyed. Then the leadership disciplines and encourage in its members the demonstration of leadership qualities. Often, because of the rotation of nurses and other staff, the goup's cohesiveness is repeatedly destroyed. Then the leadership role may fall largely on one individual, whose preoccupation at that time may be to preserve the unit and its culture. Thus, another pitfall appears. The demand upon a group's energy, in the solving of its own internal conflicts and the maintenance of its structure, may prove excessive and may detract from the primary task of treating patients or serving the needs of clients.

But any therapeutic community deserving of the title is open to constructive change. Jones (1976), discussing the therapeutic community as an 'open system', points out how a leader may delegate his power and authority, distributing it through the system, and thus become a facilitator of the process of change and growth.

Permissiveness

This expression, which has become an all too familiar part of contemporary speech, has to be redefined in terms of therapeutic community. It is ordinarily used to describe society's lax attitude to sex, violence and social deviance. In so far as this interpretation is carried over to describe the culture of therapeutic communities it is woefully misleading.

And yet, even in our context of social learning, it is all too easy for permissiveness to drift into licence, self-indulgence, and neglect, unless it is conscientiously linked to reality confrontation. Instances are not hard to find where a community's authority structure has been eagerly dismantled in the unrealistic expectation that a sense of responsibility would prevail and new opportunities for therapy arise. But the result has been a descent into confusion and discontent, followed by a painful struggle for survival. Because power and authority have been widely abused (and not least in hospitals, schools, and institutes of correction), it does not follow that they can be abandoned. Nor is it true that the less authority we use and the more permissive we are, the more effective become our treatment methods. Much of the misunderstanding of so-called 'progressive' methods stems from the reluctance of practitioners to acknowledge the importance of limit-setting and the necessity of sanctions. While discipline, to have any real significance, must finally be self-discipline, it has to be learned.

In therapeutic community terms, permissiveness means the toleration of deviant behaviour. The idea is not to accept deviance uncritically or indifferently. On the contrary, suppression by regulation or decree is avoided in order that the behaviour may be available for examination. The difficulties of living and working together and the disturbances which result are exposed in the expectation that causes can be uncovered and understanding achieved. In this sense, therefore, permissiveness reflects the capacity of group members to relate to one another in a trusting fashion without undue anxiety, and without rushing to judgment, yet accepting the need for control. As Crocket (1966b) has pointed out, to be permissive requires the exercise of authority when it is appropriate just as much as its surrender when it is not. A nice balance needs to be kept between the needs of the individual and the needs of the group.

If the therapeutic milieu is so organized that patients reveal real-life problems in an open fashion, then permissiveness serves its purpose. What results (so it is hoped) is relevant new social learning for both individual and group. Experiences are offered which encourage the ventilation of hidden feelings, expose perceptual distortions, and make plain repetitive behavioural patterns of an unacceptable kind. Successful working-through demands the sensitive handling of transference, so that the resolution of relationship problems in the group is also translated into improved relationships in the world outside: for example, with spouse, family, or employer. There is here an overlap of what has been thought to be two different sets of skills, or at least two separate points of view: sociotherapy and psychotherapy. In a way, this echoes Rapoport's plea (1960) to recognize the differences between treatment and rehabilitation. Of course, it should be remembered that Rapoport's observations were centred on Henderson Hospital in its earlier days; and it is perhaps unfortunate that the development of the therapeutic community in other locations and with different clients (sometimes originated by Maxwell Jones himself, for example at Dingleton Hospital and Fort Logan Mental Health Centre) have attracted less attention from sociologists. (An exception is the study of a deliberately rehabilitative therapeutic community by Sharp (1975).) One important illustration of the point is the recent growth of marital and family therapy in therapeutic communities (particularly those in psychiatric hospitals), where patients may be more suited to a psychotherapeutic approach than the original population at the Henderson and where families are more readily available. This offers the advantage of matching what is occurring in the artificial family of the group with the real family outside. Unfortunately, this important linkage between permissiveness and testing-out in reality may not be available in certain cicumstances like prison, where the prisoner's family may be geographically distant or excluded from participation.

The intelligent and constructive use of a permissive orientation is not always easy to maintain. Patients, particularly adolescents and sociopathic personalities, are inclined to test-out limits. The acting-out behaviour of a few patients in a unit may give rise to a high state of tension. Other patients may then hide behind defence-mechanisms, such as scapegoating, or even respond by quitting treatment altogether. It is something of a conjuring trick to keep the right proportion of support and confrontation. There may come a point when a group is failing to cope with a disruptive sub-group or individual. The decision about how to proceed may then be complicated by inflexible notions that the group, and only the group, must handle its own problems, and that to use drugs, individual psychotherapy or other techniques is an abandonment of principle. The present writer does not share that view and it is becoming increasingly outmoded. It seems more useful, when dealing with a range of psychiatrically disturbed patients, to accept that a similarly wide range of techniques may well be necessary. Some patients will survive only if given help outside the group setting and, if this is done insightfully, advantages accrue. The tyranny of the group must sometimes be resisted and the notion of permissiveness extended to recognize the legitimate individual demands of both patients and staff.

Every psychotherapist knows that only an accepting and supportive relationship encourages an individual to lower his defences and allow the opportunity for therapeutic change. But a patient's unrealistic expectations, sooner or later, must be frustrated. The acceptance and understanding which a group bestows upon an individual in the course of his recurrent mistakes and follies is transitional in nature. The therapeutic community encourages growth-learning and knows that a patient's progress may be erratic. Permissiveness means that he is not regulated into a state of conformity, but rather helped to transmute his conflict into realistic problem-solving. Yet the duty of the group or the therapist to deny and frustrate may be avoided. It is easier to be comforting and lovable than to confront and accept hostility. So patients cling dependently, nurses follow their traditional role of 'mothering', social workers hesitate to sound authoritarian, and fellow-patients are silent because 'It'll be my turn next'.

But even in the most therapeutic of therapeutic communities, the principle of permissiveness will seem at times to be in direct conflict with another fundamental principle or practice. The problem then is not one of right and wrong, but of right and right, and may be difficult to solve.

Reality confrontation

This principle, as already suggested, is closely linked with that of permissiveness. The two go hand-in-hand, and one has little purpose without the other. As patients interact they reveal socially inept patterns of behaviour which are often characteristic of them, not only in the life of the therapeutic community, but also in terms of outside relationships with family and friends. Reality confrontation implies that the individual's conduct is reflected back to him in the hope that he will accept interpretation and modify the offending behaviour. The word 'confrontation' has for most people an aura of forthright or even hostile criticism. This is unfortunate. For, while it is true that therapist and peer group cannot avoid the arousal (and being the target) of some hostility, the purpose is to give information and share feelings in an acceptable way. The task is to tell the truth in love — which is a great deal easier to say than to do.

Confrontation helps to make plain the 'games people play' and the mechanisms they use, often compulsively, to avoid their painful realities. It is the sharp end of therapeutic community practice, dealing as it must with denial, withdrawal, splitting, projection and so on. It seems to work best when the group possesses a strong ego and the individual is able to feel the support as well as the criticism of his peers. But, when the group itself is withdrawn, angry and dependent, the burden falls heavily on staff and may prove extremely difficult to carry effectively.

Main (1975) has discussed with impressive clarity the difficulties attendant upon the reciprocal, participant roles and responsibilities of staff and patients in a therapeutic community, particularly as they are revealed in a large group. He emphasizes how, when the helpful and the helpless meet, they put pressures on each other to move into a collusive projection system. Unless this is tested out against reality, there are real dangers to the personality integration of all.

In this respect, Florence Nightingale has much to answer for. While all the caring professions fall into error, the problem is perhaps most easily seen in the nursing profession. For it is nurses more than any others who are caught and taught, within the confines of a rigid professional hierarchy, to deny their own individual needs in the nurturing of others. The needy and unsatisfied part of herself, which the nurse might recognize and express, she is encouraged to disown and project into patients. The tendency then is to acknowledge only two separate categories: patients and staff, the sick and the well. Given that therapeutic communities are geared to this problem, nevertheless staff members with this kind of difficulty are readily caught up in defencefulness or collusion. This results in defective reality testing. Again, while it is true that in a therapeutic community staff and patients learn together, and consequently the staff member in difficulty will have support and opportunity for insight and growth, yet at one point in time the therapeutic machinery is under strain and may even be proved defective.

From all this it is clear that, in the goldfish bowl of the therapeutic community, reality-confrontation affects staff as well as patients. Staff performance is open to scrutiny and criticism, which gives the chance for new learning, but this needs to be handled with consideration and skill. Staff should not feel they have 'failed' if they elect to work in a different setting.

Similar difficulties occur with patients, of course, and raise the unanswered questions of selection: what sort of patients, with what sort of problems, for what type of therapy? But the dramatic clashes of confrontation versus permissiveness (which raise such queries as 'Should we have accepted this patient in the first place?' or 'What about discharging him?') generally seem to involve dilemmas over the safeguarding of values and boundaries, and the wise use of authority. The present writer (1965) has discussed these matters elsewhere. Here, one example must suffice.

Two patients, male and female, married but not to each other, form a liaison. Sexual intimacy is taking place and the relationship is recognized by all to be self-indulgent and dangerous. Discussion in groups and individually fails to have any influence. How far should this situation continue to be explored, perhaps with involvement of the spouses? Should efficient contraception be ensured? Or should discharge from the unit be effected? The difficulties are obvious.

Permissiveness is not passivity. The latter is a poor substitute for policy-making and decision. On occasion, those in the position of leadership have a duty to set limits, while seeking always to use dilemmas and conflicts as learning opportunities.

Communalism

It is apparent that the four major themes of the therapeutic community overlap and are interdependent. The principle of communalism serves to emphasize the sharing nature of the enterprise, the same sharing as occurs in the practice of democratization, permissiveness, and reality confrontation. To facilitate sharing, and perhaps to signal that the culture is accepting, trusting, and does not stand on ceremony or status, everyday duties and facilities are also shared. For example, tea and coffee breaks may be taken by patients and staff together, and dining-room and recreational facilities may be used in common. Nurses do not wear uniform and first names are generally used. All this may be seen as gimmicky and unrealistic. And window-dressing of this kind may be promoted to disguise the emptiness of the shelves inside. Moreover, the notion of togetherness may be pushed to false and unhelpful extremes which deny significant differences and individual needs. After all, the basic aim is to enhance individuality, if it is competent and adjusted to reality, not to submerge needs and personal style in grey uniformity. The pressure to conform is a two-edged weapon and it is arguable how far it may legitimately be used before it becomes oppressive or coercive. The checks and balances of group life, however, are real safeguards, particularly where staff at all levels feel free to partake in everyday activities. The therapist who is available, human, and 'transparent' may give patients a useful model. Certainly, experience confirms that the informal and spontaneous encounters of patients and staff are often more rewarding therapeutically than formal groups or reviews. The 'corrective emotional experience' may happen more tellingly at work or play if staff are alive to the opportunity.

Yet patients are often reluctant to verbalize their concern, share feelings, or clamber over their high defences. They may insist upon keeping staff members 'in role' and may resist the efforts of nurse and psychiatrist to meet them person-to-person. When such efforts succeed and close relationships are formed, transference and counter-transference problems abound. The openness and psycho-dynamic understanding of the staff group need to be well in evidence to prevent harm and ensure a therapeutic outcome.

Wootton (1977) has drawn attention to the misunderstandings and blockages to sharing as they occur in a therapeutic community. An individual's ability to engage in appropriate sharing may be contingent on knowledge of the formal and informal rules of the organization which may conflict or seem ambiguous; and, certainly, what one group member understands as relevant sharing may be judged differently by another. The matter is more complex than might appear at first sight.

Conclusion

Manning (1976c) asserts that 'the radical idea of the therapeutic community within psychiatry in the 1950s never became completely translated into action'. Main (1976), while reaffirming the capacity of therapeutic community concepts to evaluate all social organizations, confesses the absence of 'an adequate general theory of psycho-social development', and that 'much of our work is still at the level of pragmatism and intuition'. Clark (1975) points to the 'inadequacy of much professional training for therapeutic communities' and notes how communities run without expertise may court considerable danger. Practitioners of the method may find themselves locked in disagreement, forced on the defensive, or tempted to question one another's ideas and achievements. In this paper, I have added to this debate. Democratization is relative, and will vary within the constraints and goals of a community. Permissiveness and reality confrontation can be considered separate poles of a single dimension. And communalism, perhaps the least resilient concept, often masks phoney sharing by a naive staff group.

In addition to such informed criticism from within, the therapeutic community has never lacked criticism from without, much of it offered with more vehemence than understanding. Recently there has been a growing interest in general systems theory (GST) and a recognition of its relevance to group methods, family therapy, and therapeutic community practice. Systems science, by its use of fresh concepts and terminology, stimulates a new look at the whole question of therapeutic intervention. Of considerable importance is the attempt to reconcile psychoanalytic theory with systems theory or, at least, to recognize where they complement each other. This may help towards the marriage of psychotherapy with sociotherapy and bring readier acceptance of what is common to each technique. As an example of an 'open system', the therapeutic community provides a setting where such theories and practicies may be explored and exploited (see Chapter 12).

Indeed, the therapeutic community, put into practice within institutions and in outside society, has made a considerable impact in the past twenty-five years. Throughout the world the liberalization of mental hospitals owes much to this approach. Communities of many different kinds – in psychiatric units, day hospitals, hostels, schools, and prisons – continue to demonstrate the effectiveness of the model. At the same time, as an instrument of change, the therapeutic community must itself stay ready to meet new challenges and be open to new learning. The stable basis provided by a system of accepted concepts encourages further exploration, innovation, and growth.

7
The environment of the therapeutic community

Jeff Bishop

It may seem rather superfluous to be talking about the environment for an organization which has social relations as an overriding central theme, and when I say that I shall in fact be talking mainly about the planned and controlled physical environment, this may seem even more irrelevant. The aim of this chapter, however, is to show what can be gained by realizing that, as Edmund Leach says, 'societies exist within a material context. . . . But such a context is not simply a passive backcloth to social life; the context itself is a social product and is itself "structured"' (Leach, 1976). Society expresses itself through the design, planning and control of physical environment and it is essential that anybody involved in therapy understands the ways in which man consciously and unconsciously uses space, in order to bring in the environment as a positive contribution to therapy.

This chapter will describe how the environment can be used as a direct resource in therapy, how it can (if treated with care) be used as a supportive resource to the general principles of therapeutic communities, and, finally, how better decisions in the very early stages of planning new psychiatric facilities can be made through careful briefing. Much of this will be based upon work done a few years ago at a psychiatric day hospital (Bishop and Foulsham, 1973). The study was done to establish ways in which the hospital could find a better 'fit' between its organization, philosophy and functions and the available space. Because there was very little new building, one may wonder in what ways work of this sort uses the expertise of an architect. In the last few years, the architect's role has enlarged and it is important to realize that there are now a number of architects who specialize in studying how people use space; not just in terms of the technically efficient planning well known in general hospital design, but also in terms of social, psychological and symbolic systems. The sensitive architect is therefore now an essential contributor to any organization as much during the life of a building as in the design and construction stages.

Therapy settings

It has been known for some time that certain aspects of social behaviour
are constrained spatially, even without the introduction of walls,
furniture and other limiting objects. The first major piece of work
studying the spatial dimensions to interpersonal behaviour was done
by Edward Hall (1966) in the mid-1960s, followed by Sommer (1969).
They introduced the term 'personal space' to describe what was found
to be an invisible bubble which people carry around with them and
which seriously limits the type of conversation which can occur at
particular distances. This bubble has since been shown to be generally
constant within cultures (but to vary considerably between), and to be
significantly different for certain sub-groups, especially violent criminals
and those suffering from forms of psychiatric disorder. In the British
context three zones of the bubble generally operate: the intimate
(approximately eighteen inches in radius), the social (approximately
forty-eight inches in radius), and the formal (approximately nine feet in
radius). It has been shown that unless certain types of communication
occur at the correct distance, a person will begin to feel uncomfortable,
and if distortions occur during mental illness then the physical relationship between therapist and patient needs careful consideration if what
is said is literally to 'get across'.

The environmental implications of this are obvious for the simple
reason that rooms may be smaller than nine feet wide and, with the
addition of furniture, areas of less than four feet across occur frequently.
Sommer's work explored aspects of furniture arrangement and particularly seating choice, discovering that people will deliberately select their
seat and alter furniture arrangements in order to control and limit their
social encounters. One knows from experience how one can take over a
whole corner of a pub by sitting in the right chair, and the thought that
patients in group therapy ease themselves through by manipulating
the environment makes consideration of this an essential task for the
therapist.

One distinguishing feature of therapeutic communities is the large
group meeting, and at this level one further factor isolated in research
becomes worthy of consideration. In groups of people well known to
each other a phenomenon called 'social space' can be discerned, although
it has received very little attention since being identified by Hudson
(1971). Social space is really a form of 'group personal space' whereby
if an outsider enters the social space at a distance beyond that usual for
attracting interest by invasion of personal space, most members of the
group will attend to the behaviour of that outsider. Figures 7.1 to 7.3
illustrate the concepts of personal and social space and will particularly
help to explain the latter. The importance of this for large group meetings

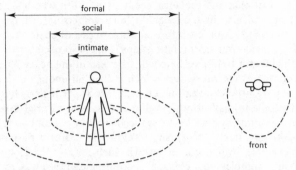

Figure 7.1 The three zones of personal space around a person and the actual shape of each zone, larger in front than at the sides and back

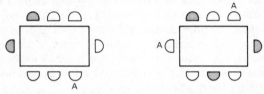

Figure 7.2 The drawings represent tables in a reference library. Sommer could predict that if the shaded seats were occupied, position A would be selected by a newcomer unless one knew others at the table

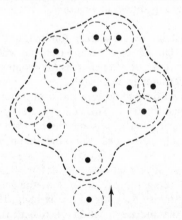

Figure 7.3 If the group of people represented by the heavy dots (and attendant personal bubbles), are well known to each other, they form a social space (broken line). Invasion by an outsider, (as with arrow) will attract attention even from those whose personal space has not been invaded, because their social space has been

lies in the fact that the therapist needs to establish whether he/she is an outsider, and also in the fact that the membership of large groups changes frequently, and therefore a whole series of spatial (as well as non-spatial) insider/outsider relationships is likely to occur.

The final factor to discuss here will arise also in the next section; this is the concept of 'territoriality', which is familiar enough at a general level to require little explanation. Lipman (1968) particularly has shown how old people in institutions develop aggressive territorial drives; and although he warns against being seduced by the concept — it is very tempting to architects (Newman, 1973) — it is likely that its most obvious examples will occur in settings such as psychiatric hospitals. Territoriality complements personal space because it is a way of 'taking over' space even during one's absence, and its implications for therapy are, quite simply, that the same group of people will behave differently according to whose territory they are occupying. There are, in fact, ways of making a place one's own other than through occupation and defence of space. 'Personalization' is the word used to describe the way people express their individual presence in space; although it serves many functions, it is mentioned here because it can be deliberately used — by patients as well as staff — to limit and define ambiguous territory, hence influencing group behaviour.

I am now going to describe briefly two particular examples of the interplay of the phenomena I have described, one example being small group therapy, the other being a large group meeting (Figures 7.4 and 7.5). In the small group shown in Figure 7.4, the following points can be made:

(A) The therapist is in a powerful, dominating position diagonally opposite the door. On the first occasion he/she will have to be there first to get this position but after that, as the group gains confidence, a less hierarchical location may be sensible.

(B) Positions 1 and 6 are reassuring and/or threatening because proximity to the therapist ('bad') is balanced by a non-frontal relationship, affecting eye-contact ('good'); personal bubbles are in fact oval, with the largest section directly ahead, therefore permitting closer contact from the side.

(C) Position 3 is relatively safe for two reasons. It enables the patient to gain 'relief' by using the excuse of something happening outside the window when pressure in the group is high. This can, however, be influenced by the precise location of 6 because glances may be construed by 6 as directed at him/her. The other reason is common to 4:

(D) Positions 3 and 4 both gain some relief because of the table between them and the therapist. Hobdell (1972) warns against this because it prevents the therapist from seeing feet movements.

(E) Positions 2 and 5 are the most 'involved', and although they are

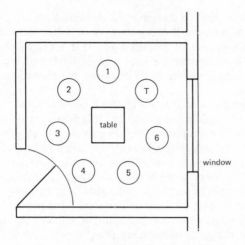

Figure 7.4 A therapy room with door, window, table, position of therapist (T), and positions of patients (1-6) marked

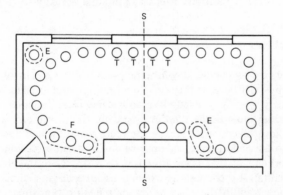

Figure 7.5 Large group meeting showing possible 'flight' positions (F), 'escape' positions (E), tendency of group to split into two (S line) and confrontation location of staff (T)

not the closest it can be important for the therapist to realize that some patients will choose those positions in order to dominate the talking.

(F) Position 4 gains another form of potential relief by being near the door. Thus, flight is potentially easy; even though other facts generally mean that someone will never actually flee, having that potential is significant.

(G) The figure is drawn, I hope, to convey an impression about the size of the room, and my feelings are that although all the necessary physical space is there the room is psychologically too small. It is also unclear whose territory is being used. If it is the therapist's this will heighten the problems of a small space. If it is neutral there are then ways in which the therapist can effect change by altering his/her position and/or importing personal items to make the room appear (at least partly) 'owned'.

In the large group shown in Figure 7.5 many of those items just discussed will occur again, although the relative advantages of some positions are weakened. The positions which do gain considerably in importance are those near the door (F). In large groups actual flight is more possible and can occur. One sees people deliberately arriving late in order to avoid crossing the room to 'trapped' positions, and (regardless of the number of chairs), some people will stand near the door. Four other aspects are important: the location of the staff and whether they cluster together (my figure shows a 'confrontation' model), the nearness to a true circle of the group shape (very many rooms tend to 'divide' into two hence creating two groups), the ownership of the space (rarely a staff room, sometimes a patient's room but, ideally, neutral), and the likelihood of some positions offering a potential virtually to hide (E).

The overall setting

The study of a psychiatric day hospital (with which I was involved) was initiated by staff because they felt there was not enough space and new conversion work was needed. It soon became clear, however, that far from needing more space there was actually too much, and what was causing the problem was the way the space was allocated and used in relation to the philosophies and organization of the hospital community. The importance of this observation is in its reference to the philosophy of the hospital. It is common to examine use of space in a directly functional manner and it therefore needs some justification to suggest that how rooms are located, allocated and used can express a philosophy. I propose to demonstrate this by describing some structures found during the hospital study, most of which contradicted the basic philosophy.

The first example is in fact the only successful one, and is about the relationship between the hospital community and the outside community. One principle of the day hospital is that of avoiding the total removal of patients from the everyday world, and of continually attempting to reinforce and enhance the individual's role in society. The new, prestige psychiatric unit in a hospital may be physically separate from the surgical areas but it is still on the campus, approached through the internal road system and stylistically 'clinical'. All these factors serve to detach the unit from its context, whereas the hospital we studied was in two large, converted old houses, totally absorbed into two residential streets and virtually indistinguishable. The fact that several local people did not even know of the psychiatric unit in their midst may be considered (idealistically) a failure, but a realist like myself can regard it as a major, and rare, success.

Within the hospital one can analyse the use of space and divide the whole into several categories of areas. The first such possible division is into staff and patient areas, according to who 'owns' rooms and even whole floors. The philosophy of the therapeutic community taken to its extreme would suggest that it should not be possible to perceive spaces as the 'territory' of staff or patients permanently, although occupancy always grants temporary ownership. In our study, however, we found certain rooms clearly 'owned' by staff and even one complete floor, including corridors. This might have been acceptable if the patients then 'owned' equal numbers and types of space, but there were actually no spaces unambiguously owned by patients, and the rooms mainly theirs were also generally less desirable and more publicly located. Being realistic again, one can suggest that there will always be some staff areas, and therefore there should perhaps be conscious attempts made to provide clear patient areas.

A second possible division of space deserves merely a small mention. The hospital we observed had a unit for autistic children, a playgroup room and one other children's room. Although it was still at the formative stage, an idea was being circulated about moving towards a whole-family treatment approach. The difficulty would have been that a very clear existing association of the children with the basement (which contained most of the facilities for children) was rather derogatory. Other factors did enhance the articulation but it would have been difficult to encourage a whole-family approach with such a severe physically separatist arrangement.

One further division of the space will be dealt with quickly before concluding with the most important one. The hospital had three groups of patients: the central core (an unfortunate term but it applied) of day-patients, a smaller group of out-patients attending mostly in the evenings, and a variable but always small group of in-patients (who were also day-patients.) There was a very clear area owned by the in-patients, and the day-patients had their own areas (although, as I have said, none was really theirs alone). The out-patients were left very much out; they merely attended for appointments, although there were attempts to get them together as a group. The real difficulty was that they, and even their therapists, were essentially using other people's rooms and had no space either of their own or which they could make their own: their transient status was, in other words, always reinforced by the physical arrangement.

The previous examples are not in any way extreme or worrying; one is merely saying that getting the environment right will be a useful minor supportive measure to the philosophies of the therapeutic community. We did, in our study, discover two phenomena which were actually worrying staff and patients. Both phenomena were related to the division of space according to ownership by department: Medical, Psychology, Social Work, Nursing, Occupational Therapy, Administration, and Cleaning/Maintenance, etc. First, it can be said that there was a large proportion of rooms easily allocatable to specific departments (either generally or to a member of the department). This in itself caused no problems and, indeed, seemed to be desired, although again it can be said to conflict with the basic principles of a therapeutic community. The problems started when one examined the location of those departmental rooms, especially in terms of centrality. During the study some reorganization was done (against our recommendation) and the staff and patients soon realized that a (quote) 'floor of seniority' had been created, and yet not every department was represented equally here.

The extent to which this problem was felt can be sensed partly from the tendency of staff from 'the other side' (the block across the garden) to come across for what one might consider unnecessary journeys, and partly from the fact that the OT department hung on grimly to a room on the 'floor of seniority' even though their usage of it was minimal (its usefulness far outweighed its usage). There can be little doubt that the existence of a grouping by seniority was against the principles of the hospital at this time, and would need guarding against carefully because the physical disposition of rooms and functional requirements can often strongly suggest such an arrangement.

The final point is also about locational aspects and again needs to be guarded against because physical arrangements often suggest it. This is the tendency (observed at the hospital after the reorganization we resisted), to create a 'wall of administration' between patients and staff, especially at the reception area. The latter affects particularly the new patient. Accessibility for patients, a friendly feeling on arrival and a system which does not involve clerical staff as 'gatekeepers', are all essential to the therapeutic community.

New buildings

It is probably rather ambitious to commit even a short section to new buildings at this point in the late 1970s, but they are still being built and one can argue that there was never a better moment to think about value for money.

I have already mentioned the fact that most new therapeutic community buildings are going to be units within the campuses of district general hospitals, and my attitude to this also came through clearly. A community location is certainly preferable but unlikely, so the question is how one can make a campus location acceptable. One way would be to detach the unit as much as possible, relate it to surroundings and give it its own access. This approach can be ruined most effectively, however, if the usual hospital visual style is allowed to march unchecked over all buildings. The clinical, medical, sterile style with an 'integrated' series of signs, is irrelevant to psychiatric units and should be vigorously resisted.

Within the units themselves there is little to say except to suggest that all the points made in the previous sections need to be considered and applied. The only other point likely to be critical is the fact that the standard plans for new units do not include the large group room so essential to the development of a therapeutic community.

Perhaps the most important point to make about new buildings is not, however, about the design solution but about the process by which it is reached. The conventional briefing process is narrow and yet also rigidly hierarchical, depending heavily on communication with the architect through a senior professional mediator, usually a doctor. The Society of Clinical Psychiatrists (Seager, 1973) supports this process, which is strongly opposed to the approach of the therapeutic community: nurses, occupational therapists and others never meet the architects; certainly patients' views are never sought. Although it must be said that the work of the average health authority architects' department is rather dull and unimaginative, there is little the good architect can do unless he breaks through the vested interests of the mediators to the real clients. It is up to those clients to demand a say and then use it.

← why not 'patient' from another T.C.

Conclusion

The danger of writing about ideas such as those contained in this chapter is that those ideas will somehow achieve the status of major factors. The physical environment cannot make a therapeutic community successful, but it can stop one from developing. To an organization wishing to use every possible resource I believe the environment is a very useful supportive system and one which can be used fairly easily. The trouble is that once it 'fits' the overall system of the therapeutic community, people tend not to notice it!

8
Therapeutic communities and the new therapies

Joel Badaines and Marta Ginzburg

The new therapies emerged from the dissatisfaction of both therapists and clients with the purely talking methods of psychotherapy. Although psychodrama, encounter (also known as T-groups or sensitivity training), bio-energetics and other body therapies, Gestalt, psychosynthesis, transactional analysis (TA) and primal therapy are known as 'new', they have their roots in the pioneering work of Dr Jacob L. Moreno. In the 1920s he developed psychodrama and thereby presented an alternative view of 'pathology' and 'treatment'. The new therapies spread into the field of psychotherapy in the late 1950s and early 1960s in the USA and in the late 1960s and early 1970s in Britain. As early as 1912, in 'Invitation to Encounter', a series of poetic writings, Moreno describes encounter as 'A meeting of two: eye to eye, face to face. And when you are near I will tear your eyes out and place them instead of mine, and you will tear my eyes out and will place them instead of yours, then I will look at you with your eyes and you will look at me with mine.'

New therapies for old

In the new therapies emotional distress is viewed as potentially healing. Energy that is freed by emotional discharge and released can be used constructively in self-selected projects. Honesty, awareness, self-initiative and bodily acceptance are the basic principles. The therapist encourages the expression of emotions rather than their understanding.

The traditional psychotherapies are limited to clarifying inappropriate and overwhelming feelings, while the new therapies strive for restoring and increasing the person's capacity to feel. Traditional psychotherapies link inappropriate feelings in the present and destructive episodes from the past. Insight or awareness in the new therapies is stimulated by emphasizing action. Doing what the person was not capable of before facilitates immediate insight. Both therapies aim to heal hurt feelings from the past.

New therapies are very potent in group settings. Cohesiveness and the sense of belonging, control of behaviour, the generation of strong feelings, interpersonal influence and feedback enhance and complement the basic principles conducive to interpersonal growth.

Moreno began to utilize psychodrama over fifty years ago. He was a contemporary of Freud, but soon began to disagree with some of the Freudian views of man. Furthermore, Moreno encouraged the acting-in (reliving) of conflict situations and focused on the 'here-and-now'. He departed radically from the Freudian view of the role of the therapist. Moreno often shared his problems, introduced humour and spontaneity into the group therapy sessions, and related to his clients in a warm, human manner. Many of the other therapies (bio-energetics, gestalt, massage) encompass this style. His departure from the strictly verbal approach in favour of action techniques, the attention to the body, the focus on the 'here-and-now' and many other psychodramatic methods have found their way into most of the other new therapies.

Essentially, all that is new about the new therapies is that they are coming into greater prominence and acceptance by both the consumer of therapeutic methods and the providers (healers). And, increasingly, their rich potential in therapeutic communities is being realized. Modifications of one or other of the new techniques are found in many communities. We will focus on the applications of psychodrama and encounter or sensitivity groups to therapeutic communities.

Simply stated, psychodrama is an action-orientated technique. An individual enacts scenes or problems related to his past, present, or future life situation, yet all in the 'here-and-now'. It is a therapeutic method which sees human interaction in practical, concrete terms. Each psychodramatic scene is an individual's own creation, spontaneously enacted. Group members present their own conflict situations or facilitate others' doing so by taking necessary roles.

Moreno suggested that living successfully in the twentieth century required us to develop a variety of roles: lover, teacher, father, husband, repairman, problem-solver, and so on. Pathological behaviour is either a disequilibrium or a restriction among roles, or a lack of spontaneous and creative adaptation in the current situation. Spontaneous responses indicate an ability to adapt quickly and appropriately to new situations. The aim of psychodrama in a nutshell is to free a person from his past stereotypes and to develop newer and more useful approaches to his present and future life situations. This summarizes the objectives of both therapeutic communities and new therapies. The Gestaltist focuses on inner conflicts and, using psychodramatic techniques, releases blocked emotions, to promote greater personal integration and clarity. The bio-energetist has a similar goal, but seeks to arouse painful repressed emotions and to release blocked energy through breathing methods and by working with the body.

Applications to therapeutic communities

The staff

The range of experience and professional training for the staff in therapeutic communities extends from the totally untrained to the highly sophisticated psychiatrist-psychotherapist. Yet many of these specialized skills may be of less value in a therapeutic community because of the nature of such a setting. A sensitivity group for staff can offer support and help them to explore their roles. Problems in staff relationships, expectations of each other, and the ambiguities that arise as staff roles blur and hierarchical structures flatten can also be dealt with effectively in this kind of group. In both a half-way house in Texas and in St Charles (Richmond Fellowship) such a group met for about an hour and a half each week; in the former, there was an outside consultant, but, in the latter, the staff met on their own. In both instances, not only did the meetings reduce staff tension and turnover; they also helped staff to maintain a reasonable perspective, give mutual support, and reduce mis-communication.

Psychodramatic sessions are used for staff supervision. A staff member may, for example, be having difficulties with a particular group that he is leading. Rather than just talking about it, the group can be recreated psychodramatically using other members of the staff group. The shared impressions and experiencing of the group in such a direct way can facilitate clarification of the problems and illustrate alternatives which can then be immediately tried out.

A similar approach is used in counselling situations. One particular staff member was having problems with one of the residents with whom he had a one-to-one counselling relationship. The counsellor 'became' the resident who balked at every suggestion and resisted all community confrontations on her limited progress. The 'scene' became realistic, the 'resident' effectively blocked all suggestions by 'the counsellor' (played by another member of staff), who rapidly became realistically angry, frustrated, and felt inadequate. Suggestions from other staff were not given; instead they demonstrated how they would cope with the situation. The (real) counsellor then was able to incorporate the suggestions into a new, and more effective, style. Furthermore, he could immediately practise it psychodramatically and get more feedback – this is impossible with more traditional methods of supervision. These examples illustrate two of the many applications of the new therapeutic methods to staff relations and supervision.

The community meeting

One feature all therapeutic communities share is the community meeting. Some are used solely for resolving practical issues, while others explore emotional issues and personal problems. Often a single issue can absorb the energy of the community; e.g., the threat of violence. Psychodramatically, a person (or group) could become 'the threat of violence', taking on a potentially violent stance. This technique forces an abstract, intangible emotional tone to become concrete. It is thereby made easier for a community to resolve. The same method is effective with residents who are making slow progress, need support, or are in some way affecting the entire community. Good judgment is required, however, as there is the risk of over-exposure and isolation. It may be more constructive if another person takes the role of the community member. Further support can be provided by a double, a person who expresses unexpressed emotions and gives support to the protagonist.

Often, issues in a therapeutic community do not involve specific individuals, but roles or functions: administrators, staff, members. The concern is with attitudes towards sterotyped representatives of these groups rather than particular individuals. As an example, in one half-way house, a frequent complaint among residents was the disappearance of many staff members between Christmas and New Year. The resident community felt deprived, neglected and uncared for. It was explored by six self-selected residents and four staff involved in a socio-drama. Residents became 'tired staff' with their own personal needs for family contact, replenishment, and social and emotional contact outside the community. Staff became more aware of (by experiencing) the need for additional support and contact during the holiday period. In socio-dramatic work, the technique of role reversal helps each 'side' to clarify the needs and feelings of the other by simply becoming 'the other'. In this example, the staff were 'residents' and the residents became 'staff' in the socio-drama.

Small groups

The new therapies also lend themselves extremely well to the smaller groups which either have a focus (relationship problems, work-related difficulties, personal conflict and growth) or are of a general problem-solving nature. Gestalt techniques, highlighting certain aspects of personality, enable the individual to become more integrated and to make clearer decisions.

71

People are not always aware of how they are perceived by others, or how they behave in certain situations, such as a job interview. The small group affords psychodramatic opportunity to recreate that interview and, again by role reversal, the resident may become aware of how suitable, in fact, his responses are. This can be supplemented with the mirror technique where other people mirror his behaviour and, instead of just making changes on the suggestions of other group members, they can be demonstrated in the psychodrama scene and then practised by the resident. If specific responses are required, such as a more as-sertive approach, they can quickly be developed through modelling, rehearsal, feedback, and practice, all in the 'here-and-now' of psycho-drama. Another way of looking at this is as a desensitization procedure. By enacting the highly anxiety-provoking situation, the person may find that he can cope more adequately.

The body-oriented methods, as well as gestalt and psychodramatic techniques, all enhance the expression and release of anger, hurt and pain. The small group may offer the trust and support which facilitate the ventilation of these strong emotions. These techniques can be very powerful and, therefore, the group leader must command careful judg-ment and exercise great care and skill.

A final example of the use of new therapy techniques in a small group concerns a resident returning to her home environment. A young woman was very anxious about leaving the community. She was returning to live with her family and felt full of uncertainties. In her small group she was invited to close her eyes, and imagine herself in bed on her third morning at home. She expressed what that felt like and, by using other people in the group as her family members, she was able to work through several important issues; how would her family perceive and treat her, and what could she do to receive the kind of responses she needed from them; use of leisure time; social contacts, and fears of rejection. At the end of the two-hour session she felt more confident, and received very real group support.

Work with individuals

Some therapeutic communities also have one-to-one staff-resident counselling for giving additional support. It also helps to preserve con-tact with the more withdrawn or quieter members of the community. Techniques such as doubling, role reversal, or the staff member playing an important other figure (parent, social security officer, employer, or boyfriend) enhance the process. Similarly, gestalt techniques for inte-gration, and body awareness techniques for relaxation and enlivening the body are very appropriate.

New therapy principles as a community philosophy

Encounter, as defined by William Schutz (1973), is a method of human relating, based on openness and honesty, self-awareness, self-responsibility, awareness of the body, attention to feelings, with an emphasis on the 'here-and-now'. By removing blocks, individual functioning is improved and conditions are created for a more satisfying use of personal capacities. It is therapeutic, educational and recreational.

Phoenix House is a therapeutic community in England using encounter methods and principles. It is a residential community in London for the rehabilitation of drug abusers. Its philosophy reads:

> We are here because there is no refuge, finally from ourselves. Until a person confronts himself in the eyes and hearts of others, he is running. Until he shows his secrets he has no safety from them. Afraid to be known, he can know neither himself nor any other — he will be alone.
>
> Where else but in our common grounds can we find such a mirror? Here, together, a person can at last appear clearly to himself, not as the giant of his dreams or the dwarf of his fears, but as a man — part of a whole, with his share in its purpose. In this ground, not alone any more, as in death, but alive to ourselves and to others. (Phoenix House, internal report 1974)

In the mythological story, the phoenix was a bird reborn from the flames that destroyed it. Similar communities are Synanon and Daytop in the USA, and Alpha House, Suffolk House, and Cranstone in Britain.

The community is structured and authoritarian, functioning as a family which both loves its members, and sets limits and demands. The community operates on the basic concepts of: honesty with oneself and others; love and concern for each other, which includes emotional demands; and the rejection of punishment of behaviour and attitudes which are destructive to oneself and others. Confrontation is a key component of the therapeutic process; damaging attitudes and self-deception are pointed out to residents by each other. This helps participants to break negative patterns of behaviour, to increase awareness and self-discipline, and to present themselves more honestly.

'Act as if', a form of role play, encourages residents to become more aware, and behave with greater responsibility and self-discipline. This contributes to internalizing and adopting new behaviour. The encounter groups at Phoenix House allow emotions built up by the pressure of the community to be expressed. They offer release for intense aggressive and painful feelings. In these groups, there is insistence on total honesty and directness; rationalizations or intellectualizations are unacceptable. En-

73

counter sessions may be run by senior residents, by ex-addict members of staff (graduates of the therapeutic programme), or by professional staff members. In the encounter groups, other techniques such as bio-energetics, gestalt, primal therapy, psychodrama are also used, according to the skills of the group leader and the needs of the group.

Occasionally, prolonged group sessions (marathon groups) are held, lasting from twelve to forty-eight hours. Here, the group remains in the room for the length of the group experience, except for short sleep breaks. The fatigue, tiredness and concentration all contribute to the lowering of defences. Marathons allow residents the opportunity of working through deep-seated, painful, unresolved issues which feed feelings of guilt and lead to self-destructive behaviours such as drug addiction.

The intensity and power that the new therapies generate are necessary tools in the healing and recovery of deeply hurt and damaged individuals. This requires a responsible approach.

Psychodrama helps residents to achieve greater independence from the community by developing and improving their ability to handle stressful situations in the outside world.

Day communities depend more on clients' motivation than residential communities. The high impact and rapid results of the new therapies make them an important tool in stimulating and developing the client's motivation to change and to commit himself to a day programme.

ACCEPT (Alcoholism, Community Council for Education, Prevention and Treatment), a self-help programme, includes psychodrama, Gestalt and transactional analysis as well as more traditional forms of help. Psychodrama enables clients to explore situations which, in the real world, precipitate drinking, and to find alternative ways of responding or of expressing the blocked feelings that reinforce the drinking habit.

An important question related to the application of the new therapies to therapeutic communities is: do these techniques complement the therapeutic process and are they consistent with the basic tenets of these communities? While the list of goals of therapeutic communities is long, it would probably be agreed that they attempt to facilitate realistic, open, honest communication and expression of feelings; facilitate meaningful social interaction with greater satisfaction and security; reduce anxiety and distortion of reality; and increase the sense of worth and self-esteem. An effective community would also mobilize an individual's initiative, and realize his fullest potential for creativity and productivity. A therapeutic community provides an environment conducive to learning new, more adaptable, behaviours and achieving greater self-understanding and awareness and increasing self-responsibility. All of these would be consistent with the basic beliefs of those who use the new therapies. The new therapies stress honesty, openness and increased awareness, they remove emotional blocks in order to facilitate better functioning, and create conditions which lead to a more satisfying life. These are also the ingredients of many therapeutic communities.

Therapeutic communities operate with principles at variance with the rest of society but, it is hoped, in better accord with the needs of the members. Psychodrama works in a similar way, temporarily removing the person from the world in which he lives and creating a safer place. An individual can experience life as he would wish to live it, and explore routes to a more gratifying life-style.

Theoretically, Sharp (1964) has proposed that patients who enter therapeutic communities cannot perform important social roles in their outside community. In the therapeutic community's protective environment, the member can begin to re-establish formerly effective roles as well as develop new techniques for coping with society's demands. In this less demanding environment, if he fails to perform these roles, he will not be ostracized or removed from the therapeutic community. The new therapies facilitate this process of new learning in a similar way by offering a safe place to explore and try new roles, or improve old ones.

Finally, one of the major dilemmas for the therapeutic community is that of helping members to take greater responsibility for themselves. It demands abdication of the traditional authority model, and at least some reduction of the hierarchical system. It is important that this happens so that members can find their own solutions to both personal and community problems.

A similar dilemma could arise for the new therapist as to how much control to take regarding the directions and outcomes of the work of a client. Moreno (1964) warns: 'The director must take great care to make no suggestion as to what course of action might be preferable. The therapeutic theatre is not a court, the auxiliary egos . . . are not a jury, and the director is not a judge. Moreover, the therapeutic theatre is not a hospital where the subjects come to show their wounds. . . . The initiative, the spontaneity, the decisions must all arise within the subjects themselves.' While Moreno was talking about a marital triangle, it is fitting advice for new therapies and participants in therapeutic communities.

9

My stay and change at the Henderson Therapeutic Community

Nick Mahony

Hullo! My name's Nick.

I was a resident at the Henderson Therapeutic Community for ten months during the year 1972-3 when I was twenty-two.

At the present time I am studying English at Sussex University (1977).

The story begins:

Alone

To feel alone in a whole crowd of people . . . surrounded by a glass cage . . . to watch impassive, unmoved, at best amused . . . out there lips move, eyes swivel, faces grimace, limbs twitch, like watching a film, surprised, appalled when addressed directly.

To be a totally smooth polished crystal . . . unfeeling, pure, unsullied . . . with no projections or surfaces for people to cling to.

Self-contained, self-sufficient, self-knowing, self-judging, self-perfecting.

Outside is the unknowable, the uncontrollable, the imperfect.

Outsiders bring disruption, the unforeseen, opposition, they let you down, they lie . . . politicians lie, priests lie, newspapers lie, adverts lie, TV lies, the courts lie, police lie, teachers lie, women lie, feelings lie, feelings lie most of all, you can't trust *them*, they lead to error, they lead to pain, people lead to pain. . . . If you let them. Close off! Expunge all weakness! Feelings *are* weakness . . . if you must feel, feel nothing but hate . . . hate is pure, hate is powerful, hating *you* are master. . . . Be strong! Be strong! Hate. . . .

Far better something cold and inanimate, waiting to have life breathed into it, to be set in motion . . . responsive, powerful, belching, furious, chrome and steel . . . unthinking, unfeeling, just the rush of movement.

And then the brotherhood . . . eyes that saw as I saw, raged as I raged, hated as I hated, defied as I defied, had chosen as I had chosen.

No longer alone . . . no longer cut off, separate, no longer directionless, faithless, hopeless ... acceptance, a new family and commitment, purpose and strength, confidence and power ... secure within our band ... a law unto ourselves ... we went our way, the world went where it would.

We were a miniature army complete with uniform, codes, rules and degrees of status; a tribal existence supporting and protecting our members, rushing out into the wider maelstrom only to grab what we could ... bikes, petrol, money, sex, drink, kicks ... then retreat back to our lair, to brood, lick our wounds, prepare for the next foray, the next adventure.

The outside ... work, work-mates, legal restrictions, conventions, morality, family, career, the future all meant nothing. Outsiders' rules didn't apply to us, only to the sheep, the mugs, the grey people who couldn't see the con, the lie.

The 'I' became a 'We', yet the 'We' reinforced and perpetuated the 'Them'. Part of our kicks was to shock, horrify and bewilder everyone on first contact ... there would be no way they could pin us down, anticipate or gauge us. They had to relate to us on our terms, we invalidated theirs. Perversity was our food and drink, we delighted in watching people draw back in confusion.

We drew an absolute distinction between Family and outsiders. We had all the resources we needed within the gang. On our forays the 'others' were fodder for our amusement, our exploitation, rape figurative and sexual. It was close to guerilla warfare, the prey and the predators.

Retaliation!

Jail or looney-bin ... not a pleasant prospect or on the face of it viable alternatives. I'd had only short stays as Her Majesty's guest and a couple of remands, but what I'd seen of prison I didn't like ... from the cult of total mobile freedom to twelve feet by nine feet with two other blokes ... Ugh!

The aforementioned looney-bin was the Henderson Therapeutic Community, but for all I knew it could have been a cross between Bedlam and Broadmoor. I had a real fear of institutions and wasn't too happy about mixing with a whole load of nuts. As for the trickcyclists, just let them try and shrink my head and they'd have a fight on their hands all right.

Selection ... a truly puzzling experience ... I went with my dad who'd backed me up during the last series of court cases ... twenty-odd people sat around in this ramshackle room asking alien questions, discussing things I couldn't see the point of, using unfamiliar jargon. I found the other prospective residents (obvious nutters) ridiculous and their 'problems' laughable ... meaningless to a rough tough hero-type like myself.

Never having played the 'madness game' I was genuinely appalled at going to live with these 'loonies' . . . outsiders and living with outsiders would have been bad enough but 'deranged' ones made my flesh creep . . . the Family's brand of perversity was something I could handle, but 'madness' meant the unknown, the void, complete anarchy, the possible end of my inner self-sufficiency, self-control, self-perfection. Would the madness, the randomness, lack of control around me rub off on me, pierce the glass barrier and result in ruin?

The other major fear I had was that of 'undergoing treatment'. . . . I had heard a lot about this phenomenon during selection and was convinced that it meant people fiddling with my brain or slicing away layer after layer of my 'me'. But two considerations persuaded me to take the plunge. First 'obviously enough' self-preservation . . . to keep out of jail . . . I'd heard via 'Release' and contacts that at the Henderson you were 'let out' at weekends and the residents I'd seen at selection didn't look too badly coerced . . . I hadn't seen any locks or bars or padded cells though there was the possibility that this was all part of a plot to entice you in. And second the vague sensation that there was all the while a part of me that had been and was still being starved, that wasn't being fulfilled, that could not emerge and develop within my current life-style to which I was now committed. Instinctively I felt the need for an alternaitve, a new direction . . . not one forced upon me, but for something to be nourished and evolve from within.

Perhaps I can articulate and identify that feeling more succinctly now than I could then, yet my message must have got across to my selectors who agreed to accept me . . . an acceptance about which my emotions were very mixed . . . fear, relief, adventure and a certain chagrin to the immense amusement of the brotherhood:

'Always said you were . . . strange, Nick; haw! haw!'

The status of being a 'menace to society' was somehow more congenial than that of a mental patient. After a while, though, I brazened with my new-found notoriety and played with it:

'Hello little girl' . . . (drool, slaver) . . . (twitching paws poised) . . . 'I'm certified . . . hee hee . . . horrifying cackle and shrieks!' It got to be something of an 'in' joke.

For the first couple of weeks at the Henderson the minutes lengthened into hours . . . a cross between Kafka and Dante's Inferno . . . the disorientation was almost total:

'Here's your bed. This is your ward, A8. He's your "ward rep." (whatever that was). There's the loo. Dinner's at 6 downstairs.'

So this was it . . . 'Home'. One enamelled national health bed with a couple of square feet of 'bed-space', a hospital ward with rows of beds separated from each other by barricades of sheets, blankets and lockers erected by their privacy-seeking inhabitants. One side of me a guy had made up his little bit of territory to look like something out of *Lawrence of Arabia*, all it needed was a camel and a bit of sand. The other side of me Dennis had a Union Jack as an awning . . . the whole scene was straight out of 'Monty Python'.

Wandering tentatively around, my fevered imagination was hard at work . . . when would 'it' begin . . . I hadn't seen any men in white coats . . . yet! Maybe this was all part of the plan . . . to soften you up first . . . to catch you off guard . . . well they weren't going to fool me . . . no, sir!

'Hi . . . you're new here, aren't you . . . coming down the pub?'

'Coming down the pub'! . . . and there was me fantasizing that my letters would be steamed open, my phone-calls monitored, scrutinized and scoured for evidence of my insanity . . . I had my code all worked out.

So it was down to the notorious 'Cally', house of ill-repute and home of liquid refreshment.

'Leading the new boy astray, eh, Mick!' greeted us.

If anything, although reassuring . . . a throwback to normal everyday life, having a pint with the lads, . . . it threw me into even greater confusion: we weren't locked in . . . we could go for a drink. What sort of set-up was this place? What the Hell was this 'treatment'? Where was the catch?

Back for 'Tens' where you had to 'sign in', and my first glimpse of a 'meeting'. I stayed mostly out of curiosity, and watched:

There was Joe crouched in the corner, his hair covering his face, saying how he'd gone up to the Downs that afternoon with a bottle of sherry and how he'd felt he wanted people to spit on him and run knives through him because he hated himself so much . . . and then Malcolm, looking like he'd just stepped out of the London Symphony Orchestra, threatening (1) to poison everyone . . . he was in charge of the catering (!), (2) to set the whole building on fire and everyone with it, and (3) to leave . . . swine that we were.

I was baffled. It had been quite an initiation into the mysteries of the Henderson. None of the meeting (my God, are they all going to be like that) made any sort of sense to me. I'd never experienced anyone doing or saying anything comparable. No one else present seemed in the slightest perturbed or signified that anything out of the ordinary had occurred. For myself I formed no conclusions, no judgments. I didn't understand what people had said or why they had spoken as they had. The phlegmatic reactions of some of the residents intrigued me . . . I felt like I was in a theatre watching a play and wasn't sure whether I should shout out 'look behind you' as the villain is just about to plunge his dagger into the hero's back. I could see that a totally unfamiliar set of norms and values were in operation, but I couldn't suss them out.

I withdrew into myself, relying implicitly on my own resources. No one had shown any hostility to me and I had returned none, yet I felt deeply suspicious, surrounded by forty or fifty perfect strangers behaving in ways diametrically opposed to my own code of conduct. I was without the support and comfort of the Family, without our shared values and norms. I was my own rock, my own stability in the midst of chaos and the unknown.

There was a period of acclimatization: getting used to the routine, the structure of the day, the meetings . . . exchanging social banter . . . trying to suss out the people and the place, trying to figure out just what the magical phrase 'getting into treatment' meant . . . being frustrated by the new patients' group drivelling on about psychosomatic illnesses, no startling revelations here . . . trying to work out who the staff were, which could be embarrassing, and what they did, did they rush off after chatting with you about something as innocuous as getting the magazine printing press fixed, and write down what you had said later to be used in evidence against you; . . . getting used to attempted suicides which really did freak me out at first, the wrist slashing and overdoses. The desire to kill yourself ran completely counter to everything I admired or tried to live up to. To me hurting yourself WAS crazy; if you were in a really foul mood and hurt other people now that I could understand, but not this, nor could I understand the 'old hands'' equanimity at these all too regular episodes.

I was rather relieved to find other 'boisterous' rough and ready residents with whom you could at least have a laugh. I pretty much discounted the rest as snivelling hippie, student types; they made me nervous, looking as if they were about to fall apart at the seams at the drop of a hat, and the 'out-of-it' kooks whom I watched carefully in case they freaked out. Physical threats I could handle but this lot attacked my mind. Talking or just listening to them, at the beginning, I'd feel as if I was being shifted, almost physically, from my ordered universe of things you could touch and see into a maze-like, nebulous universe where everything was turned on its head, intangible, like struggling in invisible and endless cotton wool. When I sensed someone 'slipping away' I was scared of being contaminated or dragged along with them. And there again there were the 'normal-seeming' ones . . . what were they in here for? Jail was my excuse, what was theirs?

Once I had semi-accustomed myself to my new environment, when the initial shocks had worn off, when it had become Doug or John or Sylvia who was angry, wretched or confused and who was shouting it, bellowing it, screaming it or taking it out on the furniture or themselves, I had a vague sensation of wanting to be helpful, though I wasn't very clear how . . . we were all in the same boat after all . . . fellow social undesirables. Yet at the same time I saw the Henderson more as a 'voyage of experience', testing myself in this unprecedented situation, grasping more tools, more techniques with which to defend myself and to exploit others, so that when I left I'd be even more powerful, more self-reliant, more ready for anything and anyone. I began to experiment with different parts of myself, bouncing myself off people and watching the reactions. An experiment . . . with no personal commitment or risk.

My 'personal' involvement became greater the more I, cautiously, accepted positions of responsibility within the community. For the first month I had deliberately and successfully avoided any at all. Then I became a 'Teller' with my boon-companion H, a rowdy, burly, Manchester United supporter. Ostensibly our job was to count the votes in the 9.15 meetings for one month, but we transformed it more into a Laurel and Hardy Vaudeville floorshow, punctuated with timely witticisms and good-humoured vulgarity.

Then I was cajoled into becoming foreman of the magazine work group. This felt a bit like the gang outside as it was largely made up of competitive, vociferous people. My mission as I saw it was to make the magazine THE number one work group and I soon had it organized like a mini-army . . . pillorying opponents in editorials, lampooning them in cartoon and satire, intimidating our competitors in the Friday general work group meeting, lining the whole of one wall like SS stormtroopers ready to leap upon (verbally) anyone who had the temerity to voice criticism of us. It was inspiring . . . we revelled in our new-found dominance and notoriety.

The next job I lusted after and got was the Henderson equivalent of chief of police . . . the RLO who kept a record of people's non-attendance of meetings, and religiously intoned these lapses in the 9.15. It was a really great feeling . . . to peer saturninely across the room at someone sitting there in blissful ignorance, secure in the knowledge that they had staved off yet another discharge vote, rivet them with a reptilian stare, surreptitiously lick the tip of my pencil and spring upon them unhappy — crocodile tears — revelation that they hadn't done last night's washing up . . . uproar, curses, threats and recriminations. Retaliation . . . the records book gets ripped off at dead of night. A complacent 9.15 sits there smugly, butter wouldn't melt in its collective mouth, nonchalantly I dip into my pocket and conjure forth . . . the secret copy. Ah, the fruits of diligence!

These were games and roles I could discharge with an inherited skill and relish. What I was less well equipped to deal with was the couple of hours set aside each week for the seemingly innocuous games organized by Ed Berman and 'Interaction'. I wandered along 'for a laugh', but for the first few times felt awkward, silly, playing 'kids' games', making a fool of myself . . . especially difficult for a tough guy like myself. We'd always had lots of rough and tumble and body contact within the family. We had complete trust in one another, no inhibitions, sleeping ten to a bed at times. But these people at the Henderson games were outsiders, strangers touching me, mauling me, catching me off guard, not self-composed, not super-cool.

I gradually began to feel happier, more relaxed during the games, more adept, less bothered by the constant touching, feeling, eye to eye contact, and lost most of my unease. It was then that I began experimenting outside the games in other areas of Henderson life. I became less rigid, less worried about making a fool of myself . . . if my chair gave way beneath me whilst I was in mid-harangue on the virtues of the magazine work group, I didn't dissolve in confusion, rush out the door or find someone small to beat up, but used the incident for a savage attack on the 'maintenance' work group for producing shoddy chairs and even shoddier workmanship, etc., etc. . . . and less bothered by physical contact.

I was ambivalent about this latest turn of events. On the one hand I considered this new ability yet another useful tool, a device to make myself more powerful, removing a source of weakness (being embarrassed), and also watching from inside and tittering when practising throwing people off balance, awarding myself points, engulfing a young girl in a lascivious bearhug (complete with sound effects), thrusting an index finger deep into someone's middle ear extracting some wax and tut-tutting while they were trying to be deadly serious, tickling people when they were trying to be angry, and so on. But also now, when someone was in a state, instead of being reduced to embarrassed inhibited inaction I found was able to hug and comfort them if they were crying, or grab them if they were 'smashing-up' and hold onto them until they calmed down.

Then there was the time when Gill's mother and father joined our 'small group' (the intensive group therapy meeting, limited to a fairly static group of eight) for a 'family group', in an attempt to heal the hurt and bitterness between them. We had reached the end. It has been very intense yet very restrained, very rigid, very abstract, very 'out there'. Everyone, especially the family, were in a high state of tension . . . there was still a great gulf between them. We were all sat around a bit dejectedly, frustrated and impotent when Warwick, our group psychiatrist, said to the family:

'If you don't touch each other now, you never will.'

There was dead silence. They looked very uncertain. Then the group as a whole, instinctively and spontaneously, stood up and created a circle round them, forming a 'group hug', with Gill and her parents in the middle. They were in tears hugging each other, we were in tears, everyone was in tears. It was impossible to remain detached. 'Wow,' I thought, maybe this was where it was at, maybe this was 'treatment'. I felt I had really got something out of the group for myself. I hadn't felt awkward or uneasy . . . it had been too important for that. I felt good all over and privileged to have been present to share their moment.

It was time to take another step, another experiment, a further commitment. At the next elections I was elected to 'Gen. Sec.' attached to the 'Top Three' supremos. That first week was pretty heavy even by Henderson standards . . . people 'cutting up', overdosing, trying to jump out of windows. John, the residents' chairman, had had enough and left. Modestly I stepped into his shoes, secretly rubbing my hands in glee . . . ultimate power.

Running the 9.15 meetings, heralding a new era of efficiency, was right up my street. Myself, Dave and Judy were all pretty determined characters, eager to usher in the Golden Age of Henderson therapy. No stone would be left unturned, no defence unassaulted, no one unquestioned. All deviants would be brought to account. We arm-wrestled with the staff . . . 'who needs you lot anyway?'

When John had left I hadn't felt all that sympathetic . . . power was power . . . as 'Top Three' you were king of the castle. So 'running things' was pretty straightforward, like being magazine foreman on a larger scale. The structure during the daytime more or less ran itself . . . everyone was kept busy attending their various meetings or activities, so any 'acting-out' was effectively contained. It was always at night-time, when people were left to their own devices in informal conditions, that they were free to ponder and brood, to FEEL, what the day-time sessions had stirred up, that people would explode, their emotions having risen to the surface and gushed out. Those in the immediate vicinity would deal with the situation, but if it was getting out of hand, they would 'send for the Top Three'.

'Nick, what do we do?'

Some sort of leadership, some sort of solution was expected from me. My help was needed in a real life crisis. I found I felt a similar sense of responsibility as I had for the Family . . . going to court with them, bailing them out, helping them out in fights. Yet these people at the Henderson were outsiders, ordinary people that I had previously discounted. But they were asking me for help.

Even though they were outsiders, still they were people I'd lived with for about four months . . . drunk with, brought out the magazine with, played rounders with, watched telly with, eaten with, laughed with, grumbled with. I'd been round to some of their homes, met some of their wives, husbands, lovers, parents. They had names, faces, histories. I'd seen some of them at their most vulnerable. . . . I couldn't let them down now. Part of it was the job, part of it was me. But even with those I didn't particularly get one with or like, although I helped them out because I was in the Top Three, afterwards, after their crisis was over I felt linked to them in some way, like I felt after Gill's family group. I still might not like them but I was powerless to do harm to them.

Instead of causing fights I was breaking them up. Instead of hurting people I was comforting them. Instead of preying upon them I became their shepherd. There was a coach trip down to Brighton, 'the deviant express'.

'All got your clean hankies, then?' I asked them ironically. 'Got your buckets and spades?'

I was being both facetious and serious at the same time . . . quite the mother hen. When they got back would they all go to bed like good little boys and girls? Would they hell! They all started squabbling and fighting, to which we, the Top Three, really felt quite indulgent.

Post-Top Three tristesse . . . a time for rumination. My ideas on the nature of strength and power were changing. Up till then my ideal of personal power was the Clint Eastwood type character . . . taciturn, self-reliant, self-confident, never-asking-no-one-for-nothing, quick with his guns and slow with his trust and affection. Now I was beginning to have my doubts. I recalled an incident that had happened a few years earlier up in Nottingham.

I was visiting some bikers up there and called into this pub. I must have entered with a characteristic swagger (it had always remained a genuine mystery to myself and my mates why we were always having fights picked with us in pubs and clubs, until my fellow Henderson residents picked up on my provocative, 'casing-the-joint' room-entering, even Stuart had performed a masterly parody) because the local aging Teddy-boys started cracking their knuckles and giving me meaningful glares.

'Here we go again,' I thought philosophically.

Then the smallest one came over and sat at my table.

'Is that your bike outside?' he asked.

'Yeah!' I grunted, guardedly.

'The one that's fallen arse over tit with petrol pissing out everywhere?'

'Jesus Christ!' I half rose out of my chair.

'Aha! Had you there,' he grinned.

Sheepishly I sat down again and we had a laugh and a joke. One by one his mates sat down, the big mean-looking ones. They listened for a while, then we exchanged names, I said I was up from the 'Smoke', and we all got on like a house on fire, leaving bosom pals, all because the frailest of them had come over and broken the ice. Who, I now asked myself, is stronger than who?

At this moment during my stay at the Henderson I was applying a totally unacceptable double standard. Weekdays I was being helpful, constructive, human, whilst at weekends it was off with the lads, on the bikes, creating havoc and leaving a trail of devastation behind us . . .

haw! haw! Something had to give. In the end the decision was made for me. First my girlfriend left me and then as a result of an internal power struggle I had to leave the gang. The earth was cut from beneath my feet. The Family was no more; most of my old mates were in jail or borstal.

I was alone.

Then bit by bit, almost grudgingly, the fact dawned on me. I wasn't surrounded by forty sticks of furniture but by Jim, Gary, H, Jane . . . I cared for them. I had helped them. I had always consistently, insistently blotted out the possibility that they might care for me, that they might want to help me . . . the big hero-type, who didn't need anyone. Now I did. I knew I did. They knew I did. What was the point in denying it?

'I need you . . . all.'

The comfort was there. It has always been there . . . freely offered, not in great outbursts, just there. I was alone yet not alone . . . I was vulnerable yet I hadn't fallen to peices. I had admitted my vulnerability but hadn't been torn to pieces. I had faced my worst. No longer did I have to close parts of myself off, shut people out. The glass-barrier was redundant . . . the crystal melted . . . the hate evaporated.

My next four months at the Henderson was a time of consolidation and experiment, not this time to equip myself with new and improved defences, but learning to do without, learning to approach people and to be approachable. I hadn't become bitter . . . the worst had happened, yet I felt freer, more relaxed, less on my guard.

I began to get closer to people, on a deeper level, to share myself with them. I used to have a tendency in the groups to look at someone speaking and think to myself: 'Ah, that's X working through his hang-ups about his mother.' Or if someone was freaking out: 'Ah, that's Y acting out her paranoia again.' In a word, seeing people AS their psycho-therapeutic roles. But actually living with people under the same roof, rubbing shoulders with them every day in a host of different contexts, they became Jane, Dave or Chris. When it was Jane crying it was Jane, not her 'hang-up', that I was holding, soothing. If Dave hurt then I hurt. If I hurt, Chris hurt.

Anyway, the groups themselves weren't the places that things 'happened'. They gave cerebral insight and stirred feelings up, but it was during the unstructured times of the day, weekends, night-time, down the pub, etc. when the intellectual insights of the day or the week or month percolated down to the 'gut'. The small group, the intense group therapy meeting, complete with psychiatrist, evoked the highest EXPECTATION, where everything was going to be explained and magically put right with a therapeutic wand, where all the high-power TALKING was to be done, yet it was OUTSIDE the meeting that the EMOTIONAL realization occurred, when things clicked into place.

Because of the expectations raised and the fixed notion that we were going to 'do the business', i.e., sort out our own and everyone else's problems, within the meetings you were on your therapeutic guard, expecting, even welcoming, criticism or unfavourable analysis of your behaviour from your fellow-members. You could always rationalize it away:

'Oh it's for my own good.' 'My, aren't I getting into treatment . . . I just sat there while he insulted me . . . a few months ago I would have flattened him! Well at least it shows people know I'm still around.'

This would lessen the impact of what was being said and greatly lose its efficacy and its value. Outside the groups it was more 'real' . . . if in a meeting a girl would say something like 'you men . . . I hate you all', I'd handle it, possibly thinking along the lines 'I remember now . . . her father did A, B or C to her when she was X years old . . . poor kid . . . can't blame her.' If I'm standing in the dinner-queue, minding my own business, thinking about food not psychotherapy, and a girl dug me in the ribs, announcing 'Damn you men to hell!' I'd blow my top . . . 'you stupid bitch'. Maybe the row would be discussed in a meeting the next day, but the test would come the next time we bumped into each other informally, over a cup of tea, down at the pub. . . . Thus the fact that we were living together made our relationships much more 'real' and valuable than if we had only met each other for a few hours a day in our therapeutic roles. Indeed, there exists a whole network of Hendersonites, ex-staff and ex-residents, who regularly keep in touch mafia-style, not to mention the numerous marriages Henderson has catalysed.

I continued to mature, to develop, to feel more confident with the 'new me'. I had proven to myself that I could accept responsibility and discharge it as I had done in Top Three and another stint as Gen. Sec. The Henderson had been the only place outside of the Family where I had been given the opportunity to 'show what I could do', where people listened to what I had to say, where I was treated as 'somebody', a person within my own right. When I first arrived I was prepared to 'do battle' with the staff, to show them they weren't going to push ME around. But no one did try to push me around. No one had any power over me; my vote in the 9.15 was as good as that of the Medical Director. There was an incident when one quite violent male resident was being restrained by a group of us. I hadn't been there very long and so wasn't clued-in to the staff policy of non-interference.

'What happened to you . . . then?' I demanded of the diminutive Okeke.

'Me?' replied the male nurse. 'I was frightened.'

I was taken aback. One of the staff, one of the 'runners-of-the-joint', admitted (1) to fear, and (2) that we were better equipped to deal with the situation. So the staff here weren't 'tin gods', omnipotent, omniscient, trying to impress, raising themselves up by trying to keep me down. They didn't treat me as a shambling, half-witted 'social deviant'. They treated me with respect, I treated them with respect. They treated me as a person. I treated them as people. I was Nick. They were Eva, Barbara and Gary. As I was learning to get closer to my peers, so I learnt to get close to the staff.

On our trips to outside agencies, lecturing on the techniques used at the Henderson and their application to the people we were speaking to, the envoys were made up of equal numbers of both staff and residents, usually three of each. Even here 'in the big bad world outside', we were equals, neither patronized nor humoured. They served as a link between what happened inside the Henderson and the life outside, a kind of half-way house testing-ground, and served to increase my confidence and make me think about life once I had left, what sort of direction would I take. Was there that much difference between chairing a 9.15 meeting, giving a lecture to NACRO trainees, or working with committees or management meetings? I had proved my worth at the Henderson; could I do so outside?

Leaving was painful but timely. I felt it was time for another step, another risk, further personal involvement and commitment. I was still grateful to the Henderson and still had a great deal of affection for everyone but I didn't feel dependent upon it. I was getting bored and frustrated with what had now become 'interminable wrangling'. I wanted to flex my muscles.

With my old Top Three colleague Dave Fowler I worked as warden of a probation hostel where we tried to apply the techniques we had learnt at the Henderson to the running of the hostel and to the process of 'rehabilitation' (Mahony, 1976).

After much bullying and coaxing from 'friends', I took up the academic gauntlet, eager to compete on 'their' terms. Here at Sussex we have our own community ... four thousand students and faculty ostensibly gathered together for the pursuit of learning, but my greatest pleasure is the constant hum of human activity and interchange ... of ideas, experiences, hopes, fears, ideals, all the fun of being young, adventurous and questioning. In all this I share. I am one of them yet not absorbed by them ... separate yet not apart.

Part II

Current issues

This major part of the book is its *raison d'être*. The aim is to air some
of the fundamental issues in theory and practice which currently pre-
occupy those involved with therapeutic communities. With prolonged
usage the early practices and concepts have worn thin in some places;
for example, the place of work groups (Chapter 17). Developments
outside therapeutic communities have offered new opportunities; for
example, the application of systems theory to the functioning of a
community (Chapter 12). In other areas very little change or development has taken place or has been needed. Thus, although family therapy
has been advancing rapidly, its place in, and impact on, therapeutic
communities remains as it was in the early days; consequently there is
no contribution on therapy with families in this book. Other developments have not been dealt with in special contributions but recur again
as persistent threads through the chapters and sections. The two most
important are (1) the American interpretation of the therapeutic community often known as 'Concept Houses', which are examined in
Chapters 10, 18 and 26 particularly, as well as in Chapter 8; and (2)
the application of the therapeutic community to day hospitals and
day centres: Chapters 14, 23, 24, 25, 26. Some developments have
unfortunately not been adequately represented here: for instance, the
demands made on the therapeutic community approach by the District
General Hospital units for psychiatry.

Theory and practice in the therapeutic community constantly interact in the slow process of development of both. Neither section is
definitive but they reflect the variety of approaches around a common
ground. Clinical case studies are necessary details from which theoretical
and practical generalities can eventually be derived. They reflect the
wide awareness now of the conflicts and problems involved in therapeutic community work which were less apparent in the early years.

Finally, research is becoming more widespread in therapeutic communities after a lull in the 1960s. This reflects both the realization that
the earlier belief that the major issues had been resolved, was mistaken;
and it reflects also growing pressure from administrators for proof of
effective evaluation.

Section C
Theory

Enthusiasm for therapeutic communities has derived largely from a delight in the intuitive practice of the approach. Theory about how to do it and why it might work has often seemed rather dampening to the zeal. It was in the early years an ill-thought-through mixture of psychotherapeutic and sociological concepts. Rigorous models of therapeutic processes in a community were missing, though slogans were common and resounding.

In the mid-1960s more fundamental attempts to find theoretical models began to appear (e.g., Crocket, 1966a,b; Edelson, 1970). Wilson has reviewed the various models that can be found in practice. He categorizes the alternative aspects as structure, function, culture and system. This provides a framework for approaching theoretical models. A functional approach is developed by Hinshelwood, who extends the notion of a social system as a defence against personal anxieties into a form of analytic practice in which the community itself becomes the 'blank screen' of the psychoanalyst.

A systems-analytic approach allows Kirk and Millard to elaborate a mathematical model of the psychotherapeutic process at the individual, group and community levels. Levels of conceptualization are a frequent problem referred to in this book (see also Chapters 18 and 20) and Crocket has employed network theory to integrate the biological, psychological and sociological aspects of community life.

These theoretical approaches are varied and difficult to reconcile with one another. They import ideas largely from outside the therapeutic community, and show the lack of sound theoretical roots once one leaves the bedrock of actual practice.

10
Ways of seeing the therapeutic community

Stephen Wilson

Introduction

During the period following the 1939–45 war, some residential institutions began to be called therapeutic communities. Perhaps because the term was indeterminate, yet had obvious connotations of fellowship, co-operation and salutary intent, it became popular. As the number of therapeutic communities increased, so did diversity of ideas, methods and practices. Institutions ranging from large prisons to small rehabilitation hostels, from psychiatric wards to houses in approved schools, all described themselves with the same name. This chapter attempts to unravel some of the ideas associated with the therapeutic community concept and organize them into several different perspectives. It is hoped that these will provide alternative frames of reference, in which the aims and activities of any particular community can be set.

The therapeutic community as an organizational structure

Social arrangements which arise at an identifiable point in time and are founded by people with certain purposes in mind, may be called organizations. They are abstract entities, by their nature unobservable, although their effects may be apparent. Nevertheless such social artefacts may be thought of as having structure.

Max Weber (1948) attempted to codify the structural features of organizations. In particular, in his concept of a 'rational bureaucratic organization', certain elements were fundamental. These included: a clear hierarchy of offices, clear functional specification of each office, impersonal duties and a unified control and disciplinary system, based on a body of rules. For Weber, rationality was essentially the process of applying general rules to particular cases and thus saving effort, by obviating the need to derive a new solution for every problem. It

93

followed that bureaucracy, as a mode of organization, was particularly antipathetic to the unique treatment of individual cases according to their merit.

Much debate has surrounded the logical status of Weber's model and its relationship to empirical reality. It is probably best considered an 'ideal type', to which real organizations can only approximate. If this is so, mental hospitals as they existed in Britain during the first half of the twentieth century may have provided as close an approximation to a 'rational bureaucracy' as one would wish to find.

Rigidly hierarchical, the patterns of administration and patient care in these institutions were largely based on a nineteenth-century lunacy act, which was rule-bound and punitive. As recently as 1972 the Hospital Advisory Service commented in its Annual Report:

> An Advisory Team may be told by senior staff that the hospital is progressive, has modern policies and has done away with outdated practices. In reality the nurses may be spending their time counting knives and forks before locking them away, instituting bathing days for patients, keeping bowel books, shaving all male patients irrespective of their capabilities or needs, and maintaining a patient's day which has not been reviewed in twenty years.

During the 1950s renewed interest developed in the relationship between the social circumstances of patients and their mental state. The mode of management of a patient was recognized as an important factor in determining his mental well-being. This view, which had been largely obscured following the decline of 'moral treatment', was supported by sociological observations made by several workers in mental hospitals. Goffman in particular was able to link together the concept of bureaucracy as a mode of organization, with the production of damage to an individual's identity.

In his elaboration of the concept of 'total institution', Goffman (1961) suggested that, in modern society, there was an important division between the spheres of sleep, work and play. Within the bounds of a 'total institution' these barriers were broken down, so that every aspect of life was conducted in the same place under the same single authority. Inside the institution, a small supervisory staff managed a large group of inmates, through a system of inflexible general rules. These were interpreted through strictly regulated channels traversing a large social distance. The effect of this process, Goffman claimed, was nothing less than the destruction of the inmate's 'self', while the prime cause was 'the handling of many human needs by the bureaucratic organization of whole blocks of people'.

Other aspects of the dysfunctional nature of bureaucracy in mental hospitals were described by Stanton and Schwartz (1954), and Caudill (1958). These studies claimed to demonstrate the harmful effects of covert disagreements between staff members, which were exacerbated by the bureaucratic organizational systems. Bureaucratic structures, according to these authors, blocked communications between occupants of different roles by increasing social distance and providing long hierarchical chains of command along which information had to travel before decisions could be made. Furthermore, through their rigid impersonal role prescriptions, conflicts of feeling among staff members were denied expression, and efforts at greater openness were subject to punitive action. This process, and not the illness, was said to be the cause of much of the disturbed behaviour observed in patients.

The idea of a 'therapeutic community' grew up in this climate of opinion. Its development may thus be seen as a search for a new organizational form, carried out against a background of increasing awareness of the negative effects of bureaucracy, and growing dissatisfaction with this mode of organization for residential care.

The war years had proved to be a stimulus to innovation. During this period, experiments were carried out by several British military psychiatrists, who attempted to reorganize the social structure of the units for which they were responsible. A reduction in the social distance between patients, nurses and doctors was sought. Maxwell Jones attempted to achieve this in a variety of large unstructured group meetings, in which all members of the unit could participate, and in theory communicate freely. Tom Main (1946) argued the need for the social structure of a hospital to become itself a therapeutic instrument, emphasizing the desirability of an emergent structure, rather than a medically dictated authoritarian regime. Further experiments after the war resulted in the establishment of a series of units which shared in general the same principles and mode of functioning.

Several features of these units were distinctive. There was an emphasis on flattening the traditional authority pyramid, so that decision-making and responsibility were shared amongst the members of the community. A non-punitive attitude was taken towards rule infringement, deviancy and impulsive behaviour. Free expression of emotion and the outward manifestation of conflict was encouraged in all community members. Problems, it was hoped, could be resolved by group discussions, occurring in a close-knit and informal context, rather than suppressed by punishment. The optimistic belief that people could learn through participating in such experiences, and benefit from having their own accounts of themselves exposed to redefinition by other group members, was characteristic of the units.

The typical features of a 'therapeutic community' thus appear to represent a polar opposite to Weber's 'rational bureaucracy'. In place of a clear hierarchy of offices there is a deliberate attempt to blur roles and de-emphasize professional qualifications. In place of impersonal duties are obligations to break down formal barriers, mix socially with institutional clients, share facilities and foster interpersonal relationships. Finally, in place of administration based on written documents specifying general rules, an effort is made to deal with each situation as it arises on an *ad hoc* basis.

In this view, the therapeutic community represents a particular mode of organization, which might be called 'anti-bureaucracy'. Bureaucracy, when applied to human caring institutions produced Goffman's 'total institution': anti-bureaucracy might then produce a 'minimal institution' or 'therapeutic community'. Both concepts can be assigned to the same logical category, and be considered to represent different cells within a typology of residential institutions.

The therapeutic community as an organizational function

In contrast to the structural perspective, in which the therapeutic community emerges as an anti-bureaucratic institution, attention can be focused upon the therapeutic function.

Here, a community may be any group of people who come together regularly and often in the same place, and hold systematic expectations of each other. A community aspires to be therapeutic if it defines its goals as therapeutic. Wide variation in this definition may occur so that psychotherapeutic, rehabilitative, educational and political goals, or combinations of these, may be adopted. Whichever way the therapeutic function is defined, the formal structure of such communities remains theroretically unspecified.

It therefore becomes possible to think in terms of a variety of therapeutic environments, distinguished by their functional aims. An optimum structure might then exist, which maximally facilitated a given function for a particular set of individuals. The breadth of this view depends upon the extent to which the term 'therapeutic' is stretched. In its widest sense the concept degenerates into meaninglessness. If a narrow view is taken, a legitimate question arises as to the way in which an organization might promote a particular function for its members.

A heuristic model for the psychotherapeutic function of a community can be derived from the psychoanalytic understanding of institutional relationships. The phenomena associated with transference, which consist of a re-enactment of infantile love situations in later adult relationships, were recognized by Freud to be easily observable in psychiatric institutions. In such places, he remarked:

> We can observe transference occurring with the greatest intensity
> and in the most unworthy forms, extending to nothing less than
> mental bondage, and moreover showing the plainest erotic colouring
> (Freud, 1912).

Events occurring in such institutions can therefore be interpreted in the light of the transference process. Thus as Freud (1912) pointed out, patients who leave in an unchanged or relapsed condition may be under the influence of a negative transference. These people have presumably projected into the institutional staff a series of hostile psychical prototypes. Others who remain institutionalized for long periods of time may, Freud suggested, be under the dominance of a glossed-over erotic transference.

The understanding of institutional relationships in terms of transference has been developed further by Elliot Jaques, with the help of Melanie Klein's elaboration of the concept. In her view (1952), transference originated in the same processes of projection and introjection which originally determined early infantile object relationships, and gave rise to the generation of an internal fantasy world. According to Jaques (1955), institutions may also be thought of as having an unconsciously agreed fantasy form and content, consisting of shared internal world elements amongst their members. Unconscious co-operation, he suggested, might give rise to institutionalized roles whereby 'occupants are sanctioned from, or required to take into themselves, the projected objects or impulses of other members'. Within institutions, then, aspects of the early transference relationship, which may be thought of as widely dispersed in the world at large, may be gathered together and organized into a phantasy structure which underpins the overt formal role structure.

The unconscious organization of such a system of social defences has been described by Isabel Menzies (1960) in the nursing service of a general hospital. In her view the organization of social defences was itself capable of enforcing the introjection of particular defence mechanisms, thus interfering with an individual's capacity for creative development and personal maturation. The coercive power of the system of conventions and expectations attached to certain roles appears to be capable of overriding individual defence systems, which seem fragile in comparison with the organizational system.

If this is so, and social defence systems are capable of radically interfering with the internal psychic structure of an individual, the possibility arises that a social system might be devised in which psychological growth is promoted rather than inhibited. The structure of the institution might then encourage the introjection of creative objects, rather than their projection and ultimate loss.

The 'therapeutic community' is thus generated in principle from the conception of institutionally structured psycho-dynamics. What the empirical structure of such a community might be remains an open question.

A hierarchical model may then be considered which incorporates some, but not all the features of bureaucracy. This type of community is represented by Synanon and its offshoots which grew up in California during the 1960s. Rooted in the self-help movement, Synanon (Yablonsky, 1965) resulted from the initiative of an ex-alcoholic, who allowed a group of addicts to squat in his apartment, and became their leader.

The atmosphere and philosophy of these programmes is different, even antipathetic to, the democratic ideology. On admission a new resident will be required to sever all his ties with the outside world. He will live and work with other residents, occupying a position in a formal hierarchy, with graded degrees of responsibility. Upward mobility through the hierarchy is seen to be possible, and is rewarded with increased status. At first, however, a new member is regarded as emotionally childlike, having to learn responsibility and earn rights and privileges.

Life within the hostel is circumscribed by a series of simple norms which are embodied in strictly enforced rules. It is incumbent upon all residents to scrutinize each others' behaviour and ensure that it conforms to the community morality. Everybody has a duty to report rule infringement, which is considered to be a sign of responsible friendship to the rule breaker. In this environment, dominated by peer-group surveillance, discovery is inevitable and a formidable array of sanctions exists which may be applied to those who deviate. These include: verbal reprimands, demotion in the hierarchy, bans on social communication, and the use of humiliation and ridicule.

In this kind of community, which is anything but permissive and indeed shares much in common with Communist thought-reform programmes, expectations both in relation to the giving and receiving of authoritative instructions are clear cut. In spite of the ferocity of the sanctions, the narrow social distance between staff and inmates seems to ensure that an institutional underworld dedicated to undermining the staff morality does not emerge. Staff members encourage idealization and actively exhort new recruits to emulate their example.

The rigid structure of the community seems to have the effect of enforcing the distribution of 'internal objects' along particular channels. Transference is highly focused in the staff, who come to represent health and the possibility of giving up addiction. Hostile and destructive impulses are acknowledged and believed to be expunged through a cathartic process of shouting and cursing, with which every encounter group begins.

The fact that the community is cut off from the outside world, that initial regression is encouraged, followed by a step-by-step progression up a ladder of status and responsibility, at the top of which presides an idealized director, seems to make it into a symbolic paradigm for moral regeneration. The powerful force of social pressure, demanding to regulate the direction of transference, is, however, rejected by many in the initial stages; they may complain that they are being infantilized or depersonalized.

People who remain for long periods of time in such programmes, however, often experience a strong sense of internal change. This may be expressed afterwards as a feeling that they have acquired self-respect, which they need to guard carefully. A sense of gratitude to the pro-gramme is often present, together with a feeling that they have begun to develop their full potential. They may feel an increased capacity for love, affection and friendship as well as guilt and regret. There seems good reason to believe that for these people, membership of the com-munity has served a therapeutic function.

The therapeutic community as an organizational culture

When the formal structure of a series of collectivities is held constant, wide variations remain in their level of functioning. Thus morale in different army units has been noted to fluctuate, although formal role relationships and external situation appear to be controlled. Conversely morale may be consistently high in both 'democratic' and 'hierarchical' therapeutic communities, although the formal structure varies considerably.

The importance of informal relationships in determining the 'culture' of an organization has been emphasized by many writers. When rules are present they may, as Gouldner (1954) suggested, be used as the 'chips' with which higher-and lower-level personnel bargain over the minimum level of acceptable performance. Where they are absent, rules may in fact be instigated at a relatively low level in the hierarchy. Thus Brown (1972) has commented on the welter of routines found in mental hospitals:

> There is little reason to believe that more than a handful of routines
> were imposed from 'outside' the ward itself; and it is unlikely that
> all could be explained in terms of the exigencies of caring for a large
> number of patients. Certainly they were not particularly efficient;

and indeed some practices seemed no more than a self-imposed search for order on the part of the staff.

While the therapeutic function of a community may therefore be contingent upon its formal structure, this is clearly not the only, nor necessarily the principal factor to be taken into consideration.

The particular set of shared meanings and expectations in regard to the details of role performance on a given unit create its culture and determine its atmosphere. In this sense culture is dynamically conceived, as resulting from a complex process of formal and informal negotiation. The community itself may be thought of as a professionalized locale or geographical arena (Strauss *et al.*, 1963) where people come together to carry out their respective purposes. The resultant order varies from day to day, according to the particular combination of rules and policies which currently obtain. This ephemeral order may nevertheless be germane to the therapeutic function. Thus, in 1953 a WHO Expert Committee on Psychiatry commented:

> The most important single factor in the efficacy of the treatment given in a mental hospital, appears to the committee to be an intangible element which can only be described as its atmosphere.

In this view of the therapeutic community the emphasis lies on the creation of a therapeutic 'culture', a set of shared symbols and meanings which give body and depth to the sketchy outlines of the formal structure. The process of constructing such a culture is not only influenced by internal organizational factors, but also by powerful external factors. Membership of professional organizations, trade unions, communal and family group ties, social class and status all play a part. Indeed Crozier (1965) found that work satisfaction within an organization was determined more by the congruence between class situation outside and the prestige of a given job within, than by any other factor.

The creation of a therapeutic culture is thus problematic, since many of the variables which appear to be important in influencing the process cannot be manipulated. The recognition of the importance of such external variables underlies the attempt to apply a systems approach to the conceptualization of a therapeutic community.

The therapeutic community as an organizational system

In this view, organizations are considered to be complex combinations of parts, which go to make up a whole. The system is located in a larger environment, which generates its input and accommodates its output.

The individual living or working within an organization is himself conceived as a low-level sub-system forming one component of a higher-level system. The term therapeutic community has then been taken to refer to a system for change (Jones, 1974) which is equated with an 'open system'. Such a system is one whose strategy for adaptation to its environment is focused less on erecting defences against penetration from the outside world and more on 'becoming competent in controlling the external and internal environment so that its objectives are achieved' (Argyris, 1970). Social system clinicians may then address themselves to the optimal functioning of the system as a whole, as well as the diagnosis and treatment of individual patients (Greenblatt, 1972).

This functional perspective fits well in the biological sphere and is therefore perhaps attractive to medically trained psychiatrists. It is easy to view organisms as functioning systems of organs and organelles. In humans, the skin forms a convenient boundary around the whole system; and a consensus on the value of life itself sets limits for the definition of normative physiological functioning.

The transposition of this frame of reference to social organizations, however, produces many fundamental difficulties. In the first place, organizational boundaries are not clear cut. Since all systems are themselves to be considered the units or elements of higher-level systems, an infinite progression exists whereby in principle the satisfactory functioning of one system may always be shown to be dysfunctional for some larger system. Ultimately no community may then be therapeutic unless it fits harmonically with a therapeutic universe.

Second, there is a danger that the *status quo* of a given community will be taken to represent the optimum or only possible reality. All observable phenomena may then be interpreted as performing some essential function for the system. This can be seen in Parsons's model of the mental hospital, which virtually turns the 'total institution' on its head. The hospital remains a place which is isolated and all-encompassing, yet the degradation and disturbing damage to identity associated with Goffman's picture disappear. In place of references to concentration camps and army barracks, Parsons (1957) finds similarities with church and kinship units. Degradation ceremonies become 'initial socialization', an essential prerequisite to therapy, and the loss of personal autonomy is elevated to a major system need. Far from being incompatible with the family, the mental hospital is seen by Parsons as a model of family life, necessarily producing, as part of its therapeutic function, 'a situation similar to that of the child in the family'.

In the third place, the continued life of any particular organization is not always valued equally by its components. Functions must be related to the achievement of specific goals and these may differ amongst individuals or groups within the organization. Implicit in the concept of a therapeutic community as an open system is an optimistic assumption that internal dissensus can somehow be modified through increased communication. The system may then reach a healthy equilibrium and function homoeostatically in relation to its wider environment.

A hospital, however, as Etzioni (1960) has stressed, is not one social group to which everybody wants to belong, nor even a small society. Conflict between individuals' purposes and goals may result from objective factors: economic, social or technological, which no amount of increased communication can overcome. In such a situation, attempts to open up communication channels and decrease social distance may simply succeed in laying bare the underlying conflict and exacerbating it.

In reality, there may be no way in which the needs of the different sub-systems can be met which is at the same time equally beneficial to all, and functional for the system as a whole. If the system itself is to become the main object of therapy, the result for the individual may consist of improved 'adjustment' to a particular system, either through coercion or more subtle persuasion. While increased understanding of the events which take place within communities may be provided by the systems approach to thinking about them, it is difficult to see how individual psychological development can be fostered by attempts to actively 'treat' the larger system. In fact it is difficult to see how such attempts can be anything more than normal political activity mystified by the rhetoric of medicine.

Summary

Four perspectives on the therapeutic community have been delineated: structural, functional, cultural and systems. The structural perspective sees the therapeutic community as a debureaucratized unit. The functional perspective emphasizes the therapeutic goal, stressing that different formal structures may be therapeutic for different types of people. The cultural perspective draws attention to the informal aspects of the therapeutic environment which go to make up its atmosphere; and the systems perspective emphasizes the interrelatedness of different organizational levels. The perspectives are not mutually exclusive. Their analytical separation may, however, be useful to community members who are trying to orientate themselves in a particular unit.

Acknowledgments

I would like to thank David Kennard and Anthony Storr for helpful comments during the preparation of this chapter.

11
The community as analyst

R. D. Hinshelwood

For the individual racked by his own symptoms, his preoccupations with his own self-image and his irrepressible demand for relief from his anxieties, entry into the therapeutic community is a stunning let-down. He finds himself part of an organization that demands his all. He is to participate, communicate, analyse everything and everybody. The hoped-for relief from his anxieties, he finds, depends on everyone's playing a part in making the community a working community; and he too must bother his head first about the community at work.

This is a crucial dilemma for the individual member. It is not a new recognition. Rees (1945), writing about the projects of some of the pioneers of therapeutic communities (Bion, 1946; Main, 1946) says 'a situation arises that reproduces the fundamental conflict between the individual and society . . . the individual is motivated by a desire to do well for himself, but by placing him in a situation where he can only operate through the medium of others, his spontaneous attitudes toward co-operation are revealed.'

If the neurotically tormented individual seeks respite from his basic problems through unrelieved attention to his own desires, hopes and distress, he is rapidly jolted on his arrival in a therapeutic community. He can pursue his own aims only through pooling his efforts with others towards the community aims and organization.

How do people pool their efforts with each other? To gain their communal ends, which include the aim of personal therapy for the individual, they must organize their community. What is the organization of such a community to be? How shall we know when it is a therapeutic one? And how shall we know when it is not?

The total institution and the anti-institution

Goffman (1968) defined the central feature of total institutions as a

103

breakdown of the barriers ordinarily separating the three basic spheres of life: sleep, play and work. There are four main features: all aspects of life are conducted (1) in the same place and under the same authority; (2) in the company of a large batch of others; (3) in tight schedules organized from above; and (4) for the exclusive purpose of the institution.

This disruption, relegation or elimination of everything personal goes on to an extensive or total extent in many kinds of institution. In the mental hospital the stripping of the personality has been formulated as an iatrogenic illness in its own right: institutional neurosis (Barton, 1959).

Such formalizing of the way of life in an institution does not necessarily completely dispel a personal 'informal' pattern of life, but it does come to be carried on as an undercurrent regarded as irrelevant and troublesome to the institution (Stanton and Schwartz, 1954).

A formal organization always appears to have a life of its own which overtakes the efforts of anyone to make it more humane. It seems to pursue actively its own ends, which are to keep things as they are; they remain '"dynamically conservative", that is to say they fight like mad to stay the same' (Schon, 1970).

As the power and presence of facelesss, monolithic institutions has grown in our society, so have the efforts to escape them. Radical and alternative institutions have been experimented with in all sorts of areas of society: public schools, revolutionary communes, kibbutzim, approved schools and prisons, therapeutic communities as well as large mental hospitals themselves. Punch (1974) has pinpointed 'this desire to escape what is perceived as the deleterious consequences of a permanent social structure in formal organizations' as giving rise to the 'anti-institution'. He continues, 'It is an attempt to live perpetually on the margin, resisting the encroachments of formalization. It is the attempt to retain the spontaneous, immediate, ephemeral joys of "communitas" against the fate of "declining" into the norm-governed, institutionalized, abstract nature of law and social structure.' Then he discusses problems of 'institutionalizing freedom' in a communal existence continually threatened, perilously balanced, and that consciously makes self-generated uncertainty a structural feature. He specifies these problems as goal-setting, charismatic leadership, the problem of succession, crisis and insecurity, and relations with the wider society.

In line with Punch's critique of the anti-institution is Turner (1969), who describes a constant dialectic between structure and communitas (formal and informal organization as described by Stanton and Schwartz, 1954):

No society can function adequately without this dialectic. Exaggeration of structure may well lead to pathological manifestations of communitas outside or against 'the law'. Exaggeration of communitas, in certain religious or political movements of the levelling type, may be speedily followed by despotism, overbureaucratization, or other modes of structural rigidification. Communitas cannot stand alone if the material and organizational needs of human beings are to be met (Turner, 1954).

It is not a question of finding an alternative to traditional structures, to conventional authority or to the institution *per se*. There is no final form. There is only an oscillation of attitudes from one to the other.

The mental hospital

Just as therapy should aim, at least, to do no harm to the individual, so also should the therapeutic organization. The harmful process in organizations is institutionalization. This was one of the major tragic features of the large mental hospital which the therapeutic community movement set out to combat. Certain vulnerable individuals who went into these places ended up in a state of almost total denudation, stripped of all physical and psychological signs of individuality. They became the amorphous humanity of the 'back wards'. The therapeutic community movement aimed at stopping this institutionalizing force, and even at reversing it so that instead of the stripping, the identity of the personality might be rendered stronger, more durable and less vulnerable than previously.

In the old-fashioned mental hospital the individuals pool their efforts in a way which does not seem to further the aim of therapy for the individuals. The aim has gone wrong, it seems to have become perverted. What can have happened?

Stanton and Schwartz (1954) studied the 'institutional dynamics' of a mental hospital. Much of what they describe goes on in an 'unconscious' way. It is only by their observational methods that they revealed how one person can affect another, who affects another, who affects a fourth. Or how anxiety in one group of people (for example, higher levels of administrative staff worried about making economies) can turn up as disturbed behaviour in another group (patients on the wards). In other words, without a special method for studying the institution, the ordinary member of it or the casual observer will find all sorts of inexplicable happenings. The origins in the institution of a lot of its behaviour and events is not apparent and is not obviously related to its aim.

Bion approached his first therapeutic community on this basis: 'In the treatment of the individual, neurosis is displayed as a problem of the individual. In the treatment of the group it must be displayed as a problem of the group' (Bion and Rickman, 1943).

It is not too strange to realize that putting a collection of neurotic individuals with apparently inexplicable difficulties together will result in a group with inexplicable difficulties. However, such groups do not lack cohesion. They do not have difficulties in co-operation over some functions. A large mental hospital is a superbly effective institutionalizing machine. The problem is that this is not intended and such groups may not be devoting themselves to their stated purpose.

H. A. Simon (1948) argues that even in the management of commercial organizations − where the rationality of 'economic man' is supposed to reign supreme − purpose is only haphazardly formulated and is at the mercy of factors that are not understood and not under the control of the decision-makers.

These references exemplify the appearance of irrational intrusions into the rational behaviour of institutions. It is not a comprehensive survey, for that would range over very many fields of social studies. Inexplicable disruptions in hospital wards, neurotic co-operation towards perverted or damaging ends, and uncontrolled factors in industrial management show the widespread occurrence of troublesome interference. Where does it come from, how does it operate, and does it bear on the organization of a therapeutic endeavour?

Isabel Menzies (1970) studied the work and organization of the nursing professional in a hospital. She noted that there was a very characteristic structure of rules and movement of nurses through them, and a characteristic culture to the work in terms of standard practice. She began to realize that this structure and culture were not necessarily adapted to the stated purpose of nursing patients and training staff. In fact she showed that they actually created problems for the stated purposes. It became clear that the structure and function was as it was because there were certain other things to achieve before the stated purposes. This 'hidden agenda' included first and foremost the need to provide for the peace of mind of the individuals doing the job. Nursing is an emotionally challenging profession. Close and physically intimate contact with those who are suffering and dying creates distress to high levels amongst nurses. Their professional structure and culture has come to be formed in such a way as to minimize this distress for the nurses. In other words the organization of the nursing profession has resulted from the pooling of the efforts of nurses over the years and centuries to give relief from distress in a demanding job. The social structure has operated to defend the individual from his own personal distress and anxiety. The use of the social structure in general as a defence has also been noted by others (Jaques, 1953; Cooper, 1967; Rosenberg, 1970).

What could this tell us about therapeutic communities? We know that the therapeutic community takes in individuals who suffer a high level of distress for much of their daily lives. Perhaps the social structure of a community operates to defend them in some way from their distress. That is to say, perhaps they pool their efforts to protect themselves collectively by establishing a social structure to ease themselves first, and only secondly to get on with the therapeutic purpose of the community.

I shall offer a theoretical model of therapeutic community practice based on the idea that there is a 'hidden agenda' in a therapeutic community which perverts the purpose towards providing ease, rather than therapy (Hinshelwood, 1972).

The model

The foundation for such a model must be centred firmly on what constitutes treatment for patients. It is basic to therapeutic communities that the social environment can make people better; we can ask: 'How does the environment make people better?'

From what I have said it is clear there could be two answers: (a) by offering participation in a collective defence system people can be protected from their personal distress and overlook it; and (b) by offering some form of therapeutic insight and confrontation with their distress and the defences against it, people can mature.

This is an important distinction. Protection against personal distress through collective defences is a dangerous option, since greatly distressed persons may pervert the social structure as well as the community task. It may even lead to serious dependency, chronicity and institutionalization.

At the least, we can say that this option (a) should be avoided, in order to minimize institutional harm to the individuals. On the other hand, option (b) seems to offer a possibility of reversing institutional harming and instead achieve some restoration of the individual. The question is, how do we do it?

In an ordinary therapeutic group the task is to make conscious the interference that unconscious wishes and needs of the individuals make in the group itself. We employ the notion of transference.

The strange events that occur in Stanton and Schwartz's account of the mental hospital, the neurotic basic assumptions that Bion found in his groups, the vagaries that Simon found in managerial decision-making, and the perversion of social structure that Menzies described in the nursing profession or Jaques in a factory, all represent some sort of interference in the stated purpose. It is interference transferred into the organization because the individual needs it to have some other purpose. To transfer needs from one kind of relationship into an inappropriate situation is the basic feature of analytic forms of therapy.

But the therapeutic community cannot be reduced to the simplicity of the therapeutic group. The therapeutic community is a living-together group, a 'natural group'. It is more than simply verbalizing. Decisions have to be made, actions taken, sub-groups established and briefed with their tasks. A social structure has to be created for the community to survive in a material way (cooking, cleaning, maintenance) and to pursue its therapy (small groups have to be administered, drugs prescribed, and so on).

What happens if we practise group therapy in a community? The first result is inactivity. Psychotherapeutic interpretation inhibits decision-making and activity; it demonstrates a loss of understanding on the part of the interpreter if he is unable to acknowledge the reality that decisions need to be made as well as analysed. The second result is then a differentiation of meetings — business meetings and therapy meetings. This differentiation has the effect of creating structure in the community.

We have already noted that the social structure is a mixed blessing. It is aimed at achieving the purpose of the community more effectively; but it is also interfered with by other purposes. The social structure can, therefore, represent a healthy state of the community, or it may represent a community interfered with by alternative purposes — in particular the need of the individuals to achieve relief of their personal distress through collective defences.

The differentiated parts of the structure relate to each other by communication across the boundaries between them. Communications which flow freely give rise to an integrated 'healthy' structure; while blocking or distortion of communications as described for instance by Cooper (1967) creates a disarticulated defensive structure (see Hinshelwood and Grunberg, Chapter 23).

The tasks then for a therapeutic community are: (a) to identify the defensive elements in the social structure, (b) to recognize the anxieties that are defended against, and (c) collectively to work through these anxieties. Clearly this entails constant examination of the social structure as it develops and as it functions from day to day. In particular, the signs will include confused, distorted or blocked communications. This amounts to a need to assess the integration and articulation of the community, or the 'community personality'.

One important feature of the community personality, in all therapeutic communities whatever other social structure they have, is the boundary between staff and members. Staff and members form two clearly defined groups with separate functions. Each group develops its own identity and the individuals have different forms of behaviour.

To promote the community purpose, there has to be responsible co-operation and good communication across the boundary.

It is common in mental hospitals for the boundary to become dislocated and distort communications. Separate attitudes arise on either side. For example, both groups may hold, with some exasperation, the following views: patients think that staff are demanding and un-sympathetic to patients who are innocent victims of circumstances and upbringing; while staff think that patients are idle malingerers who will not face up to their own problems which are all of their own making.

These attitudes can exist side by side for long periods, even indefi-nitely. They will result in quite different interpretations of events. Dialogue will be extremely hampered: staff will say to themselves 'these people behave irresponsibly, so for their own good we will lock the doors (or give Largactil injections, etc.)'; patients will say to themselves 'the staff are critical and punitive and therefore they lock us up like prisoners'. Such disparate attitudes and underlying assumptions make communication leading to co-operation and decision-making impossible (Goffman, 1968).

The central event in a therapeutic community is the community meeting. Here staff and members confront each other openly. Indeed, all the parts of the community confront each other with characteristic degrees of articulation and dislocation (see Hinshelwood and Grunberg, Chapter 23, for an extended analysis of this theme). The community meeting provides the opportunity for elucidating and comparing the attitudes and assumptions. Anxiety will rise to high levels; the collective defences are there under challenge.

The community meeting exists to release and contain openly this anxiety, not to alleviate it. The community meeting containing the boundary between staff and members is an arena for displaying dislo-cations within the community. What interferes with the articulated integration of the community? That is the focal question for the com-munity meeting; and it is 'in a collective sense' a transference. Looked at like that the practice of psychotherapy at the community level is clear. The community meeting is an attempt to 'offer' the staff-member boundary as a focus for the dislocations in the community personality; an opportunity to understand them as collective anxieties; and then an opportunity to understand the individual's own investments in the 'trans-ferred' dislocations and the anxieties he is hiding in the community.

Illustration

We can illustrate this model with a community meeting which shows a set of staff-member relationships which form a collective (paranoid) defence against the fear of being let down or abandoned. It is interesting to note how the particular personality resources of an individual can come to the fore and be 'latched onto' by others in the process of collectivization.

In a mid-week meeting, one cf the more dominant members, A, came into the room with two walking sticks and her leg in plaster. She sat down and asked another member to put a chair under her leg. She was thus very prominent and was the single focus of attention for the group during the first half hour or so, directed by the member's own monologue. Such a monologue had been a feature of community meetings for some time and A, having a talent for it, often took the role.

It had become generally accepted by the staff that a meeting dominated by a monologue was not felt to be a valuable one. What could be done about it?

After some twenty minutes or so the monologue was interrupted by a member of staff, X, who remarked on the manner of presentation adopted by the patient in this meeting. It is necessary to convey a brief impression of A. Her admission to the community followed her separation from a much loved lesbian partner with whom she had lived for some thirty years. Her behaviour in the community had been violent and provocative of violence, which seemed to be both sado-masochistic and also abreactive. Her disinhibited behaviour was regularly assisted by heavy drinking before meetings. At the meeting I am reporting, X was struck by a lessening of her violence and provocativeness. He guessed that she had not been drinking so much and related his own impression that she was easier to empathize with, to the fact that she was not drunk. X confided all this to A and to the meeting. In her masochistic way, A insisted that this was a moral condemnation of her drinking. In spite of X's protestations that, if anything, he had been trying to convey a note of approval, the condemnation was taken up by two or three others (who happened to be heavy drinkers) as a criticism of A. Clearly there was a quite delusional state of affairs arising. Although one could say there had been a slight movement away from the monologue, it had taken the direction of a persecuting courtroom pattern with an accused and an accuser and an unfriendly atmosphere. The meeting could not be said to have changed for the better – in fact, a collective defence had been recruited. There was a dislocation in the communication between X representing staff and a largish and vocal group of the members. This group seemed to be reacting to the collective view that the hoped-for sympathetic listener had been lost and was replaced by a monstrously critical judge. The trap for X was that he had become the embodiment of that judge. In this meeting the staff had the task of interrupting the monologue while at the same time appearing to want to go on listening.

Later Y, another member of staff, made an intervention that seemed more successful (at least more people joined in and more community issues were raised). It seemed to Y that although X's remark had not been successful, it was substantially accurate. Y took it up and remarked that, although A was easier to empathize with and although most other people must have suffered similar experiences to the ones she had been talking about in her monologue, in fact nobody was able to say so, or to share their own experiences with A. This was responded to by a couple of members agreeing that they had experienced similar separations from loved ones. This led into attacks on certain members of the nursing staff who were thought to lack understanding, criticism of the staff in general over confusing changes in the timetable, and to a brief reminiscence about a popular and sympathetic occupational therapist who had left the hospital the previous week. Y appeared to be drawing attention to a communication problem between groups in the meeting. Some kind of recognition of this separation enabled members at least to come together more and to talk to each other and staff about the sense of isolation. The monologue pattern demonstrated this isolation in a dramatic rather than verbal way.

The point about this meeting is the relationship between the mono-logue pattern and the feelings of separation. The correct interpretation was not about A's own mental state, but about her manifest isolation and lack of rapport actually at the moment within the meeting. The subsequent discussion had shown deep and general feelings about isolation from members of staff, anger at being abandoned or excluded, and envy that resulted in criticism and denigration of the nurses. The feeling of being let down and unsupported was symbolized by the fractured leg.

In addition, this meeting took place just prior to the summer period, when many members and staff were about to go away on holiday. The experience of what this meant to many of the members was hinted at in the apparent inability of A to get any response or to enter into a sharing of experience with the community. The community could not share her loss and heartbreak, but given the opportunity it could enter into a defensive sharing of a paranoid situation.

This meeting is not just a picture of a forlorn individual dominating others with her misery. It is also a picture of a community which has lost a belief in itself as an adequate and productive system of relation-ships. The image of a group, a social functioning entity, has gone, and for many of the sicker members of the community, this reverberates with their own feeling of no internal harmony, an anxiety about dis-appearing in unrelated pieces like the fractured or dislocated leg. Here is a picture of the 'community personality'. The parts are not integrated into the whole, the listeners are not in contact with the speaker. Consequent anger and complaints were directed at staff because it was easier to feel 'paranoid', especially with the solidarity of a group, than to experience the fear of abandonment or of going to pieces in oneself.

Conclusion

The model I have explored in this chapter starts with the need to examine the 'health' of the community personality. The social structure is a variable; its formal shape may be static but its functional success varies. Main (1977) has pointed out that the same structure in army units is vastly different at different times or with different personnel. Thus, a unit may be in high morale or low morale and this has nothing to do with the formal structure of the ranks. In this chapter I have asked what it is that gets into the social structure to make its working grate as if sand was in the bearings.

Experience of the use of the community meetings to study this question seems to reveal that a collective view of the community as a functional working entity does arise within the membership. Preoccupations with the effectiveness of its working develop in the community meetings and can be seen to touch on all kinds of personal and shared anxieties in the membership. As the example shows, anxieties within majority or dominant sections of the community can lead to the recruitment of personal resources into a collective combination of roles that provide temporary personal relief to the individuals but at the expense of communal disharmony.

In so far as they derive from the internal problems of the members, these collective pictures of the community are the equivalent of the transference in analytic forms of psychotherapy. The 'community' acts as the analyst onto which anxieties and fantasies come to be projected. Because this is shared, and because the community is a living, acting system, these projections actually come to affect the working of the community. Such self-fulfilling prophecies are the hallmark of neurotic relationships.

In a community that is founded on the attempt to provide freedom from institutional formalism, the system runs free. Individuals tend then to transfer their anxieties onto the community and hence create structures and cultures which only temporarily bring relief, without real insight or change. The initial idea derived from Bion that neurosis is to be displayed as a problem of the group has been confirmed in my experience; and the model is a useful addition to the equipment of therapeutic community personnel.

12
Personal growth in the residential community

Janine D. Kirk and David W. Millard

> Professional as well as laymen tend to offer services to the needy
> regardless of the known value of the services rendered. . . . On the
> basis of inching along, year by year, trying new methods and tech-
> niques, knowledge is built up which is both reliable and serviceable.
> Yet one limitation . . . has been the continuing absence of reasonable
> evidence that the methods used have been profitable ones (Haring
> and Phillips, 1962).

This chapter is entirely theoretical; it attempts to describe a realistic
application of ideas derived from systems theory to understanding
therapeutic processes in residential care. There is a widespread belief
that the kinds of change in people which tend to be manifest in a greater
sense of inner contentment and in increased social competence, and
which are often described as the 'growth' or 'development' of the
'personality' or the 'person', do actually occur as a consequence of the
experience of residential care. Indeed, therapeutic communities have
been described as communities for growth. But it is often far from clear
precisely how this relationship between experiences in the community
and personal growth is to be described. The present chapter sets out a
logic of that relationship.

Such a rigorous description of what occurs is needed for a variety of
purposes. It offers, first, the possibility of better-quality evaluative
research. This matter is dealt with more fully elsewhere in this book,
and it is sufficient here to note with Davies (1974) that such studies
'will absorb disproportionate research resources for little or no reward
if they are embarked upon before the hypothesized causal relationships
have been fully and rigorously explored in the light of theoretical
concepts and by means of non-experimental evaluation'; with Manning
(see Chapter 29) that the therapeutic community approach 'is not a
unitary dimension and hence "spot the winner" research explains
nothing'; and with Paul (1967) that it is more pertinent to ask 'what

treatment, by whom is more effective for this individual with that specific problem, under which set of circumstances?' To which we would add: what constitutes 'effectiveness'? Evaluative studies of this kind would reveal the extent to which knowledge was generalizable, and this information is required both by the planners of and workers within residential provisions and also by those concerned in training the staff. The use of concepts derived from systems theory is currently enjoying in the mid-1970s a considerable vogue in the caring professions, particularly in social work, but it is the view of the present authors that its contribution is much more at the level of research than directly to those other functions of planning, practice, or the training of professional staff.

A rigorous theory of the institution

We need, then, what one of us has called a 'theory of institutional functioning' which entails some theory of personality development (Kirk, 1975). The current theories which are implicitly in operation, and even some of those which are more consciously explicit, tend to be insufficiently complex (to match the complexities of real-life situations), insufficiently precise (to allow of their accurate reproduction elsewhere) and therefore insufficiently general. What is the contribution of systems concepts to this situation?

Buckley (1967) has suggested that modern systems research can provide a basis for a framework more capable of doing justice to the complexities and dynamic properties of living systems, and Emery (1969) has argued that a systems approach to the analysis of living organizations is likely to reveal 'the general in the particular'. Systems theory deals with wholes, and how to deal with them as such, and facilitates

an analysis of the complex and dynamic relations of the parts, especially when the parts themselves are complex and changing, and these relationships are non-rigid, symbolically medicated, often circular, and with many degrees of freedom, and also deals with the problems of continual elaboration and creation of structure, or more or less adaptive evolution (Buckley, 1967).

All this seems particularly appropriate to a study of residential functioning. At the same time, models derived from systems theory seem to offer a means of mapping out the variables in residential practice, in such a way as to highlight the connections among variables and give them a logical coherence (Vickery, 1974; McLoughlin and Webster, 1970).

114

It is only recently that the characteristics of living systems have come to be looked upon as objective properties that are susceptible to an independent abstract analysis within the framework of general and exact systems research. Many of the relations involved are too intricate to yield to mere verbal analysis, so that exact in this context means that the analysis must be driven to the point at which it can be expressed in terms of mathematical relations between variables (Sommerhoff, 1969). Beyond this, it is necessary to take note of a relatively new notion in the application of systems theory to the field of human behaviour. Emery (1969) says this new assumption is that individuals themselves have open systems characteristics, and can be related to each other or organizations only in ways that are appropriate to such systems. Buckley (1967) reiterates the point that personality theorists are repudiating a static view of personality, and draws attention to Allport's writings on the personality as an open system (Allport, 1960). Miller and Gwynne (1972) also recognize this:

> Dynamically, the individual may be regarded as having the characteristics of an open system. The individual lives in an environment to which he has to relate in order to survive, and it is the function of the ego, the conscious, thinking mind, to regulate transactions across the boundary between the inside and outside.

Beyond this, again, it is possible to regard the residential institution as an open system, interacting with its environment, with an input, a transformation process, and an outcome; and with the staff and inmates as its parts, or sub-systems. An important example in the literature of such an application of systems theory is Miller and Gwynne's *A Life Apart* (1972).

Although it is not a description of a therapeutic community, it is worth pausing briefly to consider this study. The authors view the residential institution as an open system exchanging materials with its environment, and having a human throughput. They suggest that what makes the institution a living system is the interplay between resources and throughput (that is, the activities through which an intake is acquired, processed and transformed into an output). The stage of residence or throughput is broken up into 'conversion processes' which require the provision of both human and physical resources. The task of the institution as a whole is understood in terms of the relationship of the activities of the three systems of intake, throughput to each other and to the environment. However, this analysis of the processes of the institutional system does not appear to us to describe sufficiently clearly the contribution of staff members' behaviour to its effective functioning.

The final point is of some importance. If we accept that residential care should become the preferred form of treatment for the clients for whom it is provided (as opposed, that is, to 'care' or 'support' or 'holding' which contemporary opinion sees as best provided outside residential centres), the institution must be conscious of, and be able to deliver, the kind of change in residents which it seeks to facilitate. This implies some degree of control over the residential processes, and such control can be guaranteed only through the input of the staff. Once the residents have been selected, their behaviour must be regarded as 'given' and is to be reacted to appropriately by staff. Only the staff member's contribution can be consciously manipulated to achieve the desired ends.

Given, therefore, the notion of the residential institution as an open system with the individual as its sub-system, and the notion of the individual as an open system in its own right, it should be possible, using models from systems theory, to map the relations between the individuals (sub-systems) and the residential institution (system) in such a way as to provide an adequate, complex and precise analysis of the processes contributing to change in the individual as a consequence of residential experience.

We must next note a number of assumptions which are involved in our use of systems concepts:

(1) Systems may be 'open' in respect of a variety of forms of transaction. We are, of course, concerned here with transactions involving information (rather than, for instance, energy or materials). Doubtless, it would be possible to provide an account based upon a systems model of the flow of food through a residential centre; but this is probably not central to the analysis of therapeutic processes in residential care. We have to translate transactions involving material things into their symbolic significance for the actors concerned, and to deal with this as information.

Similarly, the structural characteristics of the society within the residential centre become important to the therapeutic processes in so far as they are mediated to individuals as information. The actual understanding by staff and residents of the rules, roles and relationships within the institution is relevant — but not the normative description of these (as might appear in, for example, the official formularies of the organization).

(2) It is a characteristic of open systems that they interact with their environment. Although, theoretically, everything not included within the system must be part of its environment, in practice we restrict ourselves to considering the relevant aspects or substantive environment, and this may be dealt with as the equivalent of one or more discrete elements within the system. An input from the environment differs in no way from an input directed to one element in a system from another.

However, these inputs from the environment must be discrete; if connected with one another in any way they constitute part of another (or an extension of the same) system. In considering interaction within a residential centre we have, therefore, to assume that external influences upon the relevant behaviour of the various actors are independent of one another. (Of course, the question whether they are truly independent is itself the possible ground for an empirical enquiry quite other than that which we are pursuing here.)

(3) For the purpose of our argument, we have to assume that the systems are determinate; that is, that there is a consistency in the connections between input and output which can be mapped out; this does not eliminate the possibility of choice of behaviour but suggests that such choices can be incorporated into a particular patterning of activities.

The method we have chosen to follow is to start with the interaction between two individuals. Cybernetic theory provides us with models of the organization of systems which are sufficently general and complex to be applied to institutional functioning, but which are built up from simple units. If the basic model of interaction between two system elements is viable in terms of analysing and thus controlling this level of institutional functioning, it would encourage the possibility of finding both a more precise account of interaction between individuals and also of the more complex levels of institutional functioning.

Personal growth

We turn next to a consideration of the relevant concepts. Klir and Valach (1967), on whom we rely heavily in the following discussion, state that there are three types of fundamental couplings between two elements of a system: series coupling, parallel coupling and feedback coupling. The most complicated situation is obtained by combining all three fundamental types of coupling, applied to the interaction between two individuals.

It is possible to translate this relationship into mathematical formulae, if we apply symbols to each of the actions, thus:

Let us suppose that A is a resident in an institution, and B is a staff member, because this is the interaction we choose to be interested in. (They are represented in the diagram as for a child-care institution; but what follows is obviously applicable to any interaction between the people.)

I is an environmental event, e_A and e_B represent the total input to A and B respectively, t_{BA} and t_{AB} represent the transformation of the interaction between A and B, f_A and f_B represent the feedback for A

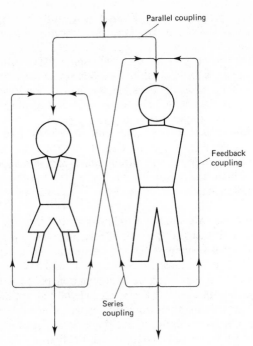

Figure 12.1

and B respectively, and o_A and o_B the outcomes of A and B respectively. Obviously, it is o_A that we ultimately wish to modify; and it is possible to express o_A in terms of all the other factors.

We express o_A in terms of the other factors, mathematically, as follows:

For A, the total input, $e_A = I + t_{BA}.o_B + f_A.o_A$ \hfill (i)

And, output, $o_A = A.e_A$ \hfill (ii)

For B, the total input, $e_B = I + t_{AB}.o_A + f_B.o_B$ \hfill (iii)

And, output, $o_B = B.e_B$ \hfill (iv)

It is the outputs from B (i.e. the staff behaviour) which we should be able to control.

Thus, from (ii), $\quad e_A = \dfrac{o_A}{A}$

substituting in (i) for e_A

$$\frac{o_A}{A} = I + t_{BA}.o_B + f_A.o_A$$

Therefore $\quad \dfrac{o_A}{A} - f_A.o_A = I + t_{BA}.o_B$

118

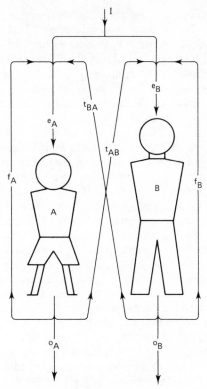

Figure 12.2

Therefore $\quad o_A \left\{ \dfrac{I}{A} - f_A \right\} = I + t_{BA}.o_B$ \hfill (v)

Likewise $\quad o_B \left\{ \dfrac{I}{B} - f_B \right\} = I + t_{AB}.o_A$ \hfill (vi)

If we then subtract (vi) from (v), we get

$$o_A \left\{ \frac{I}{A} - f_A \right\} - o_B \left\{ \frac{I}{B} - f_B \right\} = t_{BA}.o_B - t_{AB}.o_A$$

By adding $\quad t_{AB}.o_A$ to both sides, we get

$$o_A \left\{ \frac{I}{A} - t_A + t_{BA} \right\} = o_B \left\{ \frac{I}{B} - t_B + t_{AB} \right\}$$

Therefore $\quad o_A = o_B \dfrac{\left\{ \dfrac{I}{B} - f_B + t_{AB} \right\}}{\left\{ \dfrac{I}{A} - f_A + t_{BA} \right\}}$

This equation, then, gives us the outcome from A in terms of the characteristics of B and A and their interaction. That is, a measure of the behaviour of the individual resident appears on one side of the equation and all the other variables in the situation on the other side. Among these variables, those relating to the resident (A) will be 'given' so that the only means of manipulating changes in o_A depends upon variations in the values of the characteristics of the staff member (B). The principle thus emerges of specifying the choice of behaviours in B which will produce a desired change in the behaviour of A.

The next stage is to relate these mechanisms to ideas of personality growth. Higher-level living systems are complex, adaptive systems which, rather than minimize their organization or preserve a given structure, typically create, elaborate or change, their structure as a prerequisite to remaining viable as ongoing systems. There are still processes in the complex living-system-environment exchanges that tend to preserve or maintain the system's given form, organization or state, and these are known as morphostatic processes (that is, homoeostatic, or deviation counter-balancing processes), but there are also processes which tend to elaborate or change a system's given form, structure or state, and these are known as morphogenic, or deviation-promoting processes.

In order to understand these processes, we use the principles, borrowed from cybernetics, of positive and negative feedback, control, communication and information processing, and goal-seeking.

Cybernetic theory deals with systems that are purposive or goal-seeking, and Sommerhoff (1969) has suggested that the distinctive organization of living systems shows itself in the goal-directness and goal-directiveness of their activities. These goals may be specific, or may be the attainment of some general improvement in the system's capabilites or performances. The environment of such systems is characterized by 'variety', which is a 'set of more or less distinguishable elements, states or events' (Buckley, 1967). The process by which this 'variety' is transmitted is 'communication', and, in more complex systems, this communication is predominantly by information exchanges (Buckley, 1967). Feedback is the means by which a system processes this information about the environment, either by correcting for its own malfunctioning (morphostasis), or by changing to adapt to the changes in the environment (morphogenesis) (Katz and Kahn, 1969). The principle of feedback is the basic principle underlying purposive or goal-seeking mechanisms (Buckley, 1967), and is the means by which a system controls its responses to information inputs in terms of its goals. The progressive development of feedback results in increasing self-awareness in the system.

The notion of negative feedback, exemplified in the thermostat, or in the regulation of many biological processes, is familiar. We can readily find illustrations from residential life. For instance, institutions generally have an implicit scale of degrees of freedom of authority within the rules. A rise of emotional temperature might be represented by increasingly aggressive, or acting-out behaviour. The 'thermostat' in this case would be, perhaps, another member of the community who, at some point, will react, or impose some sanction 'to turn down the heat', so that the resident knows at which point his behaviour is no longer tolerated and may regulate his behaviour accordingly.

This suggests a general model for those aspects of institutional functioning related to morphostasis, that is, which tend to induce stability in the residents. This may be a healthy model, as in the case of controlling undesirable degrees of aggression, or acting-out; but it may also be unhealthy, in that the exercise of such control may be inappropriate or maladaptive, tending, as writers such as Goffman (1961), Barton (1959), Townsend (1962) and the Morrises (1963) have described for total institutions, towards apathy and institutionalization.

Therefore, we also need a model which allows for growth and development, for reinforcing those aspects of behaviour that are desirable. This brings us to the concept of positive feedback. If we imagine that the effect of the thermostat on the heat source in our previous illustration is to turn the heat up, rather than down, then any upward deviation in the temperature would be amplified; this is an example of a positive feedback loop. In this case, the former system of regulated activities no longer applies, and the system would have to change its characteristics or elaborate the structure of its component parts in order to survive. This is the basic principle of the morphogenic, or structure-building and elaborating process. Obviously, the deviation-amplifying process would be non-adaptive if, for example, positive feedback led to an increase in aggressive behaviour; but it would be adaptive if it led to growth and elaboration, which resulted in changes in the motives of individuals, in their activities and interactions; in fact, changes in the organization of the individual system as a whole (Buckley, 1967). Such morphogenic processes can be contrived by the institution, through the manipulation of both the characteristics and the behaviour of the elements we have labelled B in our model, and, through them, the behaviour of the entire system.

The morphogenic processes could in principle be mapped out by models derived from cybernetic theory, and could then be quite accurately described in mathematical terms. Before considering this, we need to look at the conditions necessary for morphogenic processes to take place, as applied to the field of residential care. These conditions have been derived from general systems theory, without prior reference to the residential situation (Buckley, 1967).

First, there should be some degree of tension between the individual (sub-system) and its environment (the residential institution), such that the individual carries on a constant interchange with environmental events, acting on and reacting to them. Obviously, tension is ever-present in the interactions of the individual with his environment in one form or another: indeed, it is the deviation within the individual from the norms of psychological experience, social behaviour, physiological functioning or the like, which generally constitutes the indication for admission to some form of residential care.

Second, there should be some source of a mechanism providing for variety, to act as a 'potential pool of adaptive variability to meet the problem of mapping new or more detailed variety and constraints in a changeable environment'. This implies that institutions should try to encourage the individual to attempt a variety of ploys of the relevant kind, by running regimes which enable individuals to experiment with as wide a variety as possible of solutions to the sorts of difficulties which have led to their admission to care; to try, for instance, a wide range of sorts of personal relating. For example, it may be that an important function of the community meeting within a therapeutic community is to introduce individual participants to a wider range of possible behaviours than are presented in other types of regime such as, for example, individual psychotherapy or behaviour therapy.

Third, there should be some set of selective criteria or mechanisms against which the 'variety pool' may be sifted into those variations in the organization or system that more closely map the environment and those that do not. Obviously, such mechanisms represent inner or psychological characteristics of the individual resident. This aspect of the necessary conditions for morphogenesis may, however, be manifest in the practice of residential caring by such procedures as reviews. In part, these are occasions for identifying the mapping techniques adopted by a resident in his contacts with staff and other members of the community, and for reinforcing staff members' capacity to assist the resident in the selection of more appropriate patterns of behaviour.

Fourth, there has to be some arrangement for preserving and/or propagating these 'successful' mappings. This, again, can be done in individual staff-resident interviews, and also in institutional settings where there is a regular, therapeutic community meeting, where there are well-thought-out plans for giving greater degrees of responsibility and authority to individuals who are growing into that kind of ability, or in small groups.

We next turn to consider the ways in which these processes may be synthesized into a completed account of morphogenesis. The principle involved is that the outcome of a simple interaction can become immediately the input for the next. Thus, the stream of ongoing behaviour may be analysed as a sequence of interactions. Systems analysis provides a method of handling such a situation. The numerical values ascribed to the observed components in any interaction may be translated into a series of mathematical matrices and the succession of such interactions may be computed by the familiar methods of matrix algebra. The elaboration of a number of individual matrices into a larger matrix yields a rigorous mathematical description of a system, a process described by Klir and Valach (1967) as producing a structure matrix. This process may be carried in the direction of lower levels of resolution (a term defined below) progressively by the merging of the various elements represented within the matrix until we are left with what is, in fact, an expression of the general structure of the whole institution.

Residential settings appear to be a particularly appropriate field for the application of systems concepts because of the relative ease with which a limit may be set to this process in terms of the boundary around them. Admission and discharge of residents provide a clear division between those processes which should be considered within this analysis and those which should not. Interactions occurring outside the institution are not relevant to its functioning except, as indicated above, in so far as they may be reduced to a single input to any subsystem.

To demonstrate how the use of this boundary enables us to set a limit to the mathematical analysis of the interactions within a residential community, we need the concept of 'levels of resolution' (Klir and Valach, 1967).

The notion of resolution, as in microscopy, implies that, with the use of appropriate techniques, the fine details within a structure may be seen — a situation described as a higher level of resolution. With high levels of resolution, the broader characteristics of a system will be lost to view; with lower levels of resolution, the details of its component elements will be lost:

> Different resolution levels, by means of which systems can be defined for a given object from a certain point of view, can be represented very well by an oriented graph (which has the properties of a mathematical lattice). Such graphs will be termed resolution graphs.
>
> Each node of a given resolution graph corresponds to a single aspect from which a single object is assessed. Each of the nodes expresses, however, the view at a different resolution level.
>
> The terminal (lower) node of the resolution graph (always denoted by S_1) corresponds to the lowest possible resolution level; no connecting line originates in it. At this level, only the behaviour of the corresponding system is known to the observer, but none of its structural properties. When passing through the resolution graph to

higher nodes (in the direction opposite to the orientation of the connecting lines) the resolution level increases.

Every resolution graph has a single starting (upper) node in which no connecting line terminates. This node corresponds to the highest desired level (Klir and Valach, 1967) (see Figure 12.3).

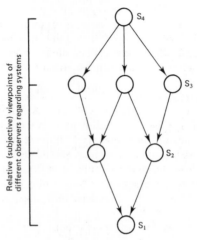

Figure 12.3

Thus, in Figure 12.3, S_1 might be held to correspond to the residential institution as a whole. Klir and Valach (1967) point out that, at this level, we know only of the behaviour of the system and none of its properties: S_2 might be held to represent an analysis at the level of all the group behaviour within the institution. S_3 might represent an analysis at the level of the one-to-one interactions, and S_4 at the level of the individual personality.

These different levels of analysis imply paying attention to different phenomena:

At the S_1 level, we may think of comparative studies of the outcome of different regimes which give no explanation of how such outcomes might be achieved. (A system of which we know only the behaviour and nothing of the internal structure is technically a 'black box').

At the S_2 level, we may think of a sociological analysis in terms of interactions between groups, viz. staff and residents, such as prisoners and prison officers (Morris and Morris, 1963), or the various accounts of structure in therapeutic communities (Crocket, Chapter 13).

At the S_3 level, there exists a vast literature describing the social psychology of interpersonal interaction.

At the S_4 level, we are concerned with the details of individual psychology and psychopathology.

Our own interest is at the level of S_3. The analysis of the individual interactions (as represented in Figure 12.2) through the use of matrices leads eventually to a matrix comprising only empty cells. At this point, we know nothing of the structure of the element under analysis, but only its behaviour. We have, at that point, passed to the next lowest level of resolution. This is a mathematical expression of the synthesis of a large number of individual instances of interaction into a more complete statement about the functioning of the total institution.

While, in principle, this process might be continued indefinitely, the residential institution provides a clear boundary by which we know when the analysis has been carried to its limit. Control over the therapeutic process ends when the resident is discharged and passes from the residential system into its environment.

The theory in practice

Finally, we turn to the practical applications of this discussion. It would be possible, with the use of, for example, rating scales of other measurement techniques, to convert this mathematical model into a meaningful theory for institutional functioning. Initially, we have to try and find operational equivalents for each of the terms in our equation in Figure 12.2. Each element of the system is a system in its own right and, therefore, has a hierarchy of levels of resolution, so that each operational equivalent may, in itself, be quite complex. That is, each of the interactions represented in Figure 12.2 by a single line may be a vector or a combination of partial inputs or outputs.

Also, within the terms of the equation, it is clearly important to compare like with like; that is, to measure variables having some internal relationship to one another. We need sets of concepts derived from a specific personality theory. Furthermore, in doing this, we must avoid the appearance of triviality, and attempt to do justice to the complexity of human beings and their interactions. Indeed, the choice of the level of complexity of the behaviour that should be observed and measured is one of the most taxing problems of an investigation of this kind.

Table 12.1 gives examples of possible real-life equivalents to the terms in our equation from two areas: those of internalization of control within the context of learning theory, and of loss and depression within the context of psychoanalytic theory.

It is obviously possible to suggest many other equivalents for the terms, both from the above suggested theories and others. The point is that if, in practice, these equivalents are to be of any use, they must not

TABLE 12.1 Examples of possible real-life equivalents for internalization of control within the context of learning theory, and of loss and depression within the context of psychoanalytic theory

		Behaviour Learning theory	Psychoanalytic theory
I	Environmental event (may be a vector of events)	Resident breaks rule	Loss
A	Personality system characteristics of resident	Tendency to act-out Aggressive Lack of self-control Behavioural repertoire Motivation	Tendency to depression Lack of affect Anxious Dependent Cognitive structures
f_A	A's internal response (may be positive or negative)	Ability to learn Ability to internalize control Susceptibility to conditioning Ability to construct preference hierarchies of needs-responses	Ability to use interpretation Ability to work through Ability to achieve insight Reduction of anxiety Increase in self-awareness
o_A	Resident's overt behaviour (may be a vector)	More or less or same acting-out More or less or same self-control	Mourning Anger Denial
t_{AB}	A's interpretation of B's response	Sees B as over-disciplinarian Respects and therefore responds to B's response Modelling/identification	Transference Ability to understand interpretation (semantic congruence/differential)
B	Personality system characteristics of staff member	Punitive Authoritarian Understanding Inability to control	Tolerant Caring Understanding Empathetic
f_B	B's internal response (may be positive or negative)	Threatened	Ability to assess significance of event Ability to interpret correctly
o_B	Staff member's response (may be a vector)	Punishment Reward Suggestion of alternative behaviour	Interpretation Sympathy
t_{BA}	B's interpretation of A's response	Sees A as troublemaker Sees A as able to control or change	Counter-transference Adjust concept of A

be too ineffable and should be quantifiable in some way. In principle, it seems possible that we could measure all these equivalents. Psychometric measures and other observational techniques which could well be applied to these purposes are, indeed, available. The theoretical approach outlined here would then form a basis for a practical investigation of therapeutic processes in residential care, based upon a coherent account of institutional functioning and such that explicit guidance might be offered to staff members concerning those behaviours which would favourably influence the outcome of care for residents.

13

The therapeutic community and social network theory

Richard Crocket

The idea of social networks developed originally at the Ingrebourne Centre, Hornchurch, as a result of a typical clinical urgency. The need was to understand the pattern of relationships established in an early weekly group programme. Why was one arrangement better than another? Who should decide it? The initiative that had changed the Centre, almost by chance, from a traditional general hospital psychiatric unit into a therapeutic community (leaving aside the benefits or draw-backs) had been the introduction of community large groups, first twice weekly and then daily. The results, not immediately but over a period of time, became dramatic, rewarding, and unexpected (Crocket, 1972). How could it be that this single innovation could have such extensive and unexpected outcomes? And, if this, what else awaited discovery by such social devices?

First efforts to answer these questions concentrated on making notes and records of who were in the groups, where they met, and what people did and where they went in between the groups. Many diagrams were drawn. These exercises focused attention on the fact that space and time were being 'used' in different ways (Crocket, 1967). And the 'using' element, although determined largely by intuition, included choices that were clearly multi-determined consciously. It was a con-tinuing dynamic process, with much intellectual rationalizing. It was clearly influenced by the surrounding environmental features of a busy general hospital. It also conformed internally to what was coming to be known as the 'medical model' in psychiatric treatment. But through-out these changes, space and time and their sub-divisions in practice provided the only firm objective social facts available for observation and for theorizing, while the interpretive perceptions of psychotherapy, translated into practical action, were giving subjective guidance to the decisions that were being taken. It was stimulating to realize that a unifying theory might be available that would bring such diverse objective and subjective elements together.

The idea of social networks

The relationships between people, as a result of which our social network comes into existence, are physically mediated. At the simplest possible objective factual level, light and sound waves connect us all and, through the brain and the central nervous system, link together the physico-chemical processes of our bodies. We see and hear and sometimes touch, smell and, perhaps, even taste, each other. As a result of associated communication (and, of course, also under the influence of other sensory experiences), we move about. In due course, we are influenced by further communication, associated with another relationship or relationships, and have cause to move again.

The relationship network is, therefore, created by movement. This is indeed, one of the basic distinctions in evolution between animals and plants. Animals have a nervous system and a muscular differentiation that enables them to move about, and plants do not. Humans have developed the most elaborate internal physiological structure of all animals to support their movements. They have also developed the most complex of societies in which to live. These societies are the manifestations of relationships between people, and it is their physical patterns as a unitary whole that we are concerned with.

If one envisages the geographical surface of the earth on which people move around, and extends one's thinking about these movements to the globe as a whole, one can see that the network is necessarily global: it extends contemporaneously round the earth, with people in different places interacting with each other and moving about, meeting, separating, meeting again and so on. The relationship nodes in this human network occur when people are together.

Even when separated from others who are familiar to us, we carry around memories and active feelings for and against people we know or have had to do with. Where we go, whom we meet and whom we avoid, are determined by these feelings: the relationship desires, fears and controls that influence us at the time. Within the neurological matrix of the brain are stored the variable complexities of general inheritance and past experience, unconscious and reflex custom, conscious memory, and capacities for planning and creative experiment, into which here-and-now experiences are continually being absorbed and integrated. And the complexity is multiplied to an unimaginable extent when this mode of thinking is extended to include the maturational and developmental changes not only of each human being during his life, but also the cerebral and muscular interaction taking place between people at the nodes of the network at any given moment.

Perhaps the complexity becomes less daunting, however, if we can perceive underlying elements in the whole that are of a more fundamental nature, just as recognizing the ubiquity of interrelating amino-acids in the micro-structures of physiology has simplified our understanding of apparently vastly different animals and their internal organs and tissues. In fact, in the global human network, the mass pattern of interaction has common features everywhere. The 'social system' derives from what people do in the course of relating to each other. 'Doing things' is exactly that – an underlying universal throughout the network. Amongst social animals there is a psychological hierarchy of movement (simple and relatively undifferentiated) up through behaviour (purposeful and integrated movement) to action (sustained social behaviour, serving not just the organism, but the system as a whole). Action is most elaborate amongst cerebral human beings and, as Huxley has pointed out, evolution is now taking place in terms of psycho-social rather than physical survival (Huxley, 1964).

Social structure results from regularities in what people do. People everywhere live rhythmically, although they usually do not stop to think about it. They are governed by the daily movements of the sun, for example. They tend, in general, to start off each day by taking up a regular pattern of action, often to do with work. They fill the day with relationship activities, and return to the same geographical spot to sleep at night. The occasion for this 'structural point' (a useful time-space notion) is very clear. Men and women make pairing relationships that have strong controlling values, expressed in the regularities of shared domestic life. 'Home' becomes not just the abstract symbol of the pair, but a shared physical reality. Once established, the structure of domestic sexual relating develops and matures, and, when children arrive, the powerful forces of attachment to 'home' from which later adult social habits (and pairing capacities) will develop are obvious.

People discharge very many roles in society other than the all-powerful sexual ones. All roles have their own associated expectations of regularities and norms in relationships. Roles are, therefore, amongst the main determinants of social structure; but the essence of social structure, common to all roles, is to be found in the movements, the behaviour and (especially) the actions of people, with their associated customary patterns.

The importance of stressing these patterns of action can perhaps be illustrated by reference to communication, which is a phenomenon we are accustomed to in everyday life. We often think of it as flowing along lines or channels like telephone wires or copper pipes, or being transmitted by means of words in speech, pages of print, and so forth. It is natural to think of people as moving from one place to another in order to pass on a message. But it is not enough to envisage communication as something that takes place within the relationship network. The movement that gives structure to the network is itself a manifestation of communication; it results from messages that influence its component parts to be where they are. Meaning does not just attach to messages that use structure. Structure itself provides a message, and is ultimately the message.

'Abstracted' and 'real' networks

The idea of social networks is not new, although quite recent. It has developed chiefly in social anthropology. Nadel (1959) and Bott (1957), for example, used the term 'network' to describe interaction between people based on role relationships and kinship respectively. Other social anthropologists have followed up this idea, and much of the relevant work has been summarized recently in a book edited by Mitchell (1970), and work by Barnes (1972). Kurt Lewin (1951) approached the idea of a network in his description of psychological field theory. Bott, however, ascribed priority to Barnes in the use of the term 'network': and Barnes has acknowledged a debt to Meyer Fortes for the latter's book *The Web of Kinship* (Fortes, 1949), and to Radcliffe-Brown (1952), who talked of social structure as a 'network of actually existing relations'.

But the use social scientists make of the notion is as a metaphor, or an analogy. What anthropologists and sociologists actually do is to look at a particular social field and abstract from it the relationships they are interested in. They then consider these relationships as if the connectedness involved constituted a physical network. It is true enough that such relationships, so long as they are observed and recorded accurately, can have a network meaning, and I have proposed the term 'abstracted networks' for these. But this kind of analysis, which is the kind of observation made in epidemiological studies also, has only limited value for the institutional therapist, whose aim must be to understand the total structure of the community he is concerned with, and which he is determining. Relationships follow on structure, as well as determining it; and by establishing a particular pattern in a treatment setting the therapist is planning for usable manifestations of relationships. The term 'real network' can usefully describe not only the total and actual physical relationship movements and mutualities, in space and time, which we create in a therapeutic community, but also the wider total and actual network realities and entities that anthropologists and other social scientists will undoubtedly be acknowledging quite soon (Crocket, 1975).

The therapeutic community as a network pattern

When a therapist who is in a postion to do so starts a therapeutic community, it is, in a sense, a creative social network experiment. He brings
people together into one place for the purpose. He chooses to do so —
there are alternatives. And once he starts he begins to have further
choices about how the community will function.

The choice to have a therapeutic community cannot be taken without the prior enabling concurrence of a number of people in society at
large. It is a small but complex part of the social system. It requires
co-operation amongst administrators, builders, bankers, and so forth,
and can start only after decisions and actions taken by others who have
been allotted or have assumed the power to establish such organizations.
Often enough, perhaps such enabling people do not know consciously
just what they are doing when they facilitate these events. Indeed, they
may not want them. But, despite this, the appearance on the scene of
an actual physical, functioning community necessarily follows on these
enabling decisions and also on the associated discharge of power within
society.

Power can be seen as the ability to control movement, behaviour, and
actions of other people. These expressions of power, narrowed down to
the context of the treatment of illness and translated into the outcomes
of what people do, can be listed as follows: (1) Decisions about policy
in discharging the primary task of the treatment organization. (2)
Decisions about what resources will be made available (such as money,
buildings, apparatus, staff, etc.). (3) Selection of individuals who will
have responsibility for treatment, and who will be allocated suitable
specified roles (and therefore power) within the organization.

These events all involve the discharge of authority and the use of
power. The system is bound together by such elements. Understandings
about authority in fact pervade society. It is not surprising that aspects
of authority are also always very prominent inside treatment communities; and that, indeed, attention is often focused on them because so
often it has been faulty internal adjustment towards authority in the
personality of the patient that has led to his admission for treatment.
It is becoming clear also that adjustment to authority on the part of the
therapeutic leader and his co-therapists determines much of the culture
of a community, and can be both liberating and inhibiting towards its
devlelopment.

Authority and permissiveness are words that cannot be discussed
extensively here, but the nature of the social interaction they relate
to is controlled by inner psychodynamic experiences in childhood
(Crocket, 1966a). There is a vast literature about this, much of it
psychoanalytic. At the present time, the conceptual system that seems

most appropriate to communities incorporates object-relations theory, because the notion of good or bad objects, splitting, and shared reality, are clearly relevant to collectivities of all kinds. An outline statement might be as follows:

(1) Mother and child are initially symbiotic.

(2) They mature and separate.

(3) The child reacts to separation by internalizing a 'good' and 'bad' fantasy structure.

(4) The available inner 'goodness' and 'badness' is projected on to external objects, and an increasingly elaborate external 'reality' develops.

(5) With maturity, inner good and bad values are modified in the light of experience of the outer realities when tested by innovative action.

(6) Resultant realities are shared.

(7) In so far as sharing confirms the validity of inner values in association with perception of external realities, subjective security, happiness and fulfilment follow.

The group transactions of a community provide very many opportunities for sharing of values, both internally in insight and externally in sharing of reality and in innovative action (by which I mean action that brings new experiences). Authority and permissiveness are continually evident. A therapeutic leader can practise the authority role only in terms of his own personality, but he can be aware of the conscious choices available, and we can summarize briefly a number of distinctions about how authority can be dispensed and used in community. The following are different modes of using authority:

(1) Authority may be received from patients, and then applied directively and without discussion through a hierarchy by staff action to individuals, supposedly for their benefit. Patients are dealt with on a one-to-one basis. This is the authority of most traditional hospital units.

(2) Authority may be similarly received and dispensed directively to groups, or to a community as a whole. This happens in institutions such as prisons, sometimes in armies, a ship, or special hospitals, where direct physical control by staff is seen as a role requirement.

(3) Authority may be accorded to a therapist by an individual patient, but delegated or reflected back to the patient by the therapist, who thus compels the individual to be responsible for himself and his own decisions. This is the permissive 'metacomplementary' authority relationship of one-to-one psychotherapy.

(4) Authority may be accorded to a responsible therapist by a group of individuals in a treatment entity, but then delegated or referred back to the group by the therapist. The group may then assume a directive authority towards its own individual membership.

(5) Similarly, the group may be directive to itself as a group, including its therapeutic leader, taking decisions in association with consensus,

and enforcing them through its leadership by power over individuals. This approaches a communistic process.

(6) Or the group may dispense its authority by delegating it back permissively to its individual members, giving them permission to do what they like as individuals.

(7) Finally, the group may be permissive to itself as a group, seeking to exist without compulsion. It is then very anarchic, in so far as, and for so long as, it does not lose its group cohesion.

In practice, therapists shift dynamically all the time in their co-therapeutic use of the authority accorded them and, indeed, it is the requirement to share authority values that makes co-therapy such an important element in treatment in communities.

The ability to conduct community affairs, and particularly the exercise of authority in association with groups, is a skill; and insight plays a large part. It operates through recognition of valid social structures and success in using them. There are very many choices in practice about splitting of structure, but only to the extent that the individual concerned is aware of his own inner need for security in discharging his role and can discuss the connection between his socially traditional or conventional dissociative behaviour and his fear of, or wish for, mutuality. It is infinitely easier and safer to split than not to split. Consensual communities are, therefore, likely always to be less common than one-to-one treatment units.

Boundaries

Returning to the notion of therapeutic communities as part of the larger social network-at-large, created by decision-taking and the exertion of power, they have certain physical characteristics. For example, they have boundaries. Most of them have a location, a territory that is theirs, a geographical space with boundaries to the outside world. They function in buildings which generally 'belong' to them in a conceptual sense. Moreover, they have a membership. So-and-so is a member of the community; so-and-so is not. Such-and-such a person used to be in the community. Such-and-such will become a patient next week. There is, therefore, a time boundary as well, both for individuals coming into the community and for the community as an entity, a beginning and an ending. All these boundaries – of territory, in membership, and in time – are physical, objective and factual. They are subject to definition, of course. And they can be variable. But they are not abstract. We are describing a part of the global human network which has been hived off, as it were, from the rest of the social network for treatment purposes, and it is the actual physical acts associated with hiving off, and the creation of the external boundaries that make it a community, and a social entity. The boundaries can be very diffuse, variable and transient but, without them, the treatment unit does not exist.

There is always also a subsidiary internal programme of smaller groups and activities, commonly on a weekly basis, this programme being subject to control and change. Such a schedule of groups, or other traditional commitments (including formal one-to-one sessions) sub-divides space, time and people to create boundaries inside the community in exactly the same way that the creation of the community itself has resulted from establishing boundaries in society-at-large, through the exertion of power.

The actual process by which a community comes into existence has features involving space and time that are common to all social institutions in the network-at-large. As matters progress and decisions are reached, so do the recognizable regularities appear. Groups of enabling people meet and separate repetitively. Work is done on buildings. At a suitable stage appointed clinical staff begin to meet together in the particular location allotted to them. Patients also begin to be advised, directed, or persuaded to go there at appointed times. The regularities of social structure are under way and a new network entity is in existence.

This process can be described at different levels, and most easily at a 'surface' level in terms of the actual people, buildings, and ensuing arrangements within the organization. It can also be described at an abstract 'structuralist' level. If we use the NHS as an example it might emerge as in Table 13.1, or Figure 13.1.

TABLE 13.1 NHS structure

NHS Surface level	The Ministry of Health exerts power,	appoints staff,	and provides accommo-dation,	within which treatment is given.
Abstact structuralist level	Authority emerging as a result of cultural interaction in society at large	enables leaders,	to create structural forms and patterns,	and use ensuing boundaries for purpose-ful ends.

Continuing with the translation of concrete 'real' events into abstract notions, once structural patterns are in being there is a continuing process by which they are maintained and made effective, incorporating

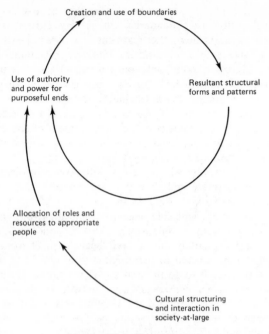

Figure 13.1 Formula A

feedback both from internal transaction in the day-to-day life of the organization, and from transactions across the external boundary. This may be shown in Figure 13.2 by a spiral construct, the loops indicating self-regulating feedback into the continuing system.

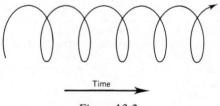

Time

Figure 13.2

The formula given in Figure 13.1, which for convenience I shall call formula A, clearly applies to many social institutions other than hospital units. For example it describes the army, the churches, schools and local bowling clubs. Possibly it applies to families. But in Figure 13.1 it can be given a clinical context by substituting the word 'therapeutic' for 'purposeful'. It becomes even more narrowly relevant if we then replace 'therapeutic' with 'therapeutic community'. We have a formula which permits a comparison between different social institutions not in terms of surface appearance but in terms of common structural characteristics of a more elementary nature; formulae A (a), A (b), A (c) ... A (n). It may be worth noting that it is the context in which the formula is applied that gives it its very diverse surface characteristics.

The traditional concepts of psychotherapy and psychoanalysis (in all their forms) provide another and in a sense a deeper structuralist formulation, because it arises within the individual's personal history. The interpretations of psychotherapy have to do with the motivations, the desires, the fears, and the transformations within individual experience (either as therapists or as patients) that result in the social application of formula A. This is where the traditional work of the psychotherapist is carried out − in the long slow meticulous process by which one person shares in and modifies the subjective life of another, and hence his behaviour.

Using the object-relations scheme outlined earlier one could add another formula (formula B), therefore, which might look like Table 13.2.

TABLE 13.2 Formula B

Infantile 'good' and 'bad' experiences	enable an individual	to share or reject	a structural form or pattern.

Again, the context in which this formula applies has very diverse surface characteristics. In business, politics, the police force, and artistic expression such as drama or music each setting is very different from psychiatric treatment. Even in psychotherapy there are large surface differences between, say, the daily fifty minutes with the couch and chair in the psychoanalyst's consulting room, and an out-patient weekly psychotherapeutic small group, or the daily large group of a therapeutic community.

In delineating formula A the effect should not be to diminish our customary psychotherapy, but to add to it by giving value to co-therapy. Such formulae indeed have meaning only as expressions of value of this nature.

Definition of the therapeutic community

Keeping formula A in mind, we are now in a position to look at the possibility of a structural definition of a therapeutic community. Definition is a continuing problem. The therapeutic community appears to be one of those phenomena we all recognize when we see it, but have great difficulty in describing in words. Definitions again are meaningful only in the context of their use. We can define descriptively, using the appearance of things, a kind of surface description. Or we can define in terms of the hidden elements which produce the surface appearance.

Therapists have little necessity in practice to define what they mean with great exactitude. Most are committed to methods of treatment which do not call for close definition as part of the task, except perhaps in so far as scientific conscience comes into play (as, of course, for some it should). But if an acceptable definition is available we should aim to find and use it.

The concept expressed earlier is fairly clear cut: that we bring a group of people together, first by organizing suitable accommodation, then persuading (or compelling) them to come there, after which we make use of the ensuing internal transactions for therapeutic purposes. One does this in the case of treatment communities by evoking feelings which, to take a short cut, I suggest have transference significance, positive and negative. In 1966 I published two interconnected definitions, one describing the essential structural characteristics of a consensual psychotherapeutic entity (the psychotherapeutic community), and the other the notion of a treatment structure based on one-to-one relationships, but supplemented by a consensual element (the therapeutic community). They were as follows (Crocket, 1966b):

In its fullest form a psychotherapeutic community is a consciously contrived large group of people, made up of patients and staff, to which both patients and staff are asked to relate for therapeutic purposes to the maximum degree possible, rather than to individual therapists.

A therapeutic community is a consciously contrived large group of people through which individual treatment is supplemented as far as possible by psychotherapeutic community relationships.

Since then I have sought to combine these descriptive definitions in one formulation, and I quote it now:

A therapeutic community or psychotherapeutic community is a treatment organization which seeks to maximize its use of total group consensus in relation to decision-taking by its individual members in the discharge of their social roles.

138

Each phrase in this condensation has to be rigorously understood: thus especially 'maximize' (within the limits and role skills of the membership, including patients); 'total group consensus' (acknowledging the requirement that all the members, not just a selection, share in consensual transactions, usually through routine large groups); 'decision-taking by individual members' (individual participants have choices all the time — they take decisions, shown in action, which are, or are not, in conformity with others' understanding, and with mutual agreements or requirements when these are recognized); and 'social roles' (a phrase which embraces the variety of rewards and expectations associated with performance, whether as patient or staff-member).

It is the co-therapeutic decision-taking of individual members, and especially collaboration in the use of authority and power by the responsible therapeutic leader, that results in a psychotherapeutic as against a therapeutic community in 1966 terms.

Although the consolidated definition offered now is likely to be valid in a structuralist sense it omits reference to many important features of therapeutic communities, and especially the bonds that develop between its members, and between its members and the community. It is true that given the structure the bonds should follow. In this sense it is not necessary to mention them. But 1966 descriptive definitions, which in essence suggested that a therapeutic community is an organization whose features result from establishing a consensual transference bond between its members and itself, have the advantage that they have methodical implications derived from psychotherapy. Because they use the elemental and well-nigh universal concept of transference they are easier to apply in a traditional professional field.

Section D
Practice

Although separated from the previous section on theory, the chapters in this section test out theoretical ideas by exploring the difficulties of implementing them in practice. Nick Manning and Raymond Blake outline in Chapter 14 some of the problems that this implementation has thrown up. Even in a relatively favourable situation, a community will generate social processes which tend to undermine collective aspirations by forming a structure distorted by the needs of certain dominant sub-groups or individuals.

The examples in Chapter 14, drawn from Henderson Hospital and St Luke's Project, are extended in the subsequent chapters. Kenneth Myers reflects in Chapter 15 on his own difficult creation of a therapeutic community ward in a large traditional psychiatric hospital, concluding that such a venture is easiest in a progressive atmosphere but that this may also result in the ultimate redundancy of such a special ward. In Chapter 16 Alan Mawson reveals some of the dangers of that age-old problem of leadership: the difficulty of delegation, the need for clarity and the consequences of 'double-talk' which he finds in the literature. More concretely, Anna Christian and Bob Hinshelwood discuss the positive contribution that real work groups (creating and sustaining the material setting of the community) can make to the integration of the individual and the community. Communities fortunate enough to employ cleaners, cooks, and maintenance staff may in fact have to create artificial 'make-work' for the less intellectual members. Such a pampered existence encourages disintegration and the destructive acting-out of the therapeutic community 'potlatch'. Finally, Kennard thinks through the consequences of various constraints on community life: the environment, the patient, the staff. All of these may extend or inhibit the development of a flexible and mature therapeutic culture and structure.

These examples of theoretical practice could obviously be mulitiplied many times over. Other chapters in this book also reveal a rich variety of experiences, particularly Section F on clinical studies. The most valuable source of information, however, is for the reader to visit a community and experience the action for himself.

14
Implementing ideals

Nick Manning and Raymond Blake

Introduction

This chapter tackles a problem rarely discussed either in the literature or elsewhere: what are the problems involved in actually putting the therapeutic communuty ideology into effect? This is a wide question, and we wish to limit ourselves here by making several assumptions. First, we do not wish to cover the problems of converting a downright hostile administrative or professional environment to our point of view. Second, we assume that our staff and residents/clients are basically in favour of trying this approach although they may well be, and probably are, ignorant of many aspects of it. Third, we assume that our resources (time, space, personnel, and so on) do not present unusual difficulties. We are, then, interested in the kinds of problem generated around the community in a not unusually difficult situation.

All too often the trials and tribulations of a community are projected onto things other than the immediate social processes. This development, ironic in such an explicitly self-reflecting ideology, of course has some reality based on the intermittent experience of a difficult environment or unsympathetic professional attitude. However, there are also difficulties, we would argue, inherent in any group of people struggling more or less self-consciously to implement a set of ideals. Essentially we see the creation of a therapeutic community as the implementation of a certain set of aims and values (the culture) by means of suitable working arrangements (the structure). As the project gets under way, the complexities (including conflicts) within the culture and structure generate unanticipated processes shaped by the needs of individuals and groups in the community. For example, the desire for leadership or dependence, or the obligation to preserve and pursue a professional career may undermine cultural objectives and distort the structure.

In this chapter we shall reflect upon these problems from our experience of two therapeutic communities which encompass opposite ends of the field in Britain. One, the Henderson, is internationally known, long-standing (thirty years), generously staffed, medically dominated, and well researched (Jones, 1952; Rapoport, 1960; Whiteley *et al.*, 1972). The other, St Luke's, is in many ways the opposite of this. It is three years old (at the time of writing), run by the local authority social services department, and less well staffed than the Henderson. However, it deals with a similar set of clients (young and relatively articulate), and subscribes to the same set of aims and values.

From our reflections we will extract ten models of community change, which help to explain the processes which shape the culture and structure of therapeutic communities. These models, listed in the last section of the chapter, will be indicated below where relevant to the discussion of the two communities.

St Luke's Project

St Luke's Project is an example of an evolving community in which we can see culture and structure developing rapidly. More specifically, the structure evolved from the interaction between a relatively stable set of ideals promoted by the leader (one of the present authors) and the raw material for a therapeutic community — space and time to meet, and a growing number of members. As this structure developed, many of the limits and distortions outlined in the list of models can be seen.

Culture

The aim was to develop a version of the therapeutic community treatment model in the Social Services. The aim of the Social Services Management was rehabilitation of people moving from hospital to society, and prevention. The clientele would be people who had been hospitalized several times. The combined aims become, as a senior psychiatrist in the borough stated: 'to break the readmission cycle' (see model 3).

The model was based on Tom Main's idea that a therapeutic community is a system within a network of systems (in common with every person from birth to death). The people referred would have disintegrated systems, relationships, responses. The work was to integrate these. The work is for change: the model was a change agent model.

It appeared essential to help the clients/patients to realize their primary responses. These responses, internally and socially, formed the focus of their symptoms. If they could realize the destructive nature of this response, they would also realize alternative choices. To realize this alternative choice, they would need to be involved and responsible in the whole process, or progression: the progression of paradox, the paradox that it requires ego strength to realize one's weakness, and to develop alternative constructive responses, personally and socially.

This process of change is existential, a here-and-now process. It is multi-dimensional, linking the present with the past and the past with the present. But change, though multi-level and needing time, is only recognized in the present. The great advantage of the therapeutic community model is that it allows multi-dimensional experiences. It also involves the persons: their response and their responsibility. It is not a treatment given, but a treatment experienced and participated in. Strength is as important as weakness.

Madness and sanity are expressed both individually and socially. They appear to be in large measure learned responses, even if they are learned at an unconscious level. Hence the aim was for an integrated model, integration of social therapy and psychotherapy. In the context of social therapy, group psychotherapy would take place, but with reciprocal interplay giving mutual enhancement.

The culture can thus be summarized as first, responsibility: you are responsible for yourself. Second, honesty: be as honest as possible. There was only one rule: no destructive physical violence to be inflicted upon another person.

Structure

The structure which developed in pursuit of the the aims outlined can be grouped into various loose areas such as selection procedures, or staff relations. Many aspects of the structure evolved in common with most therapeutic communities: the daily programme of large and small groups, and so on. And indeed the culture itself became filled out in due course, for example, with a more precise specification of the theoretical position taken in psychotherapy (the Kleinian model) (see model 2). However, we are interested here in structures which posed problems in the pursuit of therapeutic community ideals.

Selection

The profile was: neurosis; personality disorder; borderline drug abusers and sociopaths; and controlled psychotics. In fact, some alcoholics were selected who became an excessive burden on what was then a brittle group. In some cases the referring sources were not frank enough about the alcoholics. These either dropped out or were expelled. The selection profile became sharper through experience and related to the strength or cycles in the community. Selection skill became more effective as the decision-making was delegated to the community over time. This was a major development. It took place in three phases.

First, the staff discussed referrals with the community; the applicant visited; there was a discussion the following day and the applicant was asked to telephone his/her decision, yes or no. This sounds democratic. However, the staff members' opinion carried excessive weight (see model 6). The staff then decided to keep a very low profile in the discussion. The result was that the interview with the applicant developed into a deeper, more penetrating dialogue between the community and applicant. This was the second stage. However, communities have cycles. In the second year the confidence of the community was high; inflation was around. One day the Assistant Director of Community Services, who visited regularly, commented on the heavy challenge of the application interview, a point the staff (who were somewhat inflated also?) took note of (see model 1). The whole process was reviewed in the community business meeting. The third stage, the present model, then emerged.

The applicant visits on Monday. After lunch he meets the preparation group, usually three senior members and two staff. The members explain the aims, programme and culture. The applicant is invited to question, and then is sensitively questioned in turn. There is a lot of sharing of experiences between members and applicants. This leads to a sharing by the applicant of his relevant past and present situations and aims. They often comment on how 'different it is here'. 'I don't usually talk this much.' The staff will involve themselves to the minimum. The applicant knows there will be feedback on this group to the community the following day, Tuesday. On Wednesday the applicant returns, if they so decide, for the decisive meeting with the whole community. He will be supported by the preparation group members in his dialogue with the community, after which he stays for the remainder of the day, thus having experience of the Monday large, and Wednesday small groups. He is then asked to telephone his decision on Friday. (The community has decided by vote on the Thursday.)

This model was used for most of our third year. It is consistent and effective. Further, this was the period with the most difficult applicants, resulting from a major reduction in referrals due to the shortage of social services staff and a Day Hospital referring their more intransigent patients. With all the selection models, ninety-eight per cent of applicants thought unsuitable decided not to come. Only five have been formally rejected. In the majority of cases the decision is mutual. Fifty per cent of applicants became members.

In this development the phases appear to have been: (1) staff dominated; (2) community dominated; (3) balanced.

Psychotherapy

Two points stand out here as regards implementation. First, the members appear to be suffering from their original response to primary deprivation. The Kleinian model of good and bad objects and splitting appears to be the one returned to most: the fear of love because of the loss of love; the angry or frightened defence against this loss. The diagnoses may define the defence. Therapy appears to be enabling the original loss to be re-experienced and understood in contemporary terms. In this process the defence against the loss of the good object, love, warmth, and the ensuing sense of personal validity are experienced existentially. The person comes together. Splitting is replaced by acceptance, of good and bad.

Two-thirds of our members appear to have this experience in some measure, sufficient to achieve our aim of basic confidence, basic integration. This experience is concentrated as the member's leaving date nears and the loss of the community becomes a reality. When they leave, the ex-members' group is there to build further developmental stages. These are the people who successfully break the readmission cycle. Of the remainder, the one-third who drop out experience no change; or the benefits they have experienced surface some four months after leaving, judging by a sample of letters. They present our major challenge internally – and one of the main reasons for doing research.

The second point is the value of directness and honesty: telling a person exactly how they are experienced by others. This directness appears to free the integrating forces within the person so that over time they stand a better chance against the destructive ones. This process of honesty appears to upset some of the visitors, and the referring sources (see models 6 and 7). This is one benefit of working closely with the whole therapeutic or care team. 'I thought I could twist his arm,' said an angry member after a disappointing visit to her psychiatrist. In this case staff had told the referring hospital social worker they would not keep the lady if the hospital colluded with her.

There appears to be a reciprocal relationship between the staff's ability to handle splits between themselves and their ability to handle splits within the community. Likewise, there is a similar link between the culture of honesty and responsibility and the ability of the community to experience and realize its splits. The learning is reciprocal: it is a combined operation in staff and members.

Limits

There appears to be much idealizing in the therapeutic community approach. The reality of a therapeutic community based in society,

147

where the members want to operate, brings into focus sharply the limits of realistic behaviour (see models 5, 7 and 10).

For example, a sub-group of members were 'dropping pills and smoking'. This was the first of such syndromes. Some members did not realize it was happening. The staff raised the issue in the community group. A long, at times angry, frightened, and then thoughtful, debate followed. Issues covered were: the maintenance or closure of the unit; what the individuals involved were really doing; responsibility; cultural clashes, etc. (Kensington and Chelsea contains a wide range of cultures represented in the project.)

Drug abuse stopped, with very minor exceptions. No one left. Within a few weeks the community wrote out a list of Expectations. They stood unchanged a year later. They include the following:

1 Members are responsible for themselves.
2 Time-keeping is important.
3 Medication is to be responsibly reduced.
4 Maximum participation is expected in the community and in groups.
5 Part-time work/training is to be undertaken where possible.
6 Drugs and alcohol are destructive to the work.
7 Members must live in the borough which provides the money.

Cycles

The power of cycles only became apparent when the first batch of original members left. It was the Association of Therapeutic Communities supervisors' group who commented that there is a particular pain when the first members leave. It took the staff and community some two months to work through the mourning, dependency and challenge. In his book *Community as Doctor* (1960) Rapoport refers to oscillations. In St Luke's we find a dual effect. The staff aim at keeping a low profile, particularly when the community is strong. But when it is weak, in a low cycle, the staff engage more in the exploration of the weakness (see model 4). This gives a reciprocal relationship: the involvement of staff is inversely related to the strength of the community.

Staff

Staff members are the main culture carriers in a therapeutic community. For this they need a relevant structure and discipline. Their structure and discipline, or lack of it, will resonate in the community, and vice versa. This reciprocal relationship is illustrated below.

The staff programme in St Luke's, from Monday to Friday, includes:

staff sensitivity group; administration; supervision; consultant's session; training. The week starts with a sensitivity group – the touchstone of staff dynamics. It is essential and 'the heart of the process'. Staff relationships, work stress and transference issues are the main content. But administration is also vital. The staff are unhappy when they allow it to build up.

Supervision is for students mainly, but for the staff group it also provides opportunities for learning. In this process, consultancy is most important. The value of an external therapeutic community consultant and analyst is considerable. He brings objectivity and insight, which the staff team have to translate into therapeutic community practice. This latter function is one of the subjects for the training session.

This staff structure is vital. If it slips, undue stress follows (see model 5). It is a matter of keeping abreast of learning (therapy). If the staff drop behind, analytical interpretations can be demoralizing. One example occurred in a consultant session, pointing to staff anxiety which made some staff feel 'over-burdened'. The energy went through the floor. It was immediately necessary to explain part of the dynamic causing the anxiety: the staff were being made bad objects. The energy returned, but it took two weeks for the staff team to recover its normal resilient form through understanding the whole process.

This has been the only difficulty noted in a consultancy staff process which has proved most effective. It seems to highlight the sensitivity of the consulting process; the difficulty the consultant is faced with when the staff are in a brittle state; and most of all, the crucial importance of maintaining the staff structure, i.e. the programme.

External relations

St Luke's Project is a therapeutic community in the Social Services. There appears to be a greater affinity of values between the therapeutic community approach in the Social Services, with its concept of self-determination, than in the Health Service with its medical model. However, even with the imaginative Assistant Director's help, there were still important constraints, in terms of individuals and organizations (see model 7). These required the use of skills externally which are normally associated with internal working. The therapeutic community system has to relate to the network of systems within which it is operating.

Ambition was not helpful in this context. There were some near collision courses. For example, there was natural anxiety in the management about members carrying the keys of the building; and members (clients) participating in the selection of clients/patients. The original Introductory Leaflet drafted with management stated that selection would be by staff. However, in the second year management agreed to the staff's printing the actual selection model.

The middle management appeared threatened by the lack of control over the disturbed people. This situation changed by the following process: all the management visited and participated in the community, including the psychotherapy groups; it was agreed that all innovation proposed by the community would be discussed with management before implementation; management meetings were arranged with the Assistant Director present.

Some of the above issues related to the Health Service. The original attitudes of enthusiasm, doubts and suspicion among the psychiatrists have changed through a practical working relationship, generating a sense of partnership. This has resulted through communication: assessments of all members are sent to the referring sources quarterly. These combine the member's self-assessment and the staff assessment.

It would appear there is a long way to go before it is acknowledged that all the services have a common problem, and the available resources are examined in the light of this problem to see how they can be combined effectively. This would be integrating the systems. It would also be in line with the White Paper, *Better Services For the Mentally Ill* (DHSS, 1975).

Henderson Hospital

In contrast to St Luke's, the culture and structure of the Henderson have had a long time to settle down. Hence, we can study the tensions between culture and structure more objectively, in addition to personal observations. This section draws upon and extends a previously published piece of work (Manning, 1976b) in two ways: a further set of data has been collected five years after the previous set; and the interpretation of the data has been extended in the light of the authors' experience. It is worth reiterating a point made in the previous study that 'knowledge is expanded to the extent that research workers learn from and build upon previous work . . . much work continues to break new ground which makes cumulative work difficult' (Manning, 1976b). The measures used are not as sophisticated as many, yet they have been replicated over an extremely long period of time (twenty-three years), which adds enormously to their strength.

The empirical problem to hand is the comparison over this twenty-three-year period (with data available at the eighteen-year point) of how staff and residents espouse the therapeutic community ideology (culture) on the one hand, and organize their community (structure) on the other. Differences between culture and structure can then be explored by reference to the social science literature on individuals in groups and organizations.

A detailed description of the measures used in 1955, 1973, and 1977 can be found in Manning (1976b). Briefly, the cultural dimension was tapped through a 'values questionnaire', which provides a measure of the extent to which an individual's values are in accord with ideal therapeutic community values. The structural dimension was tapped with a simple measure of which groups were actually found to be most helpful to the members of the community. By inspecting the groups chosen as helpful, and comparing this with the values expressed, a number of disjunctions appear. Exploring these through informal observations suggests that social processes are constantly at work to distort or undermine the fullest expression of the therapeutic community ideology in practice.

Values questionnaire

The distribution of staff scores on the values questionnaire was much the same in 1977 as in 1973. The theoretical limits are between 0 and 42 (the higher the score, the more therapeutic community values expressed). The average scores in 1955, 1973 and 1977 were 26·7, 30·7 and 30·7 (see models 1 and 2). It was not possible to collect results from a series of *new* patients as before, but the existing patient group's average score was 29·8 in 1977 — broadly in line with the staff group, and consistent with the trend in *new* patient averages of 19·9 and 25·4 in 1955 and 1973.

Group ranking

In contrast to this consistently high score on therapeutic community values, there have again (as in 1973) been some interesting and provocative changes in the evaluation of groups by staff and patients. The 1973 findings showed that 'the staff seem to have emphasized one or two groups as fundamental. . . . A similar process has occurred among the patient group. Furthermore, differences between staff and patient evaluations have increased . . . despite the common move in values toward the ideal' (Manning, 1976b) (see models 6 and 9). This trend has in general continued, although difference between staff and patient evaluations have declined (Table 14.1) (see model 5).

The staff have demonstrated quite clearly by 1977 that they agree almost unanimously on the small psychotherapy group and the community group as the essential groups (see model 4), and also that no groups except the work group come in the first three choices of any staff member. We see also how close the distribution of the actual

151

TABLE 14.1 Total score for the four highest scoring groups (%)

| | Staff | | | Patients | | | Maximum[*] |
	1955	1973	1977	1955	1973	1977	
Small group (psychotherapy)	25	32	43	27	44	47	50
Community meeting	21	27	33	10	8	24	33
Work group	14	14	19	11	17	15	17
Ward meeting	7	4	0	3	13	6	0
Other groups	33	23	5	49	18	8	0
Total	100	100	100	100	100	100	100
No. people in sample	26	33	21	84	37	26	

[*] Maximum percentage of total score if groups are ranked in the order on the Table by everyone (scored 3 for first, 2 for second, 1 for third).

scores in 1977 is to the theoretical maximum if each staff member were to rank their first three groups identically in the order on Table 14.1.

Within the patient evaluations, we see that the low score of the community group in 1973 has been largely reversed, although it still provides the greatest point of disagreement with the staff. Overall, the distribution of patient and staff scores is broadly similar (see model 6).

The 1977 data confirm the trends detected in 1973: that staff depend heavily on the small group for therapy, and the community meeting for social control; and that patients increasingly concur with this arrangement. Other groups are unanimously judged to be of less importance. This is counter to the philosophy of a 'twenty-four-hour' programme, where 'everything is treatment', which the staff and patients espoused in the values questionnaire. This gap between ideals and reality, between culture and structure, tentatively explored through the 1973 data (Manning, 1976b), is now confirmed more firmly with the 1977 data and hence can be discussed more confidently.

To find explanations for this problem, we must examine first why the ideals and reality have changed; and second, whether this change originated within the community itself, or in the constraints of its environment. Three models were suggested to explain the 1955–73 data. Now we can expand this set to explore more possibilities, some of which have also been suggested by developments in the St Luke's Project: we can identify at least ten models of change.

Ten models of community change

These models of community change may themselves be grouped into either external constraints, or internal processes; the latter can be further divided into changes of ideals or actual practice:

Internal processes: changing culture

(1) *Idealization*. Morrice (1972) has suggested that therapeutic community values have become exaggerated over time, for example through the uncritical acceptance of slogans such as 'everything is treatment'. Limits and qualifications are forgotten, and principles such as democratization are transmuted into sacred myths. A variant of this argument is to be found in Festinger's (1956) study of a 'doomsday' prophecy cult in the USA, where he found that the 'cognitive dissonance' generated by the failure of the prophecy resulted not in the dissolution of the cult, but rather a renewed vigour in proselytizing beliefs. Hence, we might suggest that the failure of research to demonstrate the efficacy of therapeutic community principles leads to a closer adherence to ideals, and, therefore, higher scores on the Henderson values questionnaire.

(2) *Experience*. Jones (1976), Manning (1976c) and Whiteley (Chapter 2) have noted the common observation that the therapeutic community operates with principles more basically discovered in group psychotherapy and organization development. The complex interaction between the personality and its social environment, and hence the mutual influence of the one by the other, is well documented. The therapeutic community's strength was the promotion of these ideas in psychiatry, and more recently in other groups dedicated to personal growth. Therefore, to maintain momentum and develop their work, therapeutic practitioners are extending the theoretical limits of their principles further; for example, greater democracy (as in St Luke's selection procedure), or more extreme confrontation (as in Concept Houses).

(3) *Contradictions*. Even while recording the now famous themes of democracy, permissiveness, communalism, and confrontation, Rapoport (1960) acknowledged their obvious contradictory implications. Where should limits be set? Which dictate is superior to which? Are not treatment and rehabilitation ('growth' and 'adjustment') different? Subsequent critics have pursued the discovery of these difficulties (Morrice, Chapter 6; Zeitlyn, 1967), in a process common to almost all scientific progress (Kuhn, 1962): the construction of a theoretical ideal (paradigm), within which contradictions (anomalies) are steadily accumulated, until a new theory must be constructed to explain the contradictions (paradigmatic revolution). We may be witnessing, therefore, a contest between the old therapeutic community paradigm and its accumulated anomalies.

Those who support the original paradigm may cling more tightly, as revealed in the Henderson values questionnaire, while more recent formulations develop. This tension may also affect practice (see model 6).

Internal processes: changing structure

(4) *Attitudes – behaviour discrepancy*. The gap between what people say they do (or will do) and what they actually do has been a source of puzzlement for social psychologists. However, Fishbein (1967, 1971) has recently arrived at a celebrated solution. He argued that the difference between attitudes expressed (for example, xenophobia) and actual behaviour (racial discrimination), noted frequently in the literature, could be explained by informal norms which surround and constrain everyday behaviour. 'Behavioural intention' leading to actual behaviour emerges from both enduring attitudes, and more immediate norms:

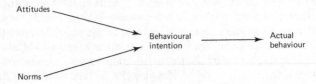

These day-to-day norms have been explored in such descriptive accounts of therapeutic communities as St Luke's above, but not yet categorized systematically. For example, while 'role-blurring' and 'multiple leadership' might be endorsed as part of therapeutic community ideals, in fact staff members observed at Henderson Hospital were quite competitive in demonstrating specifically psychotherapeutic/interpretive skill in the pursuit of stable leadership status (Manning, 1976b). The source of such counter-ideal norms may come from the personalities of staff (see model 5), or the difficulties of community work (see model 6), or more generally the environment.

(5) *Informal social life*. From the earliest studies of formal organizations (Roethlisberger and Dickson, 1939), it has been recognized that all such social institutions have an 'under-life', unacknowledged and without a formal 'map', which participants must discover for themselves. It has been one of the central tenets of the therapeutic community that such behaviour be brought into the official 'public arena' of the community meeting for analysis in the pursuit of treatment. However, even in the most ideal of 'twenty-four-hour' treatment environment, community members will have plenty of time to develop alternative 'coping' mechanisms and views (see Mahony, Chapter 9); staff may live in a hostel, or meet socially; and patients can relax when 'off-stage'; for example, St Luke's is open only in the afternoon. Indeed, the 1977

change of patient evaluation of groups at Henderson towards the staff evaluation may be closely connected with the new building. Patients now have individual rooms, which tend to preclude the germination of such a rich 'alternative' culture as the open wards of the old hospital. This under-life is connected closely with the individual needs of community members. For example, Menzies (1960) has argued that many social forms are constructed so that the individual can manage anxiety. And indeed the therapeutic community often deliberately fosters such constructions (permissiveness) so that the *way* an individual or group manages its anxiety can be explored. But to the extent that such processes escape public acknowledgment, the implementation of ideals may be undermined.

(6) *Internal contradictions*. Members of the community, in addition to spontaneously creating social life, described above, also try to manage or reconcile inherent conflicts in the ideals to be followed (see model 3). How much democracy? How much permissiveness? What kind of interpretation? Sharp (1975) has described in detail the way staff members have used 'managerial' concepts to mediate between contradictory demands, trying to maintain the *status quo*. Perrow (1965) has also discussed the contradictory pressures of the therapeutic community's social structure, goals and 'technology', which do not fit together. The problem is that of balancing a commitment to a set of ideals on the one hand with certain emergent realities of social life such as social control or authority on the other (Kanter, 1972; Punch, 1977); for example, management anxieties over the growth of democracy in St Luke's. Often such difficulties are managed on behalf of members by charismatic leadership, which unfortunately only delays the day when such charisma has to be 'routinized' (Weber, 1948). Leaders do not last for ever, and the attempts of their followers to resolve internal contradictions often results in instability, leading either to the ultimate demise of the community, or to its fundamental transformation.

External factors

(7) *Administrative disapproval*. For the Henderson, and many other communities, this means the National Health Service as reorganized in 1974. As Kennard (Chapter 18) points out, this effect depends on the permeability of boundaries. A therapeutic community which has independent hospital status is in a relatively strong position to resist direct pressures, although the Henderson and Marlborough Day Hospitals have recently been severely tested. The Paddington Day Hospital has had several such interventions, which have now resulted in radical transformation of both ideals and practice, and the removal of the Consultant Psychiatrist in charge (Manning, 1977). For a ward within a hospital,

such pressures are more difficult to resist and are correspondingly more dependent on a protective leader. Unfortunately, therapeutic communities have not been good at 'public relations' in this situation. St Luke's is, however, a model of what can be achieved (Archer, Chapter 4).

(8) *Neighbourhood disapproval*. Pressure from the local community can be as difficult for independent or social services hostels as a hostile administration. Indeed, it is more difficult to sit down and explain theoretical ideas to a neighbourhood, than to a sceptical committee. Sharp's (1975) study of such a hostel led him to reject the 'interactionist' perspective, whereby the ideals and practice of the hostel developed solely from the 'logic-in-use' of the members. This common assumption by 'sociologists of deviance', he argued, ignores the very real pressures on such a community from the environment, which distort social processes inside the community. He particularly dwelt on the issue of social control, necessary to maintain a 'quiet' community, but which subverted ideals of permissiveness and confrontation.

(9) *Professional careers*. It is commonly observed that the professionally trained doctor or nurse experiences acute role conflict in his early days in a therapeutic community. Indeed, Rapoport (1960) described the 'emergent pattern of role performance' of such an individual as a result of two pressures: therapeutic community ideology and conventional 'role prescriptions'. This model is far too mechanical. Rather, the individual (professional or not) has to remould his expectations with the help of informal advice and cues from other staff and patient members (Manning, 1975a). But this informal culture (see models 4, 5 and 6) not only serves to change the individual, but also enables the individual to undermine the community's ideals and practice. For example, doctors tend to take up leadership positions, running psychotherapy groups, and so on. This process encourages fantasies of dependence in patients, and aspirations for psychotherapeutic skill in non-medical staff who might be better used in more community-oriented activity (Manning, 1976b). These difficulties, of course, are much fewer in non-medical settings such as St Luke's, although the steady development of a professional self-image amongst social workers may bode ill for the future.

(10) *Legal obligations*. Many therapeutic communities have patient-members on probation. This symbolizes most forcefully the function of social control required of therapeutic communities, whether part of the health or social services. Here we can see the conflict between 'social adjustment' and 'self actualization' (Sharp, 1975) brought into sharp relief. It may be (and we have heard this in more than one therapeutic community) that for a person to become a better (i.e. more successful) criminal would be a fully successful 'goal-attainment' (Kiresuck, 1976). However, we suspect that most therapeutic community leaders faced with such a real-life problem would modify both their ideals and

practice to avoid conflict with a wider social obligation for control. Just as progressive schools were constrained by being *in loco parentis* from any excesses which might be construed as damaging their pupils (Punch, 1977), those communities acting 'in place of prison' or even within the prison system (Morris and Morris, 1963; Parker, 1971; Briggs, 1972), have to be suitably gymnastic to maintain a balance between their radical and conservative activities.

Conclusion

We can see from this search for distorting processes in community life that there is indeed a close interaction between culture and structure, such that the two are often difficult to disentangle. Initially the culture necessarily determines an emergent structure, but soon structural developments expand and modify certain cultural elements. Within this relationship the problem is to maintain a clear view as to overall objectives, so that constructive change may be separated from that which is destructive.

By no means exhaustive, the list of models presented in this chapter suggests some dangers to beware of. It is difficult to know which is the most significant. Generally it can be seen that different models apply to different situations. For example, professional goals (model 9) are more likely to undermine a long-standing community, with therapists 'passing through' for experience; again 'idealization' (model 1) and 'experience' (model 2) may also be a greater danger to the established community. On the other hand, the disturbing discovery that ideals are contradictory (model 3), or that intentions and actions are not automatically connected (model 4), may be more stressful for a younger, less experienced community. Only by studying and comparing these intra-community processes on a wider scale than has been possible in this chapter can we build up a more reliable and general model of the therapeutic community.

15

The mental hospital therapeutic community in recent years

Kenneth Myers

Mental hospitals have been disappearing for a long time. Their limitations have been described, in this country and the United States in the main, in learned, brilliantly evocative and sometimes fictional terms (Stanton and Schwartz, 1954; Barton, 1959; Goffman, 1961; Kesey, 1962). Tooth and Brooke (1961) provided the foundation for central policy which resulted in projections of closures of mental hospitals (Ministry of Health, 1962), and, indeed, there has been a massive reduction in the number of resident patients. Psychiatric services were to be based on District General Hospitals, and there has been a considerable increase in the number of psychiatric units, of various designs, included in such developments. For all their disadvantages, mental hospitals have provided and will continue to provide most of the psychiatric in-patient facilities in Britain.

Paradoxically, one advantage of a much-criticized characteristic of mental hospitals, their size, has enabled the whole range of psychiatric services to be provided on one campus. (It is interesting to note that this very argument was used to justify the concept of the District General Hospital, and that such large establishments no longer figure in future hospital policy.) Each new approach to treatment has found a niche in the mental hospital, and the interest in social and milieu therapies in the 1950s and 1960s was reflected not only in changes in the institutions consequent upon upgrading, opening doors, liberalizing approaches and changing attitudes (Clark's (1965) therapeutic community approach), but also in the establishment, in a number of them, of the therapeutic community proper (Clark, 1965). It is with the impact of such units on, and the difficulties experienced in, the host institution that we are concerned here.

The mental hospital, as it has developed, is the very antithesis of the therapeutic community. The rigidity of structure, clearly defined hierarchies, and laborious and inefficient communications systems, all of which are related to size, are clearly at the other end of the scale of values inherent in a therapeutic community. Such a unit prides itself on, and is defined by, its use of any — and every — social occurrence in its treatment programme, by the ways in which roles are blurred, and its encouragement of free communication. To establish within any organization a small unit with a different ethos, different structure and different methods of working is to create a disturbance. If, in addition, the staff of the host organizations have no training in or experience of the new methods, those who identify with the new unit will be seen as disloyal to their profession, as aberrant. If the new unit also deals with a clientele not usually acceptable to the host organization, there will be a tendency to reject or extrude it, and for the unit itself to encourage that tendency. All of these processes are recognizable in the large psychiatric hospital in which is embedded a therapeutic community.

Impact

When the therapeutic community is first suggested, the idea is welcomed as an exciting and new addition to the range of services the hospital provides. Discussions with interested parties in all disciplines are held in an atmosphere of optimism, although those with medical colleagues usually evoke the most sceptical responses: 'I hope all goes well for you.' 'It will be interesting to have a look at your results.' Efforts are made to find those staff members who are likely to be most interested — young, intelligent, lively men and women with outgoing personalities — and who are most likely to grace the new unit and make it a success. The unit opens on a high note, with expectations of hard, demanding, rewarding work, an awareness that what is being undertaken is, in the hospital's terms, different, in the knowledge that all eyes are on the new project, and with the perhaps naive view that it is bound to succeed because nobody within fifty miles is doing anything like it.

This was the picture at Middlewood Hospital, Sheffield, in the early 1970s, when a small ward for the treatment of personality disorders opened. Discussions started with the senior nurse administrator, the group secretary and the head occupational therapist. A ward became available, a list of potential residents was drawn up, and the two nurses appointed were sent off for a week, with the consultant psychiatrist, to a well-known therapeutic community. A pattern of functioning derived from that of the Henderson Hospital, with minor variations, was decided on. The unit opened, patients were admitted, and the built-in ambivalences and incompatibilities immediately became apparent.

The idea of working in a group appeals to students of all disciplines, to nurse students no less than others. There were many requests to be allowed to visit the ward, to attend ward meetings, to sit in on staff discussions. Attempts to explain that such requests would have to be put to the group as a whole were not well received; it was suggested that the necessity for doing so showed lack of control of the group by the nursing staff. Medical colleagues attempting to contact the psychiatrist did not readily accept that he was in a ward meeting: 'Can't he leave it?' When the telephone was not answered during the community meetings, administrators, professional and nursing, implied irresponsible behaviour by the staff group, and if a patient answered they were nonplussed and rang again later. It seemed that the new unit was enthusiastically accepted by everybody, provided that it functioned in exactly the same way as the rest of the hospital.

Criticism, spoken and implied, took over from uncomprehending curiosity. All disciplines were affected: the patients were not welcome on other wards, occupational therapists and nurses were resented by their colleagues for not working the same hours, and the consultant was introduced to a visiting psychiatrist as 'our psychopathic doctor — he runs a therapeutic community for psychopaths'.

Survival

Each discipline felt ostracized by its own colleagues. Therapeutic community staff were seen as dangerous, left-wing nonconformists, an impression that was fostered by their avoidance of uniform, left-wing political views, and refusal to accept traditional mental hospital practices without question. For example, the representative from the treasurer's department always called at the same time each week to make payments to patients. The staff group met at that time for one of its review meetings which was inevitably interrupted. Requests that the payment round should be varied so that the call was made a few minutes earlier were at first resisted, and then involved the nursing officer before a satisfactory solution was found.

Inevitably, the therapeutic community staff became a tightly knit group giving each other close personal support. There was a real danger that they would lose contact with the larger hospital community, and, in the absence of therapeutic communities within easy visiting distance, isolation, even within their narrowly defined professional specialty, became the reality. Meetings of the Association of Therapeutic Communities were too infrequent to be helpful, their content appeared to irritate rather than instruct or support, and the level of sophistication — or pseudo-sophistication — too high for a group with a relatively low level of expertise and very little support.

Worse was to come. A series of moves, from one ward to another, ensued. They were made in the name of 'the need for upgrading', or 'more efficient use of available ward space'. They were perceived by the community as punitive moves perpetrated by administrators; the fact that there were very good reasons for each move merely made things worse still. Referrals were infrequent; the small nucleus of, at one time, four patients were the most demanding and destructive of personalities. After three years of functioning, despair and hopelessness seemed to have replaced enthusiasm and optimism.

While the therapeutic community was drawing away from the hospital and deriving little, apart from hotel services, from the association, interest had been aroused elsewhere. The University Department of Psychiatry referred patients, the Department of Social Studies sent students on placement, medical students attended, and recognition by the General Nursing Council as a training ward meant that student nurses could be allocated during their last few months of training. The presence within the hospital of a unit where group psychotherapy was the main activity encouraged those who were interested to introduce similar ideas into other wards. Referrals increased again, and the staff group was asked to speak about their work in a variety of settings: in the nurse education department, to occupational therapists, social workers and various groups of professionals in training. The group's morale rose, they felt they had a contribution to make to the work of the hospital, and the mutual withdrawal was less in evidence.

Acceptance

The encouragement to survive came from outside the hospital initially. With the improvement in morale less investment was needed in preserving the group's integrity and more time could be devoted to examining ways of working, planning programmes of activity and looking at individual patients' needs. A stable and competent staff group was able to organize a week's review of its activities, to which it invited participants from other areas of the hospital. Inevitably, it recognized its weaknesses, and the strong undercurrent of despair recognizable in so many therapeutic communities was well in evidence. To the staff's surprise and pleasure, however, considerable interest was aroused in the rest of the hospital, and a lively correspondence followed in the monthly newssheet. While criticism continued, it was constructive, and while hostility was still in evidence it was no longer the dominant tone of the interaction. A weekly meeting of those interested in group psychotherapy was initiated, and while it could not be called a sensitivity group in any formal sense, it certainly fulfilled a valuable supporting role for the wider group than the staff of the therapeutic community, who no longer felt they had to adopt defensive stances to anything like the same degree.

The therapeutic community at Middlewood has been functioning for approximately five years. It was established in a large, traditional mental hospital and caused an initial, brief stir of interest. This was followed by a prolonged struggle for survival which, largely made possible by the interest of outside groups, was followed by a spread through other parts of the hospital of interest in group methods. The immediate impact was slight, but over the years it has become apparent that the community has to some extent been an agent for change.

Comparisons

It is not possible to make detailed comparisons of the evolution of therapeutic communities in mental hospitals, even though others have been described, notably at Claybury and Fulbourn (Martin, 1962; Schoenberg, 1972; Clark and Myers, 1970). The host institutions are at different stages of evolution, and, a factor of some importance, reflect local attitudes to mental health problems. Therapeutic communities which are established in hospitals already known for their liberal regimes and use of social therapies have a tendency to disappear, or for their differences to become less marked. Since the hospital itself is familiar with group methods at every level and in all settings, the therapeutic community is no longer unusual or different, survival is no longer an issue, and acceptance comes much earlier. Paradoxically, with the spread of the features of the therapeutic community to other settings — freeing communications, blurring roles, flattening the authority pyramid — the need for the therapeutic community itself diminishes, either because the specific job for which it was created can now be undertaken by a variety of other agencies, or because changing attitudes in the wider community have resulted in fewer demands for special facilities. The therapeutic community for chronically disturbed men and woman at Fulbourn had disappeared within ten years of its opening because referrals had become rare, and because disturbed psychotics were no longer regarded as a group needing provision of their own.

The therapeutic community at Fulbourn had evolved slowly, at the same pace as other changes within the hospital. It did not appear out of the blue, as a new and unexpected development. While it was certainly seen by the rest of the hospital as a growth point in the organization's progress, it also appeared to be a logical step to a staff group that had been encouraging ward meetings, increasing patient participation in treatment and acceptance of responsibility for one another. Yet, almost despite the growth of the therapeutic community, the rest of the hospital continued to change, the therapeutic community itself was closed, and in the middle 1970s Fulbourn has come to be regarded as an excellent example of what a psychiatric hospital should be. Visitors go to Henderson Hospital if they want to see the therapeutic community in pure culture.

What has been the significance of their therapeutic communities to the large psychiatric hospitals? They are easiest to establish where the hospital regime is already a liberal one, where the therapeutic community approach is already established. In such places they are logical developments of movements already started, but because the liberal regimes from which they spring do not stand still, but continue to evolve and become competent to deal with problems only the therapeutic community could at one time handle, they are overtaken by events. The face-to-face therapeutic community, for all its liberal pedigree, contains the seeds of its own destruction in an innate rigidity. As background to other treatment modalities it is infinitely accommodating, as treatment itself it is of necessity inflexible.

Therapeutic communities associated with psychiatric hospitals illustrate a variety of paths of development. At Dingleton, a small hospital serving a predominantly rural area, the whole institution illustrates what can be done in terms of facilitating communication. It provides a service to its catchment population by using therapeutic community methods, but also by extending its activities from the hospital base into the community, and its staff are involved in aspects of the wider community's life which are not, in many places regarded as the task of health service personnel.

By way of contrast, Francis Dixon Lodge, at Towers Hospital, Leicester, is a discrete unit for personality and neurotic disorders which is part of the service based on the parent hospital, but has limited and specific aims. The same is true of Ward 3, Middlewood Hospital. Whereas Dingleton has developed a role which extends beyond the institutional boundaries, Francis Dixon Lodge and Ward 3 are part of their hospitals but use therapeutic community methods.

Conclusions

The establishment of a therapeutic community in a large psychiatric hospital is a process which induces opposition, partly because of the innate resistance, in any organization, to change, partly because of the challenge it constitutes to the accepted practices of professional hierarchies. A very large proportion of the group's energies has to be devoted to defensive activities, to justification of its methods, and to finding support elsewhere that will help to ensure its survival. Therapeutic communities that do survive can influence psychiatric practice in the rest of the hospital; others become isolated and insulated, forming a strange little enclave, criticized but tolerated because they offer a service to those patients not acceptable in the rest of the hospital. It could be argued that the establishment of a face-to-face therapeutic community proper encourages the development of the therapeutic community approach in hospitals which have still a long way to go along that road, but it seems more likely that these are different, though related, streams of development.

The therapeutic community as treatment, has, despite its emphasis on free communication and its ability to examine and deal with social disturbance, an innate rigidity which makes further development difficult. It can be compared with, for example, the removal of a diseased gall-bladder. While minor improvements in the technique of cholecystectomy may be developed, the principle of the removal of a diseased organ is unchanged. (This is an analogy only, and should be seen as such.) So, with the therapeutic community, improvements in the techniques of communication and social analysis, of group psychotherapy, socio-drama and psychodrama, do not radically alter the principle of using all the available human resources in furthering treatment. It is as if the therapeutic community is a dead-end (though not a dead limb) on the tree of treatment. Further developments must look beyond the boundaries of the group, and embrace much wider issues of social and political life, of health and educational policy.

Certain factors must receive careful consideration when a therapeutic community is being established in a large psychiatric hospital.

(1) Preoccupation with survival results from mutually defensive stances which in turn arise out of the impact of an entirely different ethos on the host institution. The use of the word 'host', with its undertones of 'parasitism', is entirely appropriate, since there is sometimes an implication that the therapeutic community is troublesome, which it often is, and unwelcome.

(2) The therapeutic community is much more likely to be able to devote its energies to client treatment, and less to defending its position, if the ethos of the parent hospital is one of open communication, and where group techniques are in common use. This implies that experience of and training in group psychotherapy must form part of the experience of the staff of the whole hospital. On this foundation, the more specialized techniques of the therapeutic community can be built up, without the infinitely laborious and frustrating task of teaching about groups from scratch.

(3) The therapeutic community should be housed in a separate building. Those which exist in one of the ordinary wards cannot achieve the degree of domesticity desirable. The closeness of the hospital is often as oppressive, while the contiguity of the buildings creates an

impression that the therapeutic community is 'merely' another part of the hospital, doing similar work and subject to all the, often inappropriate, demands of administrative and domestic tidiness.

The therapeutic community concept has, of course, spread far outside the medical world. It may be that the medical setting is one of the least appropriate. Certainly, the large psychiatric hospital as we know it presents a number of problems to developing therapeutic communities which have little relevance to the problems of their clientele. While it may be appropriate to use, in psychiatric hospitals, techniques of the therapeutic community — a way of working — the highly specialized therapeutic community proper has probably little to offer the large hospital but a little prestige and an extra training facility. It may be an agent for change where the climate is right and the changes are already occurring, but it would appear that the same set of conditions must exist for the therapeutic community to take root in the first place.

16
The role of the consultant in a therapeutic community*

Alan Mawson

One element of the therapeutic community ideology is that the contribution expected from any individual member of the community should depend more on what he or she has to contribute — balanced against the needs of the community as a whole — than on conventional expectations associated with professional groups, or grades in an official National Health Service hierarchy. Presumably this principle extends to consultants.

If perhaps this book can be thought of as a community (of chapters) then the principle should further extend to the boundaries within which I can choose what I want to contribute. Boundaries there are to what I can say, but they arise ultimately from the aim of this particular book. The aim required the development of a co-ordinated structure to the book. That is, having specified the aim — to survey the points at issue in therapeutic communities in the 1970s — the editors must consider what organization of the chapters would most enable us to fulfil that aim.

When I first wrote this chapter to give as an address in the course of a conference, I was similarly constrained by boundaries. In that case it became necessary for Bob Hinshelwood, who had the leadership role in and responsibility for planning the conference, to consider how to organize that day. The particular organizational boundaries that limited my freedom to choose what I could say are expressed by the title allocated to me. They were not experienced as unduly irksome, or resented as an unjustified interference with my right simply to do my own thing, because I understand the reasons for them — I know that they are not an arbitrary imposition. Within the organizational boundaries that arise from the aim of that conference or from the aim of this book I am free to decide what I want to say, and then to say it.

My role as NHS consultant in the host community at that conference

*Based on a paper given to the Association of Therapeutic Communities, October 1974, at the Marlborough Day Hospital.

did not give me automatically the role of conference organizer. That role fell appropriately to Bob. I approach my role in the community from a different point of view.

Raymond Blake (1974) in an issue of the *Association of Therapeutic Communities Bulletin*, makes a plea for 'clarity': clarity about our principles, processes, goals and limits within the therapeutic community movement. He also wanted to see us develop a more scientific attitude, and noted the rather negative attitude of the Association to research. In the same issue he had a long and carefully-thought-out letter about a potential strategy for changing a culture and organization towards that of a therapeutic community: in this second letter he made the point that staff in institutions are not only 'culture-carriers', they are the source of the culture – for good or ill, like parents in a family. He is enthusiastic about the general concept of therapeutic communities, but honest and caring enough to be something more than a starry-eyed convert to an ideology which fails to spell out its constituent elements, or test them. In his plea for clarity he wrote that while in Roman theology it is a 'cardinal sin' to give up hope, in his system of values it was 'much worse to confuse knowledge with belief – even if it was more comfortable'.

I can think of no better way of describing my idea of what the 'role of a consultant in a therapeutic community' should be, than to say it should involve supporting these attitudes and striving to encourage them in one's colleagues:

(1) To exhibit genuine concern and enthusiasm.

(2) To demonstrate that enthusiasm for an approach does not require the suspension of one's critical faculties.

(3) To urge and urge again that individuals and groups formulate their ideas regarding aims, and on how they may be achieved. As Popper has pointed out, once formulated clearly in words, our ideas can be discussed (and argued about if necessary) without personalized dispute. Heated but rational discussion and argument, without personal ill-feeling or personal attacks, between individuals or groups, was what I missed most when I moved from the Maudsley (where it was going on all the time) to a therapeutic community where at first it seemed well-nigh impossible. Often we have *ad hominem* arguments, imputing dishonesty, conscious hypocrisy, or even 'fascism' to an opponent (or to categorized groups such as 'consultants'), rather than reasoned disagreement, and appeals to evidence.

(4) To face up to, instead of dodging, ethical issues and questions of values that arise from our approach. Having done so (or while doing so) he could and should help his colleagues to do the same.

(5) Finally, the therapeutic community consultant must be honest

with himself — and with his colleagues and patients — about issues of authority, responsibility, and power.

As individuals and as the staffs of different units, our reluctance to clarify stems from a reluctance to grasp firmly, and grapple with, the last three areas. It is easier to avoid a clear formulation of aims in observable practical terms, because to do so would involve the risk of recurrently discovering how far short of them we fall. It is easier to avoid a clear operational definition of our methods because to do so might reveal how little logical or empirical grounds exist to show that they are dictated by the goals whose efficient attainment should be their justification. Honest examination of ethical issues and values within the therapeutic community movement could reveal very deep splits and divisions amongst us. Issues of authority and responsibility are especially hot to handle: it feels safer to leave them shrouded in catch phrases. A subsidiary reason is that there is a good deal of confusion, both in the minds of individuals (including those authorities who have written about therapeutic communities) and between subgroups within therapeutic community staff. Part of the confusion springs from a disregard for semantics — but I will return to that later. I will take first the issue of aims and how they may be achieved, and then the question of authority and responsibility.

The aim of a therapeutic community

Human activities may be evaluated in either of two ways: as 'good' or 'bad' in themselves; or alternatively as means to a specified end (aim or goal). The second approach raises the question of efficiency (Nokes, 1960). For certain types of activity and organization questions of efficiency are rarely raised, and this is most clearly exemplified by the 'humane institutions' such as psychiatric hospitals or schools. For social institutions such as psychiatric units to be viable it is not in fact necessary for them to be efficient. Nokes stresses the degree to which questions of 'efficiency' seem hardly to be live issues in these settings. When their activities and organizations are examined it often appears that they bear little observable or demonstrable relation to the supposed ultimate purpose of the institution (see Chapter 19). Such concern as can be detected about the discrepancy in the ultimate purpose of the institution, and the way its activities are organized, is likely to be among new staff. This places them in a painful predicament, most commonly solved by the newcomer eventually internalizing the institution's values and view of itself for himself.

Furthermore, 'it is not merely unnecessary for a humane institution to be efficient in order to remain in existence, it is not even necessary for its personnel to have any clear idea of what it is for' (Nokes, 1960). That is to say it is rare to find any genuine clarity in the conceptualization of such institutions' aims (let alone how they could best be attained). All too often the practices and techniques of the institution are classified as legitimate or otherwise quite independently of evidence of their efficacy. Furthermore, the practices and techniques of the institution tend to be determined by considerations such as tradition, or the whims and eccentricities of those in possession of personal prestige, power and influence, rather than by their relevance to the institution's proper purpose.

I would argue that it is a prime responsibility of the senior staff in any psychiatric service, and perhaps particularly of the consultant or other 'formal leader' of a therapeutic community, to concern themselves with the aims and goals of the institution; in the case of therapeutic communities this may be a task particularly complex and beset with difficulties.

Adequately examining the aims and goals of the institution also involves identifying the covert goals: it is easy enough to ask people what goals they believe they are pursuing, and to note what they say. Even if there are substantial areas of expressed disagreement to start with it may not be too difficult by discussion or consultation to arrive at apparent consensus as to what the aims of a therapeutic community are, or should be, and even as to how they may best be attained. But at this point the advice offered by Einstein to anyone who wished to discover what a theoretical physicist did, comes to mind. He recommended, 'I advise you to stick closely to one principle: don't listen to their words, fix your attention on their deeds.'

An institution such as a therapeutic community may have as its professed aim the liberation of its patients from the limitations and constraints of neurotic illness or personality disorder, in order that they may go back into the world able to live a freer, more effective and richer life. Closer examination of how such a community actually operates (e.g., its social organization, values, rituals, what behaviour and attitudes it reinforces) may show it to be directing more energy to satisfying the staff's need to be needed and the patients' desire for a professionally sanctioned retreat from the stress of responsibility for themselves and others. In other words, a contemporary therapeutic community may operate the same sort of defensive-collusive system that characterized the old-style asylum, differing only in that the system is dressed up in a new set of socio-political attitudes and is tricked out with a different set of rituals.

Leadership and authority

If we consult the standard literature of the therapeutic community movement (for example, Maxwell Jones and David Clark, themselves consultants in therapeutic communities), we find a certain inconsistency with respect to questions of authority, leadership and the role of the consultant. On the one hand much stress is laid on such words as 'democracy', 'democratization', 'equality', 'egalitarianism', 'flattening of the authority pyramid', 'power sharing', 'decision-making by consensus', and so on. Then on the other hand, a few pages later, we find statements at a less abstract level, which seem to contrast somewhat with the first set. Let me exemplify with some quotations:

(1) The Therapeutic Community Concept ... 'involves a redistribution of power, authority and decision-making ... and a more democratic egalitarian social structure generally. The single powerful staff leader is gradually replaced by a group of leaders.' 'The emphasis on free communication both within and between staff and patient groups, and on permissive attitudes which encourage free expression of feeling, implies a democratic egalitarian rather than a traditional hierarchical social organisation' (Jones, 1968a). BUT... 'In no sense do the staff or the doctor in charge relinquish their ultimate authority, which remains latent and can be evoked when necessary' (Jones, 1968a).

(2) 'Even in clinical psychiatry there is no reason why leadership should be on the basis of the formalized authority structure and status system of the National Health Service.' 'Our aim is to provide a democratic decision-making policy in all areas of hospital functioning.' 'The democratic egalitarian structure of the therapeutic community implies delegation of authority from the central administration to the problem area itself' (Jones, 1968b). BUT... 'A daily meeting of the hospital secretary, principal nursing officer, and physician superintendent (the "Holy Trinity") ... which has come to be seen as a co-ordinated body ... takes place for half-an-hour, as well as a daily meeting of the senior staff committee, about sixteen members in all (comprising all senior trained staff), which lasts forty-five minutes. These two groups deal with all the administrative problems of the day as well as problems bearing on patient management' (Jones, 1968b).

These apparent inconsistencies can give the impression of 'doublethink' regarding issues of authority, power and leadership. Indeed, the less charitable might infer an element of hypocrisy. I would prefer to assume that these apparent contradictions reflect genuine confusion, springing from a variety of sources, of which I think I can personally identify three, and no doubt those with greater experience in the field will be able to identify others. The first that strikes me is that Humpty-Dumptian disregard for semantic niceties which bedevils much of the literature in both medicine and social science. 'When *I* use a word,' Humpty Dumpty said in scornful tones, 'it means just what I choose it to mean — neither more nor less.' 'The question is,' said Alice, 'whether you *can* make words mean so many different things.' 'The question is, said Humpty Dumpty, 'which is to be master — that's all.'

But if we are seriously interested in communicating, we have to remember that when we use a word, it must mean the same to us as it does to the person we are speaking to (or the people we are writing for), otherwise our thoughts are not transmitted intact. Furthermore, if we use a word to stand for some technical process or phenomenon, and that word also has a meaning in common usage, we run an additional peril of being misunderstood. Humpty Dumpty's scornful dismissal of such simple semantic factors is reminiscent of the way in which advocates of the therapeutic community approach use such words as 'democracy', 'equality' and 'consensus'.

The second source of inconsistency between the abstractions regarding leadership and authority and other statements by the same authors having such a different flavour, is that there must always be some degree of 'mismatch' between an 'ideology' and the psycho-social or socio-political system to which its devotees wish to apply it. With regard to the therapeutic community ideology, the difficulties born of this mismatch are compounded by the conflicts that can arise in practical situations, between different elements of the ideology, e.g., 'permissiveness' versus 'reality-confrontation'. As Rapoport (1960) has pointed out, the four principal components of the ideology are not taken in any predetermined order of priority, and can easily conflict in a given situation, making it difficult to arrive at a decision as to which principle should be upheld at the expense of one of the others. Of course common sense occasionally decides the matter, as when fidelity to the ideal of permissiveness would result in murder or impulsive suicides; but often the decisions to be considered are more complex (see Chapters 6 and 14).

The third source of the apparent inconsistency in pronouncements relating to leadership and authority is the fact that in therapeutic communities issues of where leadership, authority and power actually lie tend to be 'blurred' just like other role distinctions, without this being regarded as necessarily bad. Ironically, this is a feature that therapeutic communities share with large-scale hierarchical bureaucracies; in the latter the formal hierarchy is precisely defined and designated, but to get anyone to accept that they have, as individuals, the responsibility for, and authority to, take action or arrive at a decision, may be well-nigh impossible. The words we use to stand for concepts tend to affect the concepts themselves, and even alter our perception of the under-lying denota. The word 'blurring' does a serious disservice to the therapeutic community movement, creates unnecessary dissension and difficulties between staff within individual therapeutic communities, and can be damaging to the interests of patients. The dictionary definition of 'blurring' is 'making vague or indistinct'. But what Maxwell Jones intended was to find a concise way of representing an extremely valuable idea: the release of staff and patients from the rigid strait-jacket of traditional role expectations, in order that each individual could make the fullest contribution compatible with his particular personality, knowledge, skills and problems. Unfortunately, this does not save us from the actual or potential consequences of the particular word 'blurring', used to express an admirable idea in 'shorthand' form. Thus, when the underlying principle is extended to redistribution of authority and the sharing of power, we must acknowledge that the consequent ambiguities may give rise to unnecessary confusion and anxiety, for staff and patients alike, and can even be potentially danger-ous. Here is a good example; in it, I am the guilty party.

It was Bob Hinshelwood, and not I, who had the leadership role in, and responsibility for, planning and organizing the conference for which the paper was prepared. It included choosing the theme, planning the day and delegating to others particular tasks. Now the decision that he, rather than I, should have the role of organizer and leader with respect to the conference was agreed upon between the two of us several months before, on the perfectly rational grounds that he had seen, and played a major part in, the development of the Day Hospital here towards a therapeutic community from its beginnings; and that he had a longer-standing and more committed relationship to the Association of Therapeutic Communities. The point of the example is that after we had agreed between ourselves, I then made an error of omission of the very sort I have been complaining is typical of the therapeutic community movement, i.e., a failure to clarify where leadership and authority lay with respect specifically to the conference. The conse-quent 'blurring' of roles caused confusion in the other staff and patients involved. Was I abdicating my authority and responsibilities *in toto* to Bob? Had he staged a quiet but effective *coup d'état* and become the formal leader in all but name? I had failed to clarify adequately for them our arrangement and the reasons for it. Furthermore, it was not until a 'staff group' just nine days beforehand, that I realized I had been guilty of this omission. In the intervening months, consequences had been accruing for the patient community, the staff, myself and my relations with both of these groups: consequences which I had dimly perceived but been unable to understand at the time, and which even subsequently took some time to undo. It is a small, but good, example of the necessity of clarifying, rather than leaving 'vague and indistinct' who has authority, and particularly of explaining when and why it is distributed in ways at variance with conventional expectations.

17
Work groups

Anna Christian and R. D. Hinshelwood

The inception of the therapeutic community, being in wartime, had as its context the moulding of a war-neurotic and shell-shocked rabble into a high-morale fighting unit again. Selfless endeavour for king and country was the ethos of the Northfield Military Hospital. And rehabilitation back into industry during the period of post-war reconstruction was the inspiration of the early days at Belmont, the fore-runner of the Henderson. The work group was the pivotal event in the therapeutic community at this time (Bion and Rickman, 1943).

How odd that seems now to those of us who have wandered into this field in the last decade or so! As much as any institution in the West, the therapeutic community was affected by Marcuse's 'Freudian Marxism' and the May Revolution in Paris in 1968. Only recently the Freud statue at Swiss Cottage in London sported the graffito, 'The super-ego in your head supports the supermarket in your street.' Marcuse took over the orthodox Freudian view that the super-ego is formed from instructions and cultural values accepted by the developing individual from social agents (family, school, etc.) entrusted to do this. Marcuse goes on to explain that this is a self-perpetuating process from one generation to another. A capitalist culture will go on instilling capitalist values and capitalist super-egos in its children, who will grow into parents and teachers doing the same. This is a process that goes on quite irrespective of the economics and the changes in technological tempo that society may have gone through in the course of a generation. Consequently, he says, our super-egos stem from the time of early capitalism. The hard-working, puritanical, protestant ethic which developed, required all pleasure (especially erotic) to be sublimated in non-stop drudgery, and was appropriate to that phase of Western development. We live now, Marcuse says, in a time of plenty, when the problem is to stimulate demand, rather than ensure subsistence. So we don't need to work. Eros may be freed if we choose (Marcuse, 1955).

The growth of the Welfare State, the availability of readily dependent members of therapeutic communities, and a confused ideology have in conjunction allowed the notion of work groups to slip out of the prime focus of attention of most therapeutic communities. This focus has moved to small groups and more recently to the phenomenon of large groups with a psychotherapeutic function (Kreeger, 1975).

In some therapeutic communities, and in most from time to time, some people do become doubtful, perhaps even sickened by a tendency towards self-indulgence and an aggressive justification of idleness based on the claim to painful symptomatology and illness. This beats the therapeutic community at its own game. Often there will be calls 'to work on yourself'. In this context work means something very different. Work is here referring to some internal operation, supposed to be under the control of a conscious will, as are the voluntary muscles. But we doubt whether one can command intra-psychic change in this way. Surely one cannot command interpersonal adaptations (behaviour changes) without encouraging institutional authority over the individual, reminiscent of the demands in mental hospitals or prisons to conform.

In a living institution there must be a vital dynamic between social demand and the social refuge. They have to be opposite sides of the same coin. A therapeutic community cannot survive if it seeks a division of labour between those who care (the staff) and those who are protected (the patients). Staff must also demand; and patients can and do care (even if it may be hard to see).

Much of Marcuse's argument is valid, but not all. The occurrence of a fierce enslaving and alienating super-ego is not the achievement of capitalism, but is much more nearly a basic endowment of mankind (Klein, 1932). It seems to us that it is inherent in man to devote himself to some thing outside himself, beyond himself, to care for it and to seek to protect it and to work for its protection. The degree to which this is either a hope-filled task and potentially self-fulfilling, or gloom-ridden and tottering endlessly and oppressively on the brink of failure, is a matter of individual maturation as well as environmental chance.

So the therapeutic community must hunt for, recognize and display that aspect of the humanity of every member that is capable of care and devotions, that can acknowledge and work for something outside himself and bigger than himself. What does this mean? In effect, in the therapeutic community it means the devotion of the individual to the community itself. It is the demand of the community on the individual, and his response to protect and care for the community, ensure its good order and promote its achievements (one of which will incidentally be his own growth).

At this point we would like to review briefly various attitudes to physical activity in the context of treatment and the therapeutic community.

Rationales for work

A century ago the vogue was for 'moral treatment of the insane'. This entailed stimulating and improving activities such as farming, listening to music, a hospital chapel and other Victorian delights. It was innovatory in its time. For this was the period of attempted change in Britain and Europe (as opposed to the USA) from a custodial regime to hospital-like care (Walk, 1976). It is clear that, in thinking about treatment instead of restraint, the view was that the inmates should be allowed to acquire features of life that gave meaning to their own lives. Gradually, the therapeutic employment of patients became widely accepted, giving rise to a new profession (occupational therapy) and the development of industrial therapy workshops in this country before the last war — and earlier on the Continent.

Then the war supervened. It depended ultimately on working relationships, the morale of the group, and team spirit. This ethos pervaded psychiatric establishments and gave rise to the conception of a community that is therapeutic.

This seems now to be almost a sideline in the mainstream of the development of occupational therapy and the psychiatric attitude to employment. A more orthodox attitude is that since the devil may find work for idle hands, the social rehabilitator must be quick off the mark. The protestant work ethic here fits hand-in-glove with the medical model of treatment: work is for the patients' own good, rather like Largactil. Responsibility for work groups moved from social therapists and instructors in the early days of therapeutic communities to nurses and occupational therapists. Their traditional training developed a focus on the individual. Emphasis moved to the need for personal attention to the patient. In this mainstream view, work groups and indeed the rest of the therapeutic community regime are an instrumental technique in the hands of the professional for operating effectively on the psyche and the development of the clients.

Over the last thirty years the concept of work has drifted and what is considered therapeutic work has become completely different. It now includes rationales based on four processes: self-expression, role-learning, habit-training and acting-in.

First, the increasingly humanitarian development of occupational therapy is reflected in the rationale of self-expression. People with emotional problems need reassurance about their emotions. Usually this means anger and hate. Expression of these in the presence of tolerant others can build a subsequent confidence. The use of art and music and craft activities is undoubtedly helpful in promoting self-expression.

Self-confidence and self-respect are encouraged by demonstrating to the demoralized individual that he can make a useful or beautiful end-product (woodwork or clay pots). Incidentally, this can also lead to loss of respect for the occupational therapist as gullible and indiscriminate. Such activities, devoted to reassurance, self-expression and encouragement of creativity are neither true groups, nor are they work — we would suggest the term 'hobby groups'.

Second, role-learning is one aim of a structured work group. A group that engages in physical activity must organize itself in a realistic way. It needs a division of labour and therefore must assess skills and experience for allocating roles. This creates group tensions which must be stabilized by authority relationships and rudimentary social control. Vertical structuring of 'foreman' and 'labourer' not only presents opportunities to study all kinds of problems, but also provides a setting for social learning, the acquiring of experience and skills in different social roles.

Third, since people get up and go to work in the morning as a matter of habit and good sense, social pressure in a community to attend work groups forms a kind of behaviour therapy aimed at developing the work habit.

Finally, acting-in is the discharge of 'energy' in a safe social situation. Freud's early ideas postulated a psychic energy that came to be discharged as muscular activity. It was a means of release of mental tension but could be blocked by obstacles that resulted from past traumas. Reich extended this pseudo-physics and focused on releasing the blocks. In many of the new therapies, individuals are invited within a social group to work on themselves in this way. The release of internal tensions through physical activity such as trust-exercises, beating hell out of cushions, or clarifying fantasy relationships through psychodrama are encouraged as the new form of work.

External and internal work

Internal work on the individual's intra-psychic processes or on his range of interpersonal options is in contrast to external work that is meaningfully related to the 'community's needs'. There is a danger that internal work can become a collusion on a community scale with the narcissistic side of the individuals concerned to become perfect in mind and body and innocent of any guilt.

In these attitudes that we have termed mainstream, external activity in the external world is a pretext. A therapeutic community must also set the individual in the context of the 'needs of the group', a group which is, nevertheless, the means by which he can achieve his own treatment needs. Thus, for the individual to gain his own ends, he must devote himself to the ends of the group or community in which he will achieve his ends. The individual is a part of something that stretches far beyond him; he is part of something bigger than himself. It is in this sense above all others that the therapeutic community can, and must be, a microcosm of real society. It is only in this way that a treatment situation can realize the subtle mixture of altruism and egoism that life is all about.

Difficulties with work groups

The work group could be one of the most vivid representations of the devotion of the individual to the needs of the community which will meet his own needs. It can make the feelings of guilt turn more towards a sense of responsibility, rather than a fear of punishment. So why do ongoing tasks sometimes fail? We can look at the reasons from various aspects and preconceived attitudes.

Starting with the staff group, what effect do the different staff roles have on the effectiveness of a work group? The occupational therapist has been highly trained to 'rehabilitate', and this training has given her ideas of how to do it. The nurse has been trained to care. For all professionals there can be a tendency to work by the book. The need to feel valued and important and to be seen to be effectively caring accompanies many well-motivated nurses and occupational therapists and those of other caring professions. This can set up a competitive barrier between differing roles. Competition surrounds who is doing the best for the patients. Nurses and occupational therapists rival each other for the patients' appreciation and gratitude. They may also be in competition with the patients themselves, who in a therapeutic community have a caring role. In addition, there may be a need to attract the attention of the designated leader of the community. Such a person, who may be a doctor, may in turn feel the need to establish his own supremacy with his medical aura.

These underlying feelings and attitudes interfere with the staff's listening to the needs of the total community, and prevent the development of worthwhile activity. In the context of this competition, the work groups can be used by those who run them as a weapon in the rivalry with those who do not.

Members have their own attitudes towards work. In the group there is commonly a view that work towards the benefit of the community is unrewarding and boring. Work such as washing-up has been eloquently described by Holden (1972), who quotes one patient as saying, 'How can I be expected to do the washing-up? I feel so weak that I can't even do my own washing-up at home. I have had a complete breakdown, that's why I have come to the hospital. I need rest, I need to be looked after. I know that it has to be done – but why can't it be done by those who are able-bodied? I can't do it – if I could I wouldn't need to be here.' Members can feel exploited by the staff, whose job is supposed to be to organize things better – it is a hospital, after all. Staff can re-inforce this if they feel that their time and skill is not suitably put to good use when they involve themselves in such mundane matters. It boils down to the question of who does the dirty work.

The tack of 'you (the members) should do these domestic chores because it is good rehabilitation' is met by the member's answer that he expects to be doing bigger, better and more important work when he leaves. He says, 'You are wrong. Chores are not rehabilitation.' This can seduce certain staff into a collusive game with members over a search for the perfect job. As Meyer (1969) points out, this merely puts off the evil day when a compromise has to be made. He describes a girl who, like many emotionally deprived people, wanted to find 'work with animals. This is difficult to get, so she eventually compromised by working in a bird seed factory.' The unwillingness to make this kind of compromise may be reinforced by the attitude expressed by a member who said, 'It's the staff who do the real work.' And by the real work he meant the glamour of managerial meetings and responsibility.

Work (and the work group relationships) brings to the fore some of the reasons why members have broken down. It illustrates the inter-personal problems they have met prior to admission which eventually repeat when coping with authority figures, commitment to a task, etc. These can result in feelings of depressive worthlessness which may be the one thing the member is attempting to avoid at all cost.

The economics of the community

If work groups are set up as a pretext for alternative aims, i.e. habit-training or hobbies, they immediately become susceptible to the Marcusean criticism. The effort towards an end-product that is un-necessary means that work groups become in themselves desultory and apparently aimless. They require constant justification to the com-munity members with a contrived community value: 'work-groups are necessary, valuable, good-for-you'. Such a value does not grow out of the members' own experience of the current needs of the material reality of the community at that time.

The economics of the community make certain tasks necessary and urgent, without which the living conditons would decline below levels acceptable to a consensus of the community. It is only such tasks as these that can give work meaning in the community (Jones *et al.*, 1956).

It is our impression from acquaintance with a number of recent therapeutic communities that, other things being equal, the more necessary tasks a community has to do for itself, the greater is the community spirit and morale which feels 'healthy' to the visitor. If it is the service to the therapeutic community as a whole, in tasks that lie within the capabilities of the members, that makes for a good community atmosphere, then there may be a positive therapeutic advantage to therapeutic communities that are less well provided for financially.

Tasks necessary to the community are of two kinds: management work and physical work. The community has to be organized. It has to make decisions about its form and procedures. Limits have to be put on its members, and the breaking-points allowed for. It has in fact to be managed. When these management tasks are handed over to the community as a whole, then we have the administrative therapy of the therapeutic community. It could loosely be referred to as management of the community by the community.

When there are physical tasks devoted to the material conditions and needs of the community, these are performed by work groups. Such tasks include shopping, cooking, cleaning, maintenance work and decorating, as well as those devoted to money-raising activities such as jumble sales, crafts for retailing, and so on.

Although this chapter is concerned solely with work groups, we have mentioned the connection with community management because of an important contrast. It is a contrast between work that services the organization and work that services the material environment; and this is important because it is a vital contrast in the division of society at large.

One of the features of most therapeutic communities in this country (especially within the NHS) is that they depend on the financial resources of the State, and there is an expectation that most material needs will be met by the employment of paid cooks, cleaners and maintenance men. There are far-reaching consequences: it means that the tasks necessary for the therapeutic community as a whole that are left over for the members are usually management tasks; and these may be within the capabilities of only a smallish stratum of potential members. This is one important factor in the trend in most therapeutic communities towards a predominantly middle-class clientele, with higher IQ and with ambition to reach professional or managerial status. It would be one consequence of an under-financed therapeutic community that there would be recognition of the key tasks for working-class or lower-IQ clients.

Without feeling he has a necessary contribution to make, a member of society will suffer an apathetic withdrawal or express a form of social pathology (for instance suicide) that reflects the anomie of the society. So it is in a therapeutic community. Work that does not lead to meaningful products and necessary contributions does not bind the member into the community — in fact the reverse.

It has always been necessary in therapeutic communities to establish the visible presence of the community and of the individual's membership of it by instituting the community meeting. Without such a regular face-to-face manifestation of the community it seems to be difficult to establish the members' awareness of anything. It is the demand to belong that creates the therapeutic dynamic. But only a genuine need of the community as a whole leading to necessary contributions from members can establish a sense of belonging. In this way the community meeting has now become the only resource left to an over-endowed community to establish belonging and prevent anomie in the membership.

18
Limiting factors: the setting, the staff, the patients

David Kennard

The purpose of this chapter is to try to understand some of the constraints which operate on therapeutic communities, both from within and from outside. We are concerned here not with how a therapeutic community gets started, but with the factors which, once started, will shape its development, promoting or limiting its growth in various directions. For convenience, I shall place these constraints under three headings, according to their sources. First, there are constraints which arise from the setting of a therapeutic community. These include its location and the role it fulfils for the wider community. Second, there are constraints created by the staff of a therapeutic community, whose beliefs, attitudes and skills are usually the first and essential building blocks of the community. Third, constraints are created by the patients (or residents/clients as appropriate) whose capacity and willingness to 'enter into the spirit' will influence the way a therapeutic community is run. Before proceeding to describe these constraints in greater detail, I should like to clarify the view taken here towards the nature of therapeutic community theory and practice.

The notion of the 'ideal' therapeutic community

When, in the 1940s, Tom Main, Wilfred Bion, Maxwell Jones and others began their action experiments in psychiatric hospitals, they were guided by certain beliefs: in the need for sincerity and humility on the part of doctors, in the value of sharing responsibility for running the ward with the patients, and pooling the institution's total resources, and in the possibility of learning from all this, from the daily business of living together.

Subsequently, various routine procedures were introduced which helped to further these basic goals and became widely practised in therapeutic communities, to the point of being identified with them:

the morning community meeting of all patients and staff, the election of a patient chairman, dividing up into smaller groups for carrying out work projects and different forms of group therapy, the staff feedback meetings, and what have come to be called 'sensitivity' groups. Thus the anti-bureaucratic daring of the early innovators settled down into a particular way of doing things. In a study of one of the longest established therapeutic communities, Henderson Hospital, it was found that the staff there subscribed to views which Rapoport (1960), the investigator, was able to group into four general principles. The first two of these he called 'democratization' and 'permissiveness'. These gradually acquired the status of an ideology, such that for the past decade or more, people have been arriving in therapeutic communities and saying, 'Where's the democracy? Where's the freedom? This place is a sham, there's a hierarchy after all.' The problem with such a consolidation of practice and ideology is that it may limit the potential of therapeutic communities, by inhibiting the freedom to experiment. The expectation of having to conform to a particular, ideal type of therapeutic community, regardless of who or what the community is in business for, may inhibit precisely the qualities of courage, spontaneity, humanity and curiosity that enabled institutions to become therapeutic communities in the first place.

Though I have made a plea against the idea of a single ideal type of therapeutic community, it will nevertheless be useful to have before us some picture of what a therapeutic community is. Two quotations may help to anchor our thoughts about this. Jones (1968b): 'The institution's total resources, both staff and patients, are self-consciously pooled in furthering treatment'. Main (1946): 'The Northfield experiment is an attempt to use a hospital not as an organization run by doctors in the interests of their own greater technical efficiency, but as a community with the immediate aim of full participation of all its members in its daily life and the eventual aim of the resocialization of the neurotic individual for life in ordinary society'.

These descriptions have a particular value today, because apart from the labels 'doctor' and 'neurotic', they apply to all types of therapeutic communities, whereas more recent writings have often implied a more restricted and arbitrary definition. Thus, where democratic decision-making and an egalitarian structure are regarded as the defining characteristics of a therapeutic community, we would have to exclude communities such as Concept Houses which employ a self-conscious hierarchy in which decision-making powers are carefully graded. On the other hand, in North America many workers appear to regard the latter type as constituting what a therapeutic community is. What matters, however, is the culture rather than the structure, the informal relationships which develop within the formally prescribed limits. Rapoport's third and less often quoted principle, communalism, comes close to this: 'The functioning of a therapeutic community should be characterized by tight-knit, inter-communicative and intimate sets of relationships. Sharing of amenities, informality (e.g. use of first names) and freeing of communications are prescribed.' Rapoport's other principle, reality-confrontation, also seems to apply to all types of therapeutic communities: patients should be continuously presented with interpretations of their behaviour as it is seen by others.

Two further attributes are implied in the words of Jones and Main. One is the attitude that the work of the community is a shared endeavour, that all patients and staff, or all residents, have an active part to play in its continuing viability and success. This view clearly reflects the importation of the psychoanalyst's idea of a working alliance between the therapist and the healthy part of his patient, into a world (the psychiatric hospital) where previously the patient had been seen as a passively co-operative recipient of treatment. The other feature concerns the use made of what goes on within and between groups of people working and living together. In any treatment or rehabilitation setting there is a choice (not always recognized) of whether to try to understand and harness the group dynamics which are operating, or allow them to work informally and often unseen. The former option marks the therapeutic community approach. Treatment settings established for the specific purpose of creating these dynamics, to use them as the main agent of change, have been termed the therapeutic community proper or the psychotherapeutic community. More recently, the language of systems theory has enabled this, perhaps the most sophisticated aspect of therapeutic community practice, to be further elaborated using the concept of higher- and lower-order systems, which extend from the individual's psyche through to the community at large (see Chapter 12).

Beyond this 'common core' of therapeutic communities, many differences may exist. Communities may be democratic or hierarchical in structure, permissive or meticulous in their response to deviant behaviour, blurred or clear in their allocation of roles, of various theoretical persuasions in their understandings of personal relationships, and they may employ treatments which extend beyond the individual's psyche to his biochemistry. (This last variation, the combination in a psychiatric hospital of physical methods of treatment with a therapeutic community approach, raises particular problems to which we shall return.) Having made this brief tour of the common features of the landscape we can proceed to the task of examining some of the constraints which will determine the form and contours of a particular therapeutic community.

Constraints arising from the setting

Two types of constraint will be considered here; those created by the obligations to provide a service to various external individuals and bodies, and those arising from the environmental location.

Service obligations

A therapeutic community will be limited in its autonomy by various statutory or agreed obligations to provide a service to a number of people and organizations. The actual number and range of such obligations may vary considerably. For example, a hospital unit employing a therapeutic community approach may have the following obligations: (a) to general practitioners, social workers and others to admit at any time and contain individuals who are very disturbed or disturbing to others; (b) to the medical and nursing administration to accept staff allocated to the ward; (c) to patients' relatives to provide information and reassurance; (d) to the hospital training programmes to provide placements for student nurses, doctors, social workers, etc., and entertain visitors to the hospital. Thus deluged, the ward's attempt to develop an atmosphere of joint endeavour, close informal relationships and social awareness will be constrained by the continuing need to integrate new, sometimes reluctant individuals into its culture.

In contrast to this, a hostel or day centre operating as a therapeutic community may have been established to provide non-urgent help for a particular group of people or problems, such as drug addicts or ex-psychiatric patients. Such a community may be free to decide whom to admit and how to select them, to regulate the flow of students or visitors to suit its own needs and capacities, and to choose its own staff. Its main obligations to outside individuals and bodies may be to keep them informed of its activities and to continue providing the service for which it was established.

Service obligations inevitably restrict a therapeutic community's autonomy in deciding what its goals and functions should be, but they also provide its reason for existing. It is, for example, difficult to speak of a therapeutic community without mentioning the function it has within a society. We speak of a hospital, day centre, probation hostel, or adolescent unit – run *as* a therapeutic community, or of a therapeutic community for such and such a group of people. From the point of view of many of the individuals and organizations that have dealings with the therapeutic community, it is this that matters – the service it provides – rather than how it does it. That is an internal matter, determined by the staff.

Location

The other constraint arising from the setting is its location in relation to neighbouring places of treatment or residence. In practice, two sorts of setting are common. One is where the setting is a surrounding institution, in which neighbours consist of other treatment or custodial areas. This may make for less constraint in one way, since unusual events cause less surprise. However, other aspects require conformity. Meals are brought round at a certain time. It may be difficult to alter this or arrange that the raw materials for cooking be sent instead. Cleaning is carried out by cleaning staff to a standard expected by the overall administration. Furniture, fittings and decorations must conform to the overall scheme of the institution. On a more personal level, conflicts may arise between the staff of the therapeutic community-run unit and other staff. Thus the hospital telephone receptionists may object to putting calls through for patients, or to patients' answering the telephone; the domestic staff supervisor may decide that cleaning staff are not to attend community or staff meetings as they are paid to clean, not talk; and doctors in nearby consulting rooms may complain that noisy meetings interfere with their interviews or psychotherapy.

Many of these constraints will be absent or much reduced in the other type of setting, where a community is physically insulated from its neighbours. Many therapeutic communities function in large houses in residential districts. Here, the initial difficulty may be that local residents fear damage, attack, embarrassment or bad influence, which can delay planning permission for multiple occupancy. This done, the constraints are likely to be those of normal neighbourly conduct and the local standards of property upkeep. The degree of constraint excercised by the setting may well vary inversely with that imposed by the staff. In other words, where the staff relax conventional rules, impingement on neighbours may provoke reassertion of the lapsed rules. Senior staff, in particular, may find themselves mediators between the values of the immediate social environment and those of the therapeutic community.

On a more personal level, issues arising from the setting are ones concerning the nature of the boundary between the therapeutic community and its neighbours or parent organization. The more solid and impermeable the boundary, the less constrained will the inner community be. We may call this good insulation. To some extent, we may consider solid boundaries as desirable, since therapeutic communities are not likely to be 'good' neighbours by conventional standards. On the other hand, too solid boundaries may bring certain dangers (see Chapter 26), since there is a risk of bizarre social forms developing where values are determined solely within the group or perhaps by one leader.

Since we know that boundaries which are too easily and frequently crossed make it difficult to maintain continuing therapeutic culture, there is probably an optimum degree of permeability that might be imagined which brings about the most enlivening and creative mixture of fresh perspectives with established ones. To approach this mixture a therapeutic community should have adequate, though not necessarily total control over its boundaries.

Constraints arising from the staff

It is the staff of a therapeutic community who create it, shape it and maintain its culture. Staff attributes are probably the most important in determining the limits of development. The ways in which these attributes exert an influence can loosely be gathered under four headings: the numbers and permanence of the staff, their attitudes to treatment, the skills available between them, and the characteristics of the leader.

Numbers and permanence

While these two factors may sometimes be determined by forces outside the control of the community, I have included them here since they relate closely to other staff attributes. A larger staff group is likely to produce both a wider range of attitudes to treatment and greater possibilities for the formation of splits and sub-groups or cliques. The larger the staff, therefore, the more time, effort and skill will be needed if the resulting tensions are to be explored and resolved. In all likelihood the process will always remain far from complete. The difficulty may be increased where a large staff group contains relatively fewer members with the relevant skills and experience for this task, when compared with a smaller but more highly trained staff group. Another aspect of the size difference is the different nature of the interactions and group processes which occur in small and large groups. Where it is expected that the staff will try to deal with their interpersonal tensions through the medium of all meeting together, this will be more feasible in a group of, for example, eight than in a group of two or three times this number.

A simple but far-reaching constraint on the availability of relevant skills and on the therapeutic culture is the degree of permanence of the staff. At one extreme, well known through the work of Erving Goffman and others, is the situation where everyone — staff and patients — is so permanent that the routine follows a well-worn track. Even within a therapeutic community, long-established staff members may inhibit or discourage new staff from searching for solutions to current problems, often by indicating that any new idea has already been tried out once before, with the implication that the would-be innovator is wasting his time.

At the other extreme is the situation where a majority of the staff stay only a few weeks or months. Two sorts of problem can arise from this. One is a pervasive atmosphere of uncertainty, each person watching the other for cues and sometimes following inappropriate leads. (An example occurred where student nurses on a placement felt that the key skill which they had to acquire in group therapy was to be able to ask each patient questions about his particular problem. They saw other staff, themselves casting about for appropriate roles to play, making use of this technique and took it to be the criterion of therapeutic skill.) The other problem is the continutation of procedures handed on by earlier generations of staff without understanding the reason for them, so that they assume the quality of rituals. All aspects of therapeutic community practice are vulnerable to this danger, which can occur when too many staff feel too insecure to question or alter the way things are done. This effect resembles the problem of very long-term staff. Either extreme can inhibit the freedom to experiment. While it is difficult to suggest an optimum duration for full-time staff membership in a therapeutic community, it may be between one and four years. This span would have most relevance to key figures, since it is their combination of stability and openness to new ideas that will enable optimum use to be made of the community's total resources.

Attitudes to treatment

In any treatment situation one is likely to meet a range of attitudes, philosophies or ideologies about treatment. The growth of a therapeutic community culture will be limited where there is a wide divergence of attitudes which may exist where the community is not in control of who comes on to the staff. Those attitudes which characterize staff in different types of treatment settings have been studied by Tom Caine and David Smail, and described in their book *The Treatment of Mental Illness* (1969). They found such attitudes as radicalism, divergent thinking and a preference for staff-patient closeness to be characteristic of therapeutic community staff.

In addition to these, I should like to draw attention to what appears to be a significant basic attitude: the willingness on the part of individual staff to discuss openly, within the staff group at least, the doubts, conflicts and tensions that arise in relation to patients and other staff. This willingness to self-disclose relates to two other general attitudes, concerning professionalism and uncertainty. Where professional conduct is viewed as the antithesis of being oneself, and uncertainty or indecisiveness as unnecessary weakness, then self-disclosure will be minimal. In fostering an atmosphere of openness between staff, the model set by senior staff will be crucial. Junior staff are usually willing to be open if they see that this is sanctioned by those with more experience, but they are also likely to be influenced by those who elevate the importance of privacy and confidentiality above other therapeutic values.

Relevant skills available

Opinions seem to vary widely about the skills appropriate in a therapeutic community. At one end of the spectrum any kind of professional training is eschewed, and members of the community are seen as being sufficiently able to help one another by virtue of their experience as human beings. At the other end is the community where many staff are highly trained in psychoanalysis or some other psychotherapeutic framework. It seems true to say that one of the things which differentiates a 'therapeutic' community from any other community of people living together is that certain members are designated as therapists, or some equivalent. Such members, usually the staff, are on one level involved as members of the community. On another level they try to distance themselves from this involvement sufficiently to be able to explore and influence what is going on for therapeutic ends. The combination of involvement and standing back, an undeniably difficult task, is common to all forms of psychotherapy, and to this extent any training in psychotherapy, whether individual or group, has a relevance to work in a therapeutic community. It is probably necessary that at least two or three staff members possess this skill in some degree.

In addition to skills useful in psychotherapy generally, one skill or aptitude has a special relevance to the therapeutic community: the capacity to pay attention to and integrate a much wider range of 'systems' than we are ordinarily accustomed to dealing with. We can appreciate that a person has a brain, feelings and values, and that problems can arise within each of these systems or levels. We find it much more difficult to see how a problem in one system may affect the others. Our education and experience, as well as our limited capacities, lead us to attend to each separately. As therapists or change agents of some kind we tend to specialize in one system, with perhaps a rudimentary understanding of how it relates to, affects and is affected by neighbouring systems. In most forms of therapy, this range suffices. In a therapeutic community, we set ourselves the task of trying to work simultaneously with a far wider range and understand how they interact with one another; at a rough estimate, one could describe a continuum of seven systems:

1 An individual's biochemical and metabolic functioning.

2 An individual's subjective inner world, his thoughts, feelings and fantasies.

3 An individual as a whole, his personality, behaviour and relationships.

4 A small group of closely connected individuals, resembling a family; e.g. therapy group, staff team.

5 The total staff group and the total patient group.

6 The therapeutic community as a whole.

7 The social and geographical setting; e.g. hospital, neighbourhood.

There are possibilities for extending this at either end, or collapsing adjoining systems. The purpose of the list is to illustrate that, whereas an individual therapist would focus on level 2 or 3 with some awareness of the next level up and down, the group therapist would focus on level 4 and the organization consultant (if there were one) on level 5 or 6, the task set in the therapeutic community is to encompass at least levels 2 to 6. This connects with the reference made earlier in this chapter to the problems posed by the attempt to combine physical treatment with a therapeutic community approach. The problem is not that a person's biochemistry is more or less important than his relationships, or that the total community is less or more important than either of these. The difficulty lies in the limited span of systems to which we can comfortably attend. If we focus on one or other of the extreme ends of the above list it is probable that we will only be able to visualize or take into account systems as far away as the mid-point of the list. Systems beyond this will seem at best only distantly relevant. It follows from this that to focus centrally on the community as a whole may produce similar difficulties — in this case what may be lost sight of is the individual.

Two limitations to the development of a therapeutic community seem to arise from these considerations. One is the maximum range of systems which the staff are able to encompass. If the range is too narrow what may in practice develop is an individual or group psychotherapy centre. The other is where the focus is too far up or down from the middle of the range of systems operating. I have designated the middle system as the small groups within the community, but clearly, a different list might produce a different mid-point.

Characteristics of the leader

Much has been written about the nature and importance of leadership in a therapeutic community. In particular, the need for 'charismatic' leadership has been discussed, and a paradox has been acknowledged that, when a treatment setting becomes more democratic, the role of the leader appears to become more, not less, significant. A reason for this is not hard to find. To the extent that hierarchies, rules and regimentation protect staff from feelings of doubt and anxiety, the removal or relaxation of these devices may be manageable only where there is someone to absorb or contain these feelings when they threaten to become overwhelming. This task, which usually falls to the recognized leader, may be accomplished in different ways: by taking some decisive, reassuring action, or by adopting a calm, matter-of-fact approach. The necessary element seems to be that the leader should appear to be in control of himself and the situation, thereby inspiring some confidence in others that they too can be in control. This ability in a leader probably is a component of 'charisma'. Where a leader cannot or does not provide this for the staff it is likely that, at times of stress, restrictive or bureaucratic solutions will be sought which, once introduced, may be difficult to give up because of their success in reducing anxiety.

Another distinctive role allocated to the leader is the requirement to be two very different kinds of leader, one inside the therapeutic community and one outside. As its representative, meeting representatives from other treatment units, disciplines and groups, he must be able to fight for scarce resources, defend 'his' community against criticism or attack, appear certain of his case even when he has doubts, and not shirk from using his status to bolster his point of view when necessary. Yet, as the leader inside the therapeutic community, he must be able to share and delegate his authority, encourage autonomy among the staff and patients, accept as learning situations problems that arise through errors of judgment, and generally resist the temptation to use his status to quash disagreement. This dual, almost paradoxical role is, to some extent, shared by all leaders in democratically-run institutions, and also has parallels with the role of the father in relation to his family. Yet, therapeutic communities seem to present the task in its most demanding form. Few would come into being without an aggressive, pioneering, even defiant, stand by one or more staff leaders, yet few forms of therapy demand more tolerance, sensitivity and self-awareness on the part of that leadership.

Constraints created by the patients

The therapeutic community was developed to give patients a more active and significant role in their own treatment and that of their fellow patients, yet, compared with the effects of the setting and the staff, their influence on the way a therapeutic community runs is a relatively passive one. Willingness to co-operate, to participate, to accept the staff's philosophy, these are the ways in which patients exert influence, and even this willingness may depend partly on the skill of the staff in kindling a working alliance. Beyond this, patients who seek to create their own therapeutic community have, in effect, ceased to be patients, as happened in the cases of Synanon in the USA, and Kingsley Hall in London.

A patient's willingness or capacity to participate in a therapeutic community has usually been equated with his suitability for this type of treatment rehabilitation, and suitability has usually been considered in terms of particular categories of illness or problem. In one sense, this begs the question since, wherever there is a 'community' of staff and patients, there is a potential for making this community a therapeutic one. Nevertheless, the concept of the therapeutic community can be seen to have flourished most in the treatment of particular types of disorder, and such outcome research as has been done suggests that it has advantages over more conventional institutions for neurotics, behaviour disorders, and some psychopaths and drug addicts. (Some of the problems of evaluative research are dealt with in Chapter 29.)

The question which seems relevant to our present discussion is, what is it about patients who have been found suitable for therapeutic communities that differentiates them from others? Any answer to this probably needs to take into account four factors: the type of illness, disorder or social problem which the patient presents; his personality make-up; his motivation to change; and how he fits into the particular therapeutic community as it is at that time. The importance of these factors from a therapeutic community's point of view will be the way they facilitate, or hinder, those attributes which make a patient more or less suitable. I would like to suggest three such attributes.

The first of these is a capacity to experience a sense of group membership, to take an interest in other people's problems and allow them to take an interest in one's own, to share the values of the group or community in which one lives. Individuals who cannot do this, who are either extremely egocentric or are cut off from others by virtue of delusions, dementia or severe disability, will contribute little to or derive little from a therapeutic community. A second, related, aspect is the individual's responsiveness to social reinforcement, to the attention or rejection, the concern or anger of other patients and the staff. An individual who is either unconcerned about others' feelings and attitudes towards him, or whose response to these is undifferentiated (e.g., where all forms of attention are interpreted in the same way) may not be very suited to a form of treatment based on social learning. In practice, few individuals may be deemed totally unresponsive to social rewards and punishments, and difficulty is more likely to attach to misunderstandings about the kinds of social interaction that are pleasurable or painful. A third aspect is the patient's willingness, at some stage if not initially, to accept that it is he who is responsible for his behaviour. Refusal to give

191

up the idea that his behaviour is determined by illness, circumstances, or by the way others have treated him — to give up the role of patient, prisoner or victim — is a basic obstacle which the therapeutic community has to face.

These three attributes, seeing oneself as a member of a group, responsiveness to social reinforcement, and willingness to take responsibility for one's behaviour, can act as constraints in two ways. At the individual level they will play a large part in determining how much benefit a patient is able to derive from being in a therapeutic community. For that community as a whole, a significant constraint on its development of a therapeutic culture will be the degree to which these attributes are present in the majority of patients.

Conclusion

Every therapeutic community operates within a set of constraints, some of which I have attempted to delineate here. Often these constraints may appear to be quite severe to those working in therapeutic communities. The vision of an ideal therapeutic community may at times sustain us in the face of such limitations, yet it may also blind us to some innovative solution to a problem, and discourage us from sharing problems with co-workers in other therapeutic communities to whom, quite unnecessarily, we feel inferior, suspecting them to be nearer the pure vision than we are.

In a therapeutic community, few pieces of the puzzle are new. The patients and residents are not different from those in other institutions. The organizations which provide funds and resources, and require services in return, are usually those of the conventional establishment. And the staff are, for the most part, the same kind of people who work in other settings, perhaps with a little more sophistication in group work and larger 'systems'. What is different is the way the pieces are put together. A therapeutic community is a way of tackling the puzzle of individual disturbance and human relations that seeks a more creative and affective solution than before, principally by attempting to harness natural human responses and social forces, rather than ignoring them or discounting them as 'non-specific treatment factors'. It is perhaps basically a matter of perception: of seeing more of the pieces, seeing them in relation to one another, and imagining different ways of putting them together.

Acknowledgments

I should like to thank the following people for their helpful answers and comments, expressed either personally or in their writings: Raymond Blake, Ruth Bradley, Anna Christian, Herbert Hahn, Josephine Lomax-Simpson, Nick Mahony, Jeff Roberts, Neil Small, Steve Wilson.

Section E
Staff support and training

The staff are also people. They have their personal needs within the work situation, including their need to develop.

Isabel Menzies points out the need to clarify what the work task is. In an iconoclastic institution such as the therapeutic community, muddles are inevitably endemic. However, there may be special reasons, where staff are in contact with human suffering, for the work task to be perverted into a kind of anti-task. This may produce long-term harm in terms of confusion, declining job satisfaction and loss of morale. It is an essential role for management to ensure that the staff face a realistic job that is within their capabilities, that the social structure is a suitable 'fit' with the social technology needed to pursue the primary task (Perrow, 1965).

Feelings of failure in the task are described by Hinshelwood, who notes that they can be passed around between staff and clients in an exchange system which can be mapped out. Such an exchange system of emotions is contrasted with the exchange system for knowledge and experience which is the more appropriate currency for both therapeutic community work and for supervision. He suggests that a non-elitist movement can avoid a centralization of expertise by forming a network of supervision exchanges like the exchange systems of some primitive decentralized societies which serve to integrate the whole grouping.

Hawkins argues that therapy for the clients of a therapeutic community is a self-learning process, a form of education. There is, therefore, a common principle which runs through the therapy and training aspects of a therapeutic community. This is especially so as staff have to use themselves as part of the technology to be applied and hence training requires the experience of self-learning for staff as well as clients.

All these contributions point to the human element in the resources of the staff. That element can be maximized or it can be neglected. This may be the major factor in the degree of efficiency displayed by an institution working with 'human material'.

19
Staff support systems: task and anti-task in adolescent institutions

Isabel Menzies

Introduction

Most of us as we achieve some seniority in our professions have to assume managerial responsibilities in institutions. This shift is not always easy since there are inconsistencies between the two roles, but it must be made effectively for many reasons, not least being the contribution of good management to staff support. Rice (1963) has said that the effective performance of a primary task is a major source of satisfaction and that in so far as behaviour is adult and reality-based people are loath to surrender such satisfaction.

The responsibility of management for effective task performance is a contribution to staff support, both through positive job-satisfaction and through protecting staff from the anxiety, guilt and depression that arise from inadequate task performance. My concern is not so much with positive activities of management as with the difficulties that beset good management, particularly in institutions that care for people.

Primary task

The primary task can in theory be defined simply as the task which the enterprise must perform in order to survive. But from the point of view of efficient institutional performance it must also be clearly defined in practice. Quite simply, unless the members of the institution know what it is they are supposed to be doing, there is little hope of their doing it effectively and getting adequate psycho-social satisfactions in doing so. Lack of such definition is likely to lead to personal confusion in members of the institution, to interpersonal and inter-group conflict and to other undesirable institutional phenomena which I will return to later, all of which reduce the satisfactions of membership.

In some institutions task definition is quite simple; e.g., in commercial

197

institutions it is to make profit, since without making profit they will not survive, although the precise methods adopted to make profit may be more open to debate and subject to change in changing circumstances.

Many professional workers, however, have to function in institutions where they do not have the luxury of such an easily definable primary task and where attempts to achieve adequate definition are often countered by pressures from outside the institution. Clearly such factors also make effective task performance and related task satisfactions harder to achieve. Such institutions may be referred to collectively as the humane institutions. They have also been described as 'people-changing institutions' (Street *et al.*, 1966). They have a number of problems which we can now consider.

Multiple tasks

Frequently there is no single task which has overall primacy, but any one of two or more may take priority at a given time in given circumstances. A very good example of this is a teaching hospital, which has many tasks. The care of patients may feel like the primary task but, in fact, it has to yield primacy on occasion to the training of medical students. Large formal ward rounds may be good for students but are rarely regarded as good for patients. Further, since teaching hospitals are also nurse training schools there may be conflict between patient care and the needs of nurse training, and conflict between medical and nurse training needs. Mediating the variable primacy of tasks in such institutions is no easy responsibility and calls for frequent decisions about moment-to-moment primacy at all levels in the organization often without adequately defined managerial policy. It also makes it more difficult to sustain adequately the feeling that the total organization is effective and to provide adequate support through job satisfaction for its members, since the level of performance of each task tends to be reduced by the legitimate demands of the others.

Confusion in task definition

The human institutions, dealing as they do with human beings as their throughput, are also unusually subject to influence from the wider community in terms of task definition. This can also lead to confusion and doubt. Various penal institutions provide a good example of such confusion. Public pressure orientates them in at least three relatively incompatible directions: punitive, custodial and therapeutic. The incompatible objectives are often reflected internally in the attitudes and personal objectives of both staff and clients. They result in inadequate task definition, sometimes explicit and always implicit. At present institutions, both for criminals and delinquents and for psychiatric patients, are tending explicitly to adopt definitions orientated to the therapeutic and rehabilitative, but this by no means prevents the implicit infiltration of custodial and punitive objectives. The overt and covert conflict between the task definitions makes effective performance of the explicitly stated tasks difficult and often leads to staff feeling unsupported in their roles, to low job satisfaction and to high stress. Such institutions show up badly in institutional morale indicators such as staff turnover, student wastage, sickness and absenteeism, not to mention system-provoked bad behaviour by clients.

Inadequate resources for task

Professional workers are often ambitious in what they would like to do for their clients and so tend to define the tasks of institutions in fairly ambitious terms. Unlike the profit-making institutions, which just go bankrupt and die if they set objectives beyond their means, humane institutions can often survive in this state, even if not functioning well. Adequate therapy for the total population of clients jointly served is an over-ambitious objective in terms of the total resources the community can devote to such clients. However, in the separate institutions staff tend to pursue such objectives as ends in themselves. They do not relate the defined task or objective to possible means, or may not be in a good position to do so. The result is chronic overwork, chronic disappointment in results, painful and fruitless struggles with resource-dispensing authorities, low satisfaction and high stress. Yet the alternative, a more realistic definition of task in relation to likely resources with less beneficial results with clients, is also painful, or even intolerable. It is possible that confrontation would lead ultimately to a greater sense of support and job satisfaction through performing a less ambitious task more effectively.

Society as a whole throws this problem back on the humane institutions. It fails to define objectives realistically in relation to means or to face the problem of allocating resources differentially to different needs. The dominant societal attitude is that everyone should have what help they need or even want, an attitude reflecting Aneurin Bevan's basic orientation to the National Health Service (Ministry of Health, 1944): every patient has the basic right to all the treatment he needs. One can sympathize with the objective, but if one is realistic one must admit it cannot be achieved because resources will not allow it. The failure of society at large to face this problem confronts the humane institutions with the need to do it for themselves; and in so doing often having to meet the disapproval and excessive demands of society.

Scarcity of resources may make desirable the devotion of more resources to the best 'bets' and only limited objectives such as good custodial care for the others. Such discrimination is hard to face in the institutions concerned without society's support. The result is more ambitious objectives everywhere and the chronic inadequacy of resources to achieve them, unless management is very tough.

Difficulty in precise definition

For the humane institution it is indeed difficult to define its task precisely and in other than the most general terms. Take, for example, the therapeutic communities. Their objective is therapy. What exactly does that mean? How clear is the typical therapeutic community about the precise change it hopes to achieve in its client population? The problem is clearly stated by Street and others (1966), where all the institutions described are orientated to producing more effective members of society but what they mean by that differs considerably.

Or take schools. The objective can be described as education, but what does that mean? Every pupil, parent and teacher is likely to have his own personal definition of this objective, often not easily subject to verbal formulation. Even on the more academic side, the struggle with curricular reform suggests a possible multiplicity of objectives. How much more difficult to define the wider task of schools in educating pupils for life in general or even in a particular society. How precisely is the educational system or even a particular school to define that task? The solution of this particular problem is not aided by the fact that society in general is confused. Moral and value systems, life objectives and career prospects are all in a state of flux. Developments in schools seem to reflect uncertainties in the situation. Education for effective community participation seems now to be hived off in schools under the concept of pastoral care, care for the human needs of all pupils or special care for disturbed pupils. To me this represents an opting out by the school system from an important aspect of its primary task because of the difficulty of relating education to a confused society and also because that society itself is perhaps over-dominated by an unrealistic caring philosphy regardless of resources. It would be a terrible criticism of an educational system to say it is educating its pupils for dependency.

Redefinition of task into anti-task

There is, thus, a danger of primary task being implicitly redefined when the task as originally and perhaps more realistically defined becomes too difficult, or when societal pressures against realistic task definition are too great. In other words, task may implicitly slip over into anti-task; e.g., the educational system not being realistically orientated to maturation and preparedness for life in society but to providing for dependency needs which may be anti-maturational. In an institution for deprived boys to which the author was consultant, real educational difficulties and the related difficulties for staff in achieving educational progress had encouraged an implicit redefinition of the educational task in terms of therapy. The real therapeutic effect of being able to read, write and to do simple arithmetic and of making a contribution to life in the community was in danger of being ignored.

Such difficulties do not relieve managers from the responsibility of achieving adequate task definition. They only demand more toughness. It remains crucial that staff should know what they are expected to achieve and should have adequate management support in doing so, which may also imply support in not doing things which may be desirable in themselves but are realistically impossible or too expensive.

Socio-technical systems

The performance of the primary task of an enterprise requires an appropriate organization. Such an organization has two aspects: (1) the choice and application of an appropriate technology; and (2) the choice and application of an appropriate social system, what Trist and others (1963) have called a socio-technical system. The most appropriate socio-technical system is that which gives the best fit to primary task performance. The basic model is an open system where the organization imports material from the environment, converts the material into something different and re-exports it to the environment. In the case of humane institution the most significant import is, of course, the human import of clients who must be 'converted', i.e. changed, and sent back to the outside environment hopefully more able to sustain life there effectively.

Problems in establishing socio-technical systems, though not peculiar to humane institutions, are usually more intense there. For example, a system appropriate to custodial care is likely to be inappropriate to carrying out therapy and vice versa.

The technology

Further, the humane institutions often have to function in conditions where the available technologies are themselves hard to define and depend on the actual qualities and behaviour of the people who operate them. We are ourselves the instruments of technology. It is usually more difficult to define what a person does than a machine. Clear and realistic choice between technologies may, therefore, be difficult or impossible. For example, the precise effects of different therapeutic techniques are hard to establish by follow-up study, and one often has to function without clear guidance as to the success of different techniques or technologies. The choice of technology is, therefore, much subject to the personal idiosyncrasies of the people concerned, to their beliefs and hunches and their own models of human interaction.

There is the risk then that the choice and detailed application of technology may be inappropriately influenced by the human needs of the permanent members of the institutions and be less than appropriately related to effective primary task performance. One can be aware of this problem in theory but it is difficult to guard against its effects in practice.

The social system

Primary task performance requires a social system that relates technology to task and relates the people and groups who carry out different parts of the task to each other. Task and technology together do not wholly prescribe the nature of the social system although they put significant constraints on it and may rule out certain types of social system. The chosen social system is likely to reflect strongly the psychological and social satisfactions that members of an institution seek in their membership and work in the institution. These needs are of different kinds and are both positively task-orientated and potentially anti-task. In so far as they are task-orientated, they include the satisfactions arising from being able to deploy oneself positively and fully in relation to task, co-operating effectively with others and experiencing both personal and institutional success in task performance. People require such satisfactions and their realization is an essential aspect of staff support. Such co-operation by the members contributes towards a social system orientated to the effective use of technology in task performance.

Unfortunately for task performance, members of institutions are also likely to seek satisfaction of personal needs that are anti-task; very often they need to mitigate the stresses and strains of the task itself and of confrontation with the human material on which the task is focused. In other words, members try to establish a social system that also acts as a defence against anxiety, both personal anxiety and that evoked by institutional membership. Jaques (1955) has referred to 'a socially structured defence system'. This will appear in all aspects of the institution both formal and informal, in attitudes and interpersonal relations, in customs and conventions and also, very importantly, in the actual formal social structure of the organization and its management system.

The social system is a mixture of elements, some orientated to primary task performance and some to other implicit objectives, which we can summarize under the term 'primary anti-task'. Good management must obviously be orientated to sustaining task-orientated elements and discouraging anti-task; but management in the humane institutions is in more trouble than in the institutions that process things.

There are a number of reasons:

(1) The distinction between social system and technology is not clear. The social system is itself part of technology, and as part of the experience the institution provides for its clients it has a therapeutic or anti-therapeutic effect. It is important, therefore, that the social system provide a genuinely therapeutic model for clients orientated to helping them develop and cope more effectively with the world outside.

The management system is a significant part of the model, as I realized when working as management consultant to an approved school. A main preoccupation there was the need to develop better ego-functioning in boys with primitive, unintegrated egos and, among other things, to provide effective models for identification. We tended to see both the management system in itself and the functioning of individual managers within it as such ego-models, with therapeutic or anti-therapeutic potential; and much work has been done in trying to realize the former. For example, we have worked at clarifying the boundaries of sub-systems and the authority within and across their boundaries, and ensuring that managers were really responsible for the staff within their own sub-systems and did not have to operate with staff over whom someone in another system had authority. This is a confusing situation only too frequent in humane institutions; e.g., the confusion between the medical and nursing hierarchies in hospitals and the exact location of authority between them. We also aimed at maximum delegation down the hierarchy to increase the opportunity for staff in direct confrontation with boys to act with management authority, a model of good management-cum-ego functioning.

(2) A danger may arise in the interlocking of the social and technological systems in humane institutions when the social system and particularly the managerial structure become excessively infiltrated by attitudes and behaviour derived from professional attitudes to therapy. The institution may become too permissive, too non-directive, and lacking firmness and boundary control. The staff may, in fact, both lack for themselves and fail to give to clients the firm, authoritative management which is a necessary feature of both staff support and client therapy. Very frequently, it seems, the explicit or implicit model for operating units is some version of the family, which may be inappropriate. It denies the reality that this is a work situation which needs management with clarification of roles, responsibilities and relationships. Further, the so-called family model often denies the reality of the family. A well-functioning ordinary family is likely to have a complicated and

effective management system even though it would not be described in those terms and is often not noticed because it is implicit and stable over long periods. In institutions the same effect can only be achieved by making explicit the managerial functions and relationships.

(3) The effects on staff of the human 'material' they work with are especially great in institutions whose clients are people in trouble. The clients are likely to evoke powerful and primitive feelings and fantasies in staff who suffer painful though not always acknowledged identifications with clients, intense reactions both positive and negative to them, pity for their plight, fear, possibly exaggerated, about their violence, or harsh, primitive, moral reactions to their delinquency. The acknowledgment and working through of such feelings is not easy although it is in itself an important part of staff support and primary task performance to do so. In so far as feelings cannot be worked with personally or institutionally, they are likely to be dealt with by the development of defences against them; and in so far as they relate to institutional phenomena they will tend, as I suggested above, to become institutionalized through collusive, implicit interaction between members. They come to be built into the structure, culture and mode of functioning of the institution and through that impair task performance.

The danger is that, since the anxieties defended against are primitive and violent, defences will also be primitive. The author has described this elsewhere in a study of the defensive system in the nursing service of a general teaching hospital (Menzies, 1970). Such social defences are inevitably anti-task. They relate the institution to its members, clients and task, in a way which is not fully realistic. They may deny the full implications of the client's problems, often preventing the full deployment of staff's capacities. Anti-therapeutic systems of interpersonal relationships between staff and between staff and clients are built up. They are also resistant to the change and development in institutional functioning, which is essential in a changing society to ensure effective task performance.

Such problems are illustrated in an organizational model which is only too common in humane institutions, and which the approved school where the author worked struggled to change. It is common for resources directly used by or on behalf of clients to be controlled centrally and dispensed in kind by someone like the matron. Several things tend to follow. Such resources are often rather scanty in relation to need and this is likely to lead to complaints against the person-in-role who dispenses them, who may well become notorious for her meanness and lack of understanding of need. Staff more directly involved with clients may well go into collusion with them in developing a paranoid system defensive against the pain and difficulty of confronting the problem of scarce resources with clients, and opt out of their own responsibility for the situation. Such a situation is anti-therapeutic in that it stabilizes a paranoid defence system in clients who are prone to that anyway, and militates against the opportunity to develop more ego-based confrontation with the reality of scarce resources, surely a problem in real life in the community at large. The author was invited by the matron to help her in dealing with a situation she was coming to find intolerable: the image projected on to her or more correctly her role. Effective dispensing of food resources was very difficult and she felt she was not carrying out her task effectively. What we gradually evolved was that the control of food resources was delegated downwards and across sub-system boundaries into the residential units, who were given the money for food to be dispensed as they saw fit. The matron no longer controlled the resources but took up an advisory and service function to the housemothers. The central store became a shop which housemothers could use or not as they saw fit and which had to compete with other shops. The central kitchen provided ready cooked food at the housemother's request and for which she paid. Very interesting and, hopefully, positive developments resulted. The paranoid defence system was greatly weakened. Housemothers were now in a position to confront scarcity with boys. Their previously under-used capacities were more fully deployed, their authority and professionalism increased. Staff satisfaction increased from doing a realistic job well with subsequent increase in staff support. And, incidentally, food was no longer seen as being in such short supply.

Defence systems are in the end likely to be anti-supportive to staff. This is not only because they reduce the level of staff performance and the satisfaction from it, but also because they tend to the personal diminution of staff. Comments about such personal diminution were common among the nurses in the teaching hospital; they were grieved by it and felt unsupported in their efforts to discharge their responsibilities efficiently.

(4) Clients may intervene in the development and maintenance of the socio-technical system in a way that is powerful and anti-task and provokes related powerful, anti-task, reactions from staff. One formulation of this is the concept of the anti-task sub-culture. It can develop quickly and powerfully and can also be sustained over long periods, if staff do not intervene in a task-orientated way. Too often, indeed, staff collude with it because of the difficulties of confrontation or because they get satisfaction from it themselves. They do this minimally by denying the existence of the sub-culture or, if aware of it, by trying to keep it as a separate encapsulated entity. At worst they may be drawn into it; for example, meeting violence or threats of violence by harsh punishment, or themselves being drawn into homosexual acting-out.

More subtly they can react by establishing or trying to establish another sub-culture to counter the first, which is, however, equally anti-task. Rice (1963), following Bion (1961), has described this feature of group and institutional life. Interesting developments took place in the approved school when it had had an unusually large intake of boys reputed to be potentially violent and where there had also been several unusually severe outbreaks of violence. Staff felt threatened, not only by the boys' violence but also by the temptation to counter-violence they experienced in themselves. They were working at the problem in a task-orientated way but also subtly developing a sub-culture to counter violence, i.e. a move to provide unusually and probably unrealistically, for dependency needs: dependency to counter violence. This succeeded in concentrating the problems to an unrealistic extent in those staff whose job it was to meet real dependency needs in domestic provision, and who became distressed because they could not meet the unrealistic demands on them by other staff perhaps more than the demands made by boys, to provide for dependency. This was not, of course, contributing much to a solution which could only be found by staff and boys confronting the violence together. It was, of course, also anti-staff-support because it was defensive rather than task-orientated.

(5) The real task of humane institutions can in a sense be described as relating to dependency needs; for example, in adolescent institutions dealing with young people in trouble or meeting educational needs. Neither task can, of course, be effectively accomplished only by gratifying dependency needs, but the dependency needs are there and the institutions must relate to them somehow. These institutions have, therefore, as their work task a function that is close to an anti-task phenomenon. This puts them at risk. Their efforts to function on a realistic work level will be unduly infiltrated by phenomena that derive from anti-task group dynamics. The effectiveness of task performance will thereby be reduced, for example, by gratifying dependency needs rather than by struggling for maturity, towards independence and realistic functioning. Both staff and client are diminished by such situations and will feel unsupported in their performance of their common task with likely negative reactions. Elizabeth Richardson (1973) quotes a staff member at Nailsea School who thought the behaviour problems of upper school pupils might be related to the lack of appropriate courses rather than simply the problems of the pupils as people. This is an interesting comment which suggests that behaviour difficulties in any school may be linked with the relative failure to carry out the primary task of education effectively. If so, neither pastoral care nor school counselling for individual pupils are likely to improve matters much. Work orientated to better task performance might.

It seems, therefore, that the management of humane institutions has an unusually difficult task in ensuring the best fit between socio-technical systems and primary task. This calls for an unusual degree of management skill from people who do not easily see themselves as managers.

Conclusion

This chapter has stressed the importance of effective institutional management as a major factor in staff support. We have concentrated mainly on the particular aspect of management, that is its responsibility for effective task performance. Incidental mention only has been made of other aspects of good management that support staff, for example, clarification of roles, task and responsibility and the relationships involved in them, and the support arising from being given fully challenging tasks with the authority to carry them out.

In discussing the importance of primary task performance, attention has been mainly concentrated on the difficulties that hinder effectiveness rather than the positive means that achieve it. This choice was made deliberately since it appears that there is less understanding of interference to task than of positive activities in management, not the least because the negative features are indeed hard to cope with and we are tempted to deny them ourselves.

A very important characteristic of good management seems, therefore, to be a developed capacity to keep oneself and others out of the kinds of difficulties discussed: to struggle with task definition, to get it as precise and realistic as possible and to sustain the values that go with it, to protect the institution and its staff from undue pressures across the boundaries, to mitigate anti-task phenomena such as in the socially structured defence systems or sub-cultures, to effect such institutional changes as are desirable for task effectiveness, and to reconcile the needs of task and the psycho-social needs of the members of the institution, both staff and clients.

This may perhaps be seen to advocate a somewhat ruthless preoccupation with task. The management of an institution requires some measure of that ruthlessness but this concern for task need not and should not necessarily be linked with lack of concern for people. In the main, it is likely to prove the contrary. Much of the task-orientated activity, is, in fact, directly good for people. For example, striving for adaptive and mature defences rather than primitive and counteracting the development of destructive sub-cultures are rewarding for people. Above all, such task-orientated activities facilitate the support given to staff through belonging to an institution that functions well and gives both the rewards for work well done and the rewarding relationships that go with them.

207

20
Supervision as an exchange system

R. D. Hinshelwood

Introduction

Like wealth and military might, expertise seems to accumulate in the hands of a small section of society. What part then does expertise play in a non-elitist, decentralized ideology such as the therapeutic community movement?

During the last few decades, decentralizaton has been attracting increasing interest and perhaps we must recognize that we are relatively inexperienced in organizing for it. New approaches have to be borrowed or thought out from scratch.

The therapeutic community movement in this country has stood against traditional forms and, however muddled up till now, is trying to explore alternatives, What are the implications for setting up training in therapeutic communities? I should like to make two points on this: first, what it might be dangerous to do; and, second, what it might be worth exploring and trying to do. I shall then go on to describe in some detail the outline of a role that I have developed and filled in a psychiatric day centre, run by a local authority social services department.

Traditional elitism

The traditional model for training is to provide courses for people to learn about set topics. There is nothing wrong in itself with this system; in fact, it is the kind of model that automatically springs to mind, and can be effectively and efficiently organized and carried out. However, there are certain implications. It seems to me it does spring so easily to mind because we are accustomed to think in terms of those who know and those who don't know. (See in Chapter 24 Grunberg's description of a community split into two sub-groups, one which thinks and knows, and one which feels and suffers.) The running of courses, the granting of degrees and the qualifying for membership of learned societies rest on this traditional elitist split. It is undeniable that there are differences, sometimes very great ones, in knowledge and experience, but there are dangers in expressing this in permanent structural forms. Such a boundary of elitism can acquire quite disordered emotions between the two sub-groups formed; mystery and mystification can lead on to exclusiveness and passivity, smugness and envy, superiority and paranoia. These polarizations may be a cost worth paying in many professions and institutions, but they are inconsistent with the ethos and approach in therapeutic communities. There, the experience that needs to be acquired is the experience that the patient has of himself. That cannot be taught from a designated central elite. It is an internal exploration going on in all members of the community. There has to be contact and diffusion rather than confrontation between the experienced and the inexperienced — and this intention must be catered for structurally.

Decentralized alternatives

There are cultures in the world that work largely decentralized systems. It may then be possible for our culture to learn from them alternative methods for our own. In addition, some of the large mental hospitals have with some success managed to decentralize and establish administrative therapy or therapeutic community approaches.

What can be learned from social anthropology and from the experience in large mental hospitals is that it is not enough simply to disestablish central authority. That leads to fragmenting of the whole organization (Springman, 1976). Central authority has to be replaced by some other cohesive force or system, located in the periphery (see Lewis (1974) for an exposition of the role of trance states and magical figures in integrating diffuse decentralized societies).

The Kula in the Trobriand and neighbouring Pacific islands is a highly elaborated exchange system of two kinds of gifts (necklaces and bracelets). These items are exchanged ritually throughout the whole of a large culture necessarily decentralized because of island habitations. The items are never possessed personally, but travel constantly round and through the many sub-communities, thus uniting the whole and making the unity apparent by their constant return through the circuit.

It is also very common in decentralized primitive societies to have elaborate rules of marriage and kinship. In this instance, the exchange commodity which keeps different clans in firm relations with each other is the women themselves who are exchanged in marriage (Lewis, 1976).

In those mental hospitals that have developed best along therapeutic community lines an exchange system can also be seen in operation. The exchange commodity in this instance is verbal material, communication (Martin, 1962).

I deduce from this evidence that the feature of an effective and sur-
viving decentralized system is a tangible and commonly acknowledged
exchange system between the peripheral parts. How can this apply to
training, supervision and support systems in therapeutic communities?
The peripheral parts are the therapeutic communities themselves and
the individuals making them up. It follows that the kind of training
organization most in harmony with the aims of therapeutic communities
would be based on some exchange system between the working therapeutic communities.

The Training Group of the Association of Therapeutic Communities
has considered these kinds of exchange in some detail; for instance,
there could be exchange placements of staff between therapeutic communities for experiential learning purposes. Second, those who hold
training positions in their own communities might provide an objective
external supervisor role for other, neighbouring communities. Perhaps
this could be on a reciprocal basis, but a more generalized network of
exchanges would give more protection against the damage of elitist
splitting (see Lévi-Strauss (1949) comparing generalized with discon-
tinuous exchange systems).

I shall turn now to my experience as an external professional in
contact with the internal processes of a community as they appear in a
weekly staff meeting that I attend. This meeting represents an exchange
between the community and some outside expertise. I shall describe in
a systematic way the kinds of exchange that go on in this professional
format. I shall then present process material of an actual session to
demonstrate a much more profound area of often hidden exchanges of
feeling. It will be clear that a skilful supervisor can use the emotional
exchanges of anxiety to inform the professional exchanges of expertise.

The role of the external supervisor

What is the function of supervision? In my own work I visit a day centre
run as a therapeutic community proper, under the umbrella of a local
authority social services department. As the Consultant Psychiatrist I
attend one staff meeting a week to review the preceding week. The staff
group consists of the full-time leader and his part-time deputy, plus one
or two social work students on placements.

First, I will describe the functions which I have worked out with the
staff group over the course of two and a half years for the role of the
external supervisor. And then I shall move on to discuss some of the
processes of the meetings I attend as I see them from the position of
the external supervisor, whose field of view is clearer but narrowed.

There are three areas in which a supervisor can be involved: psychiatry, sociotherapy and psychotherapy. These are broad categories, but only the third has been important in the work I am describing. As a psychiatrist, I have to overcome a general social deference to the medical elite which is reflected in the staff in this community only as a gentle but determined rejection of the 'medical model'. In spite of this the community has to live with medication, which most of the members have had and are taking.

Staff seek advice on the nature and effects of this medication. I have supported wholeheartedly the no-medication aim towards which the centre works with varying degrees of success. Medication is a medium for exchange. Prescriptions are one reason (excuse) for members to go to see or renew contacts outside the centre, and they may do that for various reasons: rejection of the centre, hopelessness, or anxiety about their progress, etc. It is also one of the means by which staff keep discussion going with the referral network. Drugs represent an extraordinarily versatile exchange commodity providing incentive for communication between a variety of groups with each other, doctors with patients, staff with clients, clients with clients, staff with doctors, and so on.

Sociotherapy is the normal social exchange system and represents the community's concern for its own life, culture, structure and management. It is a significant part of the therapeutic regime, but this staff group has rarely sought opportunities to discuss these sorts of issue.

The cornerstone of this community is its psychotherapeutic attitude at all levels. In Chapter 18, Kennard describes a stack of seven levels that can be focused on. It is a central problem of therapeutic communities to decide at any given moment what level should be the prime focus. There is a great deal of work to be done on this and to attempt to elucidate critieria for changing level. There are four levels which have emerged as most relevant in the supervisions I am describing: individual psychopathology; group dynamics; inter-group relations; and community themes.

Individual psychopathology

In the review meeting the majority of the time will normally be spent discussing the individual cases. This takes the form of a presentation of a clinical situation involving that individual — really a description of his characteristic object-relationship as it comes to be expressed in or towards the community. This is discussed and modified in the context of the family and childhood background (usually as the individual interprets his own history). And that individual's perception of his position in the community is explored as a here-and-now infantile experience and as it distorts his reality of the actual community.

Over the course of months this kind of discussion will occur several times for some patients, and the degree of change in the individual (or the degree of error in our formulations) can be assessed. Incidentally, some such repeated formulations of this kind might be the basis for a research evaluation of the work (perhaps forming the basis of a Kelly grid).

Group dynamics

As no or very little individual psychotherapy takes place, discussion of the individuals is based on impressions and evidence from higher levels of focus, and the review meetings turn to the features of the small and large groups. The small groups are the most personal and intimate of what are termed the community events. It is possible in the review to analyse the process of the groups and to establish a dynamic theme. In practice, in this community there is relatively little attention paid to the dynamics of the group as a group and to 'group transferences'. This reflects the strongly person-orientated culture of the community on which its particular warmth and friendliness depend. With this atmosphere of intimacy the staff members running the small groups, often on their own, may feel in danger of being drawn too much into the emotional interactions. Consequently there is a reluctance to examine in detail the relations to the members of staff in whatever role they are put by the group members; this threatens to become too personal in the supervision. Instead, the supervisor is limited to encouragement and support of the group leader. These transference roles are easier kept for discussion in relation to the large group where the staff operate together and can support each other.

Inter-group relations

Inevitably in a multi-group system the various groups are affected by each other (Higgin and Bridger, 1965). The two small groups from time to time polarize away from each other; for instance, one may be seen as much stronger and appropriate for more difficult cases, while the other is felt to be weaker; or one seems to be the location of everything depressing and depressive while the other becomes lively and 'manic'. Such features are important and are discussed in the review meeting when they arise. They must lead to attention being paid to the division between the staff members who run the small groups.

Community themes

One of the main tasks of a therapeutic community which seeks to employ a psychotherapeutic method is to attempt to clarify community themes that are predominant at any one time. For example, towards the end of a summer holiday period when A was away the community appeared to behave as if he represented the strength of the community, and those who were left felt a degree of weakness or impotence. Such a fantasy has consequences, such as the tendency to shelve decisions and issues; and also a tendency to polarize individuals into those who are strong and those about to break down.

The review meeting is used by the staff to help to elucidate these themes. As an external supervisor 'coming in' I have the opportunity to explore and put together the various levels. It normally follows the order I have used here, and this seems to follow a kind of natural development of the discussion; details progressively broaden out to higher and higher levels of focus.

I have described in some detail here the kind of expertise which is the commodity exchanged in supervision sessions in which I am the 'expert'. Heath (1976) accepts that 'there will sometimes be social markets in which services such as advice will be purchased with approval and compliance (the latter being the equivalents of money in social markets)' (p.27).

Staff relations

It is important to emphasize that the discussions I have referred to are based on second-hand material. That is to say, the staff select, elaborate and work over their memories and reports of what has gone on. This is partly conscious preparation for the review meeting but it is also partly under less conscious influences that derive from relations between the staff and the dynamics of the review meeting itself.

Relations amongst the members of the staff team are the focus for another meeting in the programme of the centre (sensitivity group) which I do not attend. This feature of the work of the centre has not therefore been a prominent part of the function of the psychiatrist. The extent to which direct work with staff relations should be part of the role is probably very variable. Skynner (1974) suggests it may only be rarely, and then with particularly favourable staff groups.

However, staff relations are important. They can give rise to difficulties and they do come into the review meeting at times. Basic to psychotherapy is the phenomenon of transference. In a living-together community this can become intense. Transference relationships arise between any two sets of people in the community. With the members who often go through periods of very urgent and at times explosive transference relationships, the staff individually and as a team take the brunt of desperate demands for relief and reassurance. But it is expected of the staff that they will not engage in any acted-out or collusive relationships with members except on a level that both can regard as mature. This constraint on members of staff is severe in the intensity of the therapeutic community, especially for the young or the inexperienced. It is a function of the supervisor to assist the staff in observing this constraint.

It has seemed to me that the hardest of these transferences for the staff to cope with are those connected with despair as they are experienced in relation to the staff or the community. I believe this to be true of all therapeutic communities, and indeed true of all psychiatric and personal social services which have to deal with large numbers of demoralized and despairing people. Therapeutic communities manage on the whole to avoid falling into a slough of despond (typical of the large mental hospital) by creating a sense of Messianic evangelism in the cause of a radical new approach (see Hobson, Chapter 22). It is not altogether to the benefit of members to be seduced out of their despair into a mission of this kind, yet it is the case in almost all of the therapeutic communities that I know of. It seems to me it is the function of the supervisor to be aware of this 'collective defence' against demoralization, and to keep attempting the impossible task of confronting the often less than optimistic reality without demoralizing the staff or the community. In short, he must point out failures and limitations without destroying morale, which is so constantly under threat from many sources. In general, I have adopted the policy that these should not be openly explored in the review meeting; and that if the staff are expected to exercise special constraints they may also need some personal privacy. This is particularly relevant where both members of staff are in their own personal therapy.

For the supervisor to explore staff relations or the anxieties hidden within the staff group makes naturally for a rise of tension within the group. However much this may build a stronger staff team in the long run, it is not of course welcomed by them in the short term.

Supervision is inevitably a hard situation — for both supervisor and staff. It is important to recognize that staff relations will be influenced to some extent by the presence of the supervisor. In the review meeting I am part of the staff group. I have mentioned the possibility of being a demoralizing influence, given the conditions of the work — and this undoubtedly happens at times. I have quite often felt that my contributions to the review meetings have been welcomed as much because I give status as for the content of what I actually say. One of the frustrations is that I often feel in the dark about exactly how my contributions and supervision are put into practice (if they are). I do indeed get feedback the week after on occasions but, in general, I do not get an impression of one meeting following on from the previous week's. This is inevitable in this work; the life of any therapeutic community goes forward at great speed and, as for very young infants (which often the members are at heart), a week can be a lifetime. However, it seems there may be ambivalence to me as the supervisor, who does not have to suffer the confusions and struggles of actual clinical work as directly as the other staff; and although it may add status it is clear on occasions that having a psychiatrist also creates rivalry and fears of criticism.

An illustration

I shall now present material demonstrating the manifestation of anxiety in the community which emerges in the review meeting. The atmosphere of the review meeting illustrates the crisis in the community and the demands the staff are making on the supervisor, not just for his experience, but for direct relief from the immediate anxieties washing over them from the community members.

In one review meeting, a member, N, was coming towards his leaving date and recently was more and more of a problem for the staff as he became more tense and it seemed that they had to admit failure with him. He seemed intractable. Our discussions about him on previous occasions had helped little. He seemed at the centre of frustration of the whole community and this was taking on a more and more attacking quality.

At first we tried once again to get to grips with the nature of his anxiety, but this seemed unconvincing in this meeting. N was quoted as saying it was time to stop talking and start doing. I realized that we should not be talking about his anxiety but trying to understand what he was doing with it. I began to point out how he tried to make the staff anxious. This was a rather obvious remark which did not go down well, for it seemed to confirm the rather persecuting attack on N for his harmful effect on the community, which was suffering anxiety at his hands. I pursued the point for a while but felt increasingly that I was making empty statements. We were getting into a stalemate position. I was feeling frustrated and annoyed that my words of wisdom were not falling on more fertile soil; and the staff were getting irritated with me for advising them on what they already knew. Clearly, I was not being much use as a supervisor at this point.

What I realized then — rather belatedly — was that we were recreating a stalemate in this meeting that resembled the stalemate the staff had been reporting with N. In trying to put them on the right lines, as I thought, I was experiencing the same frustration as the staff were with N. I realized I was on the wrong tack. I tried to grasp this and indicate that he might experience their help in a way that they had not intended. In particular, their insistence that he should 'take responsibility for himself' and 'experience his own freedom' may have been felt by N as if the staff were washing their hands of him because they couldn't take any more.

At this point the staff admitted that they couldn't stand him and they referred to another member, O, a woman about whom they felt similarly. They told me a dream of hers: she looked out of her window at the square where she lives, which is surrounded by a wire fence. Inside the fence there was a white Volkswagen in which there were some black men whom she thought were criminals. As she looked, one of them got out of the car and came towards her; she thought he was going to mug her. It seemed that this represented a black criminal side to her that, although she whitened it, was not adequately kept in bounds and threatened to invade and damage her mature self.

It now seemed possible to move on to the community level, as more than one member was conveying the fantasy that it was impossible to contain within bounds certain black or bad parts of themselves. N's fear that the staff could no longer take any more of him correlated with O's dream.

I thought then that I could clarify what was being done with the anxiety. It seemed as though the staff were required to confine and contain these bad things and also to contain the anxiety about them. However, N seemed to be in despair that the staff would be able or willing to cope with what was required. His stubbornness seemed to derive from a nightmare desperation about where to turn. Two of the members of staff agreed, albeit with a personal sense of depression as they felt they had failed N. The earlier persecuting attitude towards him disappeared.

However, harmony was not restored — the third staff member now came in explosively. He forcefully pushed to the fore the hostility and sadism in these two members, who were humiliating the staff by controlling them and manipulating them with anxiety.

There were two ways of understanding this new occurrence. First, the staff had split and an exchange had taken place at the emotional level of the group. The two staff had swapped anger for compassion, while the third staff member had accumulated all the anger to bursting point. Second, what I had done was to challenge the accepted staff and community attitudes to these members, and by so doing I had taken ground from the authority of the third member who, as leader, gives support and sanction to these attitudes. I had, in effect, shown him up as having failed by giving a wrong lead — which he then tried to reassert.

Like a hot potato, the sense of failure had been handed round and round. Let us trace out its route. As the time limit came up for N the staff began to feel they had failed to achieve insight and change in this man. This was then attributed to his own failure. He became more and more distressed as he accumulated more and more of the staff's frustration with him. His explosions did not help as this only aggravated the staff's feeling of having failed with him — he was passing it back to them with considerable thrust. The staff next brought it to me where I at first tried to advise on the failure with this man. This accentuated the sense of failure in the staff. Instead of understanding that they felt a failure, I had increased it. They resisted this so that it was me, next, who felt the frustration of failing to make headway: finally it had passed on to me.

I had to clear my own way out from under this, but who could I send it to? It seemed clear that my job should be to stop the buck from passing on. It is not enough merely to advise, it is necessary also to handle the immediate emotional context of the staff-supervisor relationship so that advice is usable. I did not do too good a job: the staff split and the sense of failure ended up in overpowering proportions in the staff leader again.

Conclusions

I have presented some material from this actual review meeting with the aim of demonstrating the problems that arise. Every supervisor will have his own style of working, and this will manifest itself in different ways with each different supervision relationship. The session I have described is therefore in no way exemplary but contains difficulties and errors. I should like to pinpoint three related problems that occur in the exchanges.

Batting versus sharing

Substantial parts of the session have the appearance of a contest, in which frustration and disagreement were batted back and forth between the supervisor and the staff. It indicates a situation which both sides are finding hard to confront: a failure of the work and of the supervision. This is in contrast to a sharing of the same experience, where both sides can say, 'I know what it feels like'.

Advising and containing

The advice given by the supervisor is often unhelpful – not because it is always wrong. Even when right it can seem to be out of touch, or more often critical and persecutory. This is particularly a risk where the staff are reporting from a persecuting situation; they can easily begin to feel got at from both directions. In contrast is the supervisor's ability to contain. He can give the staff the feeling that his advice derives from empathy and experience, an I-know-how-you-feel attitude, and the impression that he is struggling along with the staff to contain the problem. It is one prime function of the supervisor to put into words something that the staff have not yet grasped. He may do this himself or he may help the staff to do it for themselves. But essentially it is a process of getting something from a feeling state into words, so that it can be worked on more fully. It is the process of getting it into words which is the containment of supervision.

Projections and symbols

Evidently words can accomplish two different effects. They can evoke a feeling in someone else and can be used with that intention. Alternatively they can be used as symbols to give a picture of a feeling or an emotive situation. And the intention then is to work on or elaborate the pictures conveyed in this way for some common purpose. In the former case it is for relief of some unpleasant emotional state, while in the latter it is to confront and learn from an experience made tolerable, however uncomfortable. In the reported material the supervisor had to try to change the verbal activity from one in which the sense of failure was being passed around, to one in which this could be talked about. The mode of coping with the sense of failure could then be understood.

It seems that this is an essential conversion process, from something intolerably unpleasant (from the members) into something unpleasant but now tolerable. The factors in this conversion process are sharing, past experience and verbal symbolization.

The emotional life of a community consists to a large extent of a wide-ranging exchange system for unpleasant emotions. In my view such a system usually contains special individuals who act as a kind of sump into which negativity and bad feelings tend to drain, and who become scapegoats or prophets of doom. At the other extreme are people, of whom the staff and especially the supervisor should be one, who can convert such exchanges into a symbolic mode. Using an analogy from economics, I am describing a society in which there is both bartering and a monetary system.

The example has dealt with the rather desperate search for a means of coping with failure. In my view emotions connected with failure have a very special significance, especially in a community which accepts people who have clearly failed in some conventional sense in their lives. The accumulation of these feelings in one section of the community relieves the rest who can 'escape' into a feeling of adequacy whenever necessary. Such a process creates a body of spuriously adequate experts who are in a position to establish an elite grouping. Such is the kind of division that can occur between staff and members of a therapeutic community: those who know are cast above those who don't know about 'personal problems' (see Grunberg, Chapter 24). It is also the kind of division that can steal between the staff and their supervisor. Such a process as it happens needs to be contained within verbal symbols and traced back to its origins in the difficulties and the feelings of inadequacy in the work itself.

21

Staff learning in therapeutic communities: the relationship of supervision to self-learning

Peter Hawkins

In therapeutic community conferences, discussion groups, working parties or training sessions, the same central dilemmas about training constantly reappear. 'What sort of training should therapeutic community workers have?' 'What professional background best equips a staff member for work in a therapeutic community?' 'Does a professional medical or social work background hinder or help a therapeutic community staff member?' 'Should there be or, indeed, can there be a centralized approved training for therapeutic community workers, a Royal College of Social Therapists?'

The answers that arise are always less exciting than the questions, such as: 'The only real training is to work in a good therapeutic community,' or 'Good training comes from a good supervisor.' These answers only pose more questions about what makes for a good therapeutic community and what is good supervision.

In this chapter, to avoid getting stuck with the usual dilemmas, I am going to change the context in which these questions are debated. I contend that the whole therapeutic community process, and not just the staff training, is essentially educational and involved with supervised self-learning, rather than a medical institution involved with cure, or a social work institution involved with problem-solving and taught rehabilitation. Given this thesis, before considering the particulars of staff training, it is necessary first to consider the nature of the learning processes within the communities and what factors enhance greater learning. Then it is time to look at how these factors can be incorporated into community structures; and then to discover staff training methods which are congruent with the total community learning.

Education comes from the latin 'e-duco', to draw out from, and as such is significantly different from teaching, which implies more of an input process. The use of education as a reference point avoids replacing the mystique of medicine with a new mystique of socio-therapy or psychotherapy, where the client can still hold on to the belief of something being 'done to him'. It also puts the responsibility firmly on to the client within the community, and the staff member within the staff group, to be the main active agent in their own learning and growth. Within this context of education it can be experienced by everyone that both staff and clients are engaged in a mutual process of discovery and learning, rather than there being a polarization between pre-trained experts and clients in need.

The significant education opportunities that most therapeutic communities can offer are: time out from normal social pressures, to be able to stand back and reflect on one's own intro- and interpersonal dynamics; the possibility to try out different roles and ways of relating, without failure having lasting consequences; the chance to be involved in planning, deciding, and executing change in your immediate social environment, whatever your personal standing or experience; the opportunity to interact with a large variety of people in different contexts and with fewer social constraints than is normal; a larger amount of both positive and negative personal feedback of how others experience you and of how you affect others; and an environment which is constantly challenging and questioning, rather than just accepting the *status quo*.

So far there has not been enough careful study of the inter-relatedness of the various areas of learning within a therapeutic community and development of suitable models and theories of the precise educational process. The literature is dominated by theories that concentrate on just one aspect of the learning process such as personal insight, or behavioural change. What is needed is a balanced unifying concept of the various personal learning processes and its particular application to therapeutic communities. The most useful model to date has been developed by people working in the existential, humanistic fields of psychology and sociology, and is most usefully developed by Charles Hampden-Turner (1971):

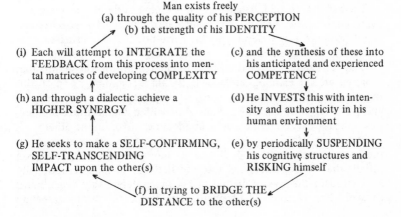

Man exists freely
(a) through the quality of his PERCEPTION
(b) the strength of his IDENTITY

(i) Each will attempt to INTEGRATE the FEEDBACK from this process into mental matrices of developing COMPLEXITY

(c) and the synthesis of these into his anticipated and experienced COMPETENCE

(h) and through a dialectic achieve a HIGHER SYNERGY

(d) He INVESTS this with intensity and authenticity in his human environment

(g) He seeks to make a SELF-CONFIRMING, SELF-TRANSCENDING IMPACT upon the other(s)

(e) by periodically SUSPENDING his cognitive structures and RISKING himself

(f) in trying to BRIDGE THE DISTANCE to the other(s)

Each of these eight stages, to which I shall be referring throughout this chapter, corresponds with a different area of necessary learning. Stage (a) calls for the confrontation of the individual's fantasies with reality, and stage (b) for intra-personal reflection and insight. Stages (c) and (d) require the opportunity for strength building, and taking charge of one's own life; taking on of potent roles and of leadership; and of challenging the individual to be more open, direct and authentic in his relationships to others. Stages (e) and (f) involve the challenging of false ego defences and the development of the ability to listen empathetically to others; to see oneself and the environment from another's perspective. In stages (g) and (h) it is necessary to have the opening to experience oneself as politically effective in bringing about change in the immediate environment, not by brute force but by effective interchange with others, the experience of being heard and valued but not necessarily agreed with. The last stage requires not only a high level of constant feedback within the community but a constant reflection by the whole community of all the processes it is involved in.

This model is not monadic but describes a growth process which is, by necessity, involved with the interface between an individual and significant others. Therefore a prerequisite is an investment in the community by the individual. If all these stages are active in an inter-personal relationship, then the learning that develops is for both, and is described by Hampden-Turner as proceeding in two interlocking spirals or 'a double helix'. However, if learning is over-emphasized in one of the eight stages at the expense of the others, then this leads to rigidity rather than growth and to unbalanced personality. Over-concentration on insight without equally developing the later stages of the cycle leads to introversion and self-obsession, while over-emphasizing behavioural change and demonstrated competence helps the individual to develop a mere social veneer.

The same type of inbalance in the learning cycle can also occur in whole communities such as those which are dominated by ego-surrender and regression without developing the corresponding other stages.

Having developed a clear understanding of such 'psycho-social learning' processes, the next stage is to elicit from this the factors that promote greater learning and growth within a community. To do this the theoretical understanding needs to be juxtaposed with the experience of living, working and training staff within therapeutic communities, so that each acts as a dialectical reflecting mirror on the other.

In a paper (Hawkins, 1977) delivered at an American conference on therapeutic communities, I illustrated how the two most common pitfalls that staff trainees fall into are that of becoming emotionally submerged in their work or that of becoming defensively over-clinical to avoid any personal involvement. The former is characterized by becoming over-identified with clients, being unable to set limits, and an inability to stand back and reflect on the processes that he is involved in. The latter is seen when staff trainees become unable to meet clients on a person-to-person basis, desperately hold on to a false persona of adequacy, and retreat into administration. In the paper I talked of how each trainee and indeed each community must be helped to steer a fine balance between the Scylla and Charybdis of emotional submergence and clinical detachment. In the terms of Hampden-Turner's model this is both to be able to invest by periodically suspending cognitive structures and risking oneself, and also to be able to integrate the feedback from being involved, into mental matrices of developing complexity and a greater quality of perception.

The primary task of a good supervisor must be to help a trainee to keep his balance between involvement and reflection, and to use the dialectic between cognitive understanding and emotional involvement to stimulate growth. Jourard (1968), during his experience of training therapists, has found that the most creative learning takes place at moments of impasse, when previously held beliefs of the trainee have been confounded by actual immediate experience. At this moment, Jourard suggests that the role of the supervisor is to avoid the temptation to explain away the impasse, but to challenge the trainee 'to grope' for a new awareness, or in Hampden-Turner's terms, use the dialectic to bring about 'a higher synergy'.

It is my experience that it is not possible to pre-chart a way of avoiding the pitfalls for a new trainee, and that learning is dependent on a staff member's having the room to make his own mistakes. However, supervision should balance this leeway by quickly pointing out, in a decisive manner, the process as the trainee gets enmeshed in it. This can be further enhanced by the supervisor's being able to respond from his own experience of learning, or from that of previous trainees. Once again, it is a principle of groping for the right balance in supervised self-learning, rather than taught prescriptions.

Along with the room to make one's own mistakes must go the space to discover one's own strengths and effective ways of working; the opportunity to develop stages (b), (c) and (d) of the learning model. This in its turn must be balanced by maximizing the feedback that the staff member gets from clients, colleagues and supervisor. The supervisor should constantly question the assumptions, theories and practice of the trainee:

In good training, after the fashion of Socrates, the skilled and compassionate dialectician will challenge every assertion and belief of his pupil until the pupil feels he is going out of his mind (Jourard, 1968).

By so doing the supervisor ensures that the learning in stages (b), (c) and (d) of the model is balanced by stages (e) to (i).

This balance, between confirmation of the trainee and constant questioning, is part of a larger balance which is necessary for learning: between acceptance and challenge and between security and disequilibrium. In his many research studies Carl Rogers (1961) has shown that validating acceptance by therapists, counsellors and teachers greatly enhances the learning of the client or pupil. However, unquestioning acceptance leads to complacency; therefore trust and security need to be balanced by a sense of disequilibrium and an atmosphere of constant challenge which leads the learner on in the process of discovery. The balance is once again all important:

> A real danger . . . is when we bring a person up to a point of discovery and, just as he is about to make the discovery, we tell him what it is. We deny him the discovery experience (Blumberg and Golembiewski, 1976).

From this foundation of principles which underlie learning and factors which promote growth, a methodology of training can be built. For the practice to be congruent with its theoretical principles, it cannot be a rigid fixed system, but one that develops and changes in response to experience and is flexible in changing to the needs of various conditions and different learners.

The first deduction that can be made from the above thesis is that whatever academic training or theoretical learning the trainee brings to a therapeutic community, the most important learning will take place while the trainee is involved in the experience of working and relating within the community. A case can be made for staff to learn a therapeutic discipline before starting at a community, so that they have a system to transcend and can learn from the interaction between their pre-taught discipline and their actual experience. Also it may be said that without pre-training the staff member is too susceptible to raw experience, with nothing to measure it by. It is my experience that a pre-training, in whatever professional field, does not necessarily provide a better starting point in staff learning than does varied life experience, from which the staff member has built his own value system and means of understanding human change and dynamics: each is equally prone to rigidity and defensiveness is liable to emotional submergence.

What is of crucial importance is some form of in-service training which provides spaces within the involvement, where the trainee can temporarily remove himself from the intense pressures of community life and stand back and reflect on what is happening. This in-service training can provide intellectual frameworks in which to make sense of community and personal experience, as well as perspectives which challenge the trainee to review his experience. It can also be a forum for seeing personal experience in the light of the experience of other trainees working in different communities.

The Richmond Fellowship, London, runs a two-year, one day a week, in-service training for all its new staff working in its twenty-seven communities, whatever their previous training, although certain qualifications allow staff to exempt themselves from certain sessions. In repeated years it has been found that students in evaluation sessions have stated that their most significant learning has come from the opportunity to compare different approaches to similar situations with staff from other communities. This sharing has led trainees to question approaches of their own community which they have previously taken for granted. The courses that have been judged less effective, by the students, have been where the trainers have failed to create a link between their subject matter, be it group work or sociology, and the personal and community experience of the trainees.

However good an in-service or pre-service training scheme is for therapeutic community workers, the main nexus of learning will be actually in the therapeutic community, where space for reflection upon experience must exist in the very heart of the community, and not just in weekly visits to a college. Every experience, be it a group, an individual encounter, or a work activity, should have its own reflective process built into it, thus increasing its learning capacity.

The best established process for reflection upon an immediate activity in therapeutic communities is the staff post-group which follows either the community meeting or a small group. In this forum the sharing of perceptions of what was happening in the group can stimulate each staff member to re-examine his way of perceiving other individuals or group processes. Also everyone can receive feedback on how his activity in the group was experienced by and affected others. The management of effective learning in a post-group is a difficult exercise, in order to prevent its slipping over into competitive interactions of criticism and defence, or into complacent, non-questioning mutual reassurance. To promote the greatest amount of learning, several processes have to be kept in balance. First, there must be the accurate recall of what actually happened, what was heard and noticed, and the separating out of actual perception from emotive or interpretive responses to it. Second, there is the sharing of the individual's subjective experience of the group, in which staff members should be confirmed in their experience rather than have their experience disqualified. Finally, there is the necessity to make cognitive sense of the processes of the group, and to synthesize both the objective perceptions and the subjective experience.

The Marlborough Hospital therapeutic community (Foster and Christian, 1977) recently decided that the whole community should have the opportunity to take part in the reflection process of the post-group on the daily community meeting. After the community meeting they had a short break for coffee and then returned to the group to review the previous meeting. This experiment highlighted some of the dilemmas inherent in the post-group process: that ideally reflection and experience should not be artificially separated but be constantly co-existing; and if you do separate them and have a group to reflect on the experience of the previous group, how do you prevent the reflection on the group from just being a continuance of the same process? (See Chapter 24.)

It is easier for a staff sub-group in the protection of their own office to reflect upon the life of the community; but are they not avoiding the greater opportunities for dialectical learning and feedback that the community affords, as the Marlborough experience suggests? How to take up the larger challenge without being submerged by the process?

In the early history of training groups run by Kurt Lewin in the United States, the whole learning process was revolutionized and intensified by the trainees' requesting to take part in the post-groups held by the trainers. The result was 'emotional, involving, almost explosive, but a fantastic learning experience for those (including the trainees) who took part' and through this 'the principle of feedback was discovered' (Rowan, 1976).

Another essential form of reflection is staff supervision, a place where every staff member can take stock of what is happening and have a recognized space to look at his own process. There will continue to be great debate, within and between communities, about how this should be organized, but what is most important is that the supervision system actually reflects the practice of the community. Therefore, in a community that combines individual counselling or therapy with group work, it is necessary to have both regular group and individual supervision. I have mentioned above how the role of supervisor differs from that of teacher, but it is also important that the supervisor is learning for himself, challenging himself to find new answers, and fully entering into the dialectical synergistic learning process.

In a senior staff training programme at St Charles House of the Richmond Fellowship we have introduced, alongside group and individual supervision by senior trainers, a system of rotating peer-group supervision which has helped to loosen further the learner-expert polarization within the community.

Also within this training programme we have introduced a multi-level feedback-assessment system, whereby the trainee will first write a self-assessment of his own learning and performance and will then share this, along with his feedback on the programme, to the whole staff group including fellow-trainees. This will be followed by his receiving feedback from all the other staff and trainers, which will be so structured as to ensure that both positive and negative feedback is given, Finally, his individual supervisor will write an assessment taking into account both the self-assessment and the group feedback, and this assessment will be shared with the trainee.

Both these systems have been developed in consultation with various groups of trainees, in order to maximize the psycho-social learning of all concerned. The same challenge exists in supervision and feedback structures as it does in post-groups: how to involve the whole community more actively within the whole process, and also how to make feedback a constant incorporated part of the community process as well as being concentrated in certain group and individual settings.

Also built into the learning of a therapeutic community must be opportunities to sharpen the quality of perception (stage (a)) through other forms of feedback, besides those that are verbal and interpersonal. To this end the use of taped or video-taped groups and individual sessions is invaluable, but where these facilities are not available, and in addition to them when they are, clarification of perception can take place by the use of role-played situations. In role-play the staff trainee has the opportunity to experience playing the roles of others (stages (e) and (f) and also witnessing others playing his role, as they see him playing it (stages (h), (i) and (a)).

These are just some of the methods of increasing psycho-social learning in staff training, but the most important aspect is that all methods used are constantly questioned, re-evaluated and re-created by everybody involved, so that they are constantly new, dynamic and alive to changing situations. Ideally a therapeutic community is 'a place of mirrors' for all involved, where the mirrors are not two-dimensional reflecting screens, but four-dimensional, ever-changing people with their own alive learning processes.

Thus, once the whole conceptual basis of a therapeutic community is placed in an educational context, it necessitates staff trainers who constantly study the learning processes of the community and who make sure that the learning-growth cycle of the community is both balanced and maximized. Further to this they have to develop the art not of teachers but of skilled dialecticians in order to enhance, supervise and learn in conjunction with, the self-learning of the staff trainees. The role is both complex and exciting, frustrating and challenging. There are many pitfalls, which are similar to those that Blumberg and Golembiewski (1976) describe for 'T' group leaders. They warn of the dangers of being too directive, providing too much information, being too clinical, becoming too personally involved, mistaking frustration and floundering for learning, and forgetting their power. There can be no final prescription about how best to learn or organize learning within therapeutic communities, only an open sharing of the learning that each individual has found effective in his own search and development. To this end, this chapter is not meant as an answer, but as part of an ongoing debate.

Section F
Clinical case studies

This section complements Section D on practice. Difficulties in practice can be learning situations and can be approached in two ways. They can be approached theoretically by referring to the ideal model to see what was done wrong; or the difficulty may be explored in the details of the actual situation where it happens. These five chapters take a detailed look at a variety of difficult problems.

Hobson complements the earlier Chapter 16 on leadership. He looks in depth at the emotional context that the leader of a therapeutic community has to live in. Such a leader is at the eye of a storm and has to ride huge waves of idealization followed by denigration. He describes how this leaves the leader as well as the community in an exhausted state, with the serious expectation that the venture may cease altogether.

Such a lethargic, apathetic disease of the community is reported by Hinshelwood and Grunberg, who also trace out the serious threat to the existence of the community — in this case because of arson. They see a positive solution in paying close attention to the structure of the community. In fact, they define the focus of attention for the community as the effort to examine and service the structure, or the community personality as it is called.

Angela Foster takes up the need for close scrutiny of structure by describing the boundary phenomena that occur between the therapeutic community and the outside world, comparing a residential community with a day community. This chapter, together with Chapters 23, 24 and 25, form an interlocking complex of contributions largely from one particular therapeutic community, the Marlborough Day Hospital. In a sense they form together a single case study of one community; and various incidents and events crop up and are highlighted from different angles and points of view.

Sheena Grunberg takes the study of consensus in large groups to a depth of analysis not before appreciated. Again, her emphasis is on structure. The structure of thinking in a large group is related to the social microstructure of the group itself: thus she describes how a fragmented quality of thought is associated with deep splits between those who are believed to know and those who don't know. Macrostructural changes in space and time can vary the quality of thinking by altering the opportunities for splitting the group.

Decision-making in this community is looked at from a political angle by Anne Crozier, who gives examples of the power of patients versus the staff in situations where emotions are raw and exposed on both sides. Brief mention is made of the Paddington Day Hospital, where a structural experiment has been in process for several years but appears to have foundered on the problem of democratic decision-making.

All five articles in this section reflect a preoccupation with the subtleties of social structure and how they affect leadership, anomie, the sense of belonging, thought itself and political involvement. It is possible that the minutiae of structure will become a major area of concern and growth in the study of the therapeutic processes of a community.

22
The Messianic community

Robert F. Hobson

The wounded surgeon plies the steel ...
Old men ought to be explorers
    (T. S. Eliot. *East Coker*, I, 147 and 202)

This chapter is a personal confession, a peculiar fragment of an auto-biography. Yet some of the tentative formulations which have emerged during eighteen years of hopes, disillusionments, frustrations, joys and sufferings in a therapeutic community could be of some value to others working in similar and yet different situations.

In an attempt to make sense of the term 'therapeutic community', we are assaulted by a plethora of nebulous terms: 'administrative therapy', 'social therapy', 'milieu therapy', and 'therapeutic community proper'. Between what are sometimes referred to as 'real therapeutic communities' there are wide and crucial differences, and yet these are inadequately described and poorly defined. A cursory glance with a critical eye at the voluminous literature, supplemented by anecdotes whispered in private groups of devotees, suggests that we just do not know what goes on. We know far too little to justify the current 'progressive' fashion in English mental hospitals, where so-called 'community methods' are being introduced widely. There are too many words and too few facts. Some important facts are the effects of the confusion on the personal lives of staff as well as of patients or clients.

There is an urgent need for careful studies of different types of community therapy. In recent years disciplined investigation has been begun in an effort to relate changes in patients to therapeutic variables, but most of us who have attempted such 'hard' research into problems which are not merely trivial or peripheral remain unimpressed by our results (Hobson and Shapiro, 1970; Hobson, 1974b). It is not merely a matter of technical and methodological difficulties; we lack coherent psychological theories which are needed to guide useful research. Psychoanalysis won't do. Present-day behaviourism won't do. Nor will any of the other 'isms' which emerge from the psychological laboratory, the sociological fog, or the solitude of the agonized existentialist. We do not know what to try to describe anecdotally, let alone what or how to measure. Indeed, we do not have anything approaching a psychology of personal relationships.

I have referred to this chapter as a personal confession. Yet every psychologist, however scientific he might wish to be, is himself a part of his subject matter. Although his tone of voice and literary expression suggest scrupulous objectivity and sublime disinterestedness, every statement he makes is a personal one (Polanyi, 1958). The psychotherapist brings his whole world into the consulting room, the hospital ward and the lecture room. But that is not to say that formulations which emerge from personal experiences are merely idiosyncratic. With the proviso that experience often only serves to confirm a man in his mistakes, it is possible that what I have to say is relevant not only to other hospital wards and units of various types, but also to august professional bodies, including societies devoted to the promotion and study of therapeutic communities; and maybe to the wider society in which we are living and partly living. I am telling my own story about many other human stories — and that is an important activity in science.

My main message is that we do harm. Much of what I have to say is about failure and damage. These topics have been barely touched upon, and are nowhere thoroughly explored, in the extensive, largely optimistic, and not seldom apocalyptic, literature in this field. I hope that this article might assist others in diagnosing what I have termed the 'therapeutic community disease' (Hobson, 1974b).

The therapeutic community disease

At the risk of over-simplification, and with some ironic metaphor, I shall arbitrarily describe three stages of development of the disease in the life-history of a particular type of therapeutic community. This broad formulation of phases, which are far from clear cut, is based mainly upon my own experience in the development of a therapeutic community called Tyson West Two at Bethlem Royal Hospital, although I have drawn upon a great deal of unpublished information about many other units of similar, although not identical, type. I shall term these three phases 'the coming of the Messiah', 'the Enlightenment?', and 'the Catastrophe'. They have been immediately recognized by many colleagues who have suffered and succumbed, or partially recovered from the malignant growth.

The coming of the Messiah

A dedicated, enthusiastic leader brings a message of brotherhood in a new society. Usually, he is a sincere idealist with a fascinating charisma. Carrying the light of democracy into the darkness of a traditional hierarchical mental hospital, he attracts a small body of followers and, at the same time, arouses fierce opposition from the Establishment. When, with the help of a certain shrewd political manipulation, he forms a therapeutic community, his 'mana' power, his magic, increases. Although he speaks of himself as 'just one member of a group', he becomes for his intimates virtually an incarnation of an archetypal figure − usually a Saviour Hero but sometimes a Great Mother. To others, he is a dangerous revolutionary or even the Devil. The charisma may gain admiration but it also excites envy − more overt in the energy, more concealed in the disciple.

What might have been an ideal is now an idealization.

By an ideal, I mean a goal accepted as being unattainable and yet worth striving for, with a realistic recognition of a necessary failure − very different from the despair of feeling a failure as a person. We need to say constantly 'I fail'. To say 'I am a failure' is blasphemy, the collapse of an idealization mistakenly adopted as an ideal.

An idealization involves a splitting between 'illusory good' and 'illusory bad'. The Leader and his colleagues collude in an idealization of himself and of the UNIT (now spelt in very large capital letters), which is often personified. The good UNIT is engaged in a battle with the powers of darkness: the 'badness' outside, which is embodied in the rest of the hospital, the traditional psychiatric establishment, or the world at large. The unit is under attack.

It is important to realize that attack occurs in fact as well as in fantasy. That is one reason why the idealized splitting is difficult to recognize; there are 'good' reasons for resentful battles: rumours of dreadful happenings (usually of a sexual and aggressive nature), petty administrative interference, and so on. Communications are distorted and members of the unit, cut off from their professional colleagues 'outside', react by counter-attack or by further withdrawal. I shall use the term persecutory anxiety, by which I mean a mounting mutual attack associated with illusory idealization and splitting. It is an interpersonal term. It can occur between individuals or between groups. In the case of a therapeutic community, the self-perpetuation of the increasing attack and counter-attack is reinforced by numerous factors. Some, amongst many others, are as follows:

(a) There is the development of an esoteric 'in-group' unit language.

(b) An exhilarating sense of cohesion develops not unlike that experienced by some of us in small ships during the war, where I was first visited by the idea of a therapeutic community. This cohesion is to be distinguished from what I shall later term a differentiated 'aloneness-togetherness'. In the 'all-togetherness' there is some 'pseudo-mutuality', a fear of recognizing personal differences which are potentially divisive. But that is not to say that the state is altogether 'pseudo'.

(c) The symptoms of many patients improve strikingly – for the time being.

The 'Enlightenment?'

'Enlightenment?' (in inverted commas with a large question mark) occurs when some of the above-mentioned processes begin to be recognized intellectually. A danger to which even experienced analysts are prone, not only in their work but also in professional societies, is to make formulations about themselves, sometimes with a pretentious dogmatism. We forget that what is unconscious *is* unconscous. There is a great temptation for inexperienced staff to join in this prestige game of self-explanation.

With dawning recognition that an egalitarian 'democratic' ideal has thinly disguised a destructive, albeit subtly concealed, power-game, there is now a good deal of talk about the 'badness inside'. Debates occur about definitions of 'role', 'status' and 'authority'. Such concepts are certainly of the utmost importance. The sickness lies not in what is talked about but in how the conversation develops, not in the content but in the manner. A sign of great danger is a tone of voice implying a subtle satisfaction, 'now we know ourselves'.

This rationalizing tendency often serves to exacerbate the persecutory situation. However, as well as great dangers of disintegration, there are potential positive possibilities. During the 'Enlightenment?' the persecution occurs within the unit group where, if it is recognized with passion, it can conceivably be dealt with. Rivalries and destructive alliances (e.g., patients versus staff, or sub-groups of each) can represent a relative disintegration which leads to a new differentiated and yet integrated state (Hobson, 1959, 1964). But, often, the disease moves into a third stage.

The Catastrophe

The unit can disintegrate and collapse. A number of therapeutic communities have done so with very serious consequences. The existence of Tyson West Two was maintained at a cost – a cost many of us are no longer willing or, indeed, able to pay. This cost could be conveyed only by telling many stories. But these would inevitably involve recognizable persons and I can only make a few broad generalizations.

Serious psychological breakdowns occur, especially in prominent members of the staff. Imagine the situation of a leader. His charisma has been wearing thin. Suddenly he sees anew his Brave New World, established with personal emotional sacrifice, devoted clinical work and complex political manoeuvring. It is an illusion. The image of the unit, and of himself, is shattered. He experiences in his body the destructive impact of the split-off 'shadow' which he has done his best to recognize. Maybe this does not happen to properly analysed leaders. It can be avoided if the leader leaves soon enough to spread the gospel honestly elsewhere before moving on once again, although he can leave a trail of destruction behind him. Perhaps these days we know enough to prevent it — but this I doubt.

The continued persecuting situation can be damaging to patients and staff in many ways, too diverse to be elaborated here. Recurrent disturbances occur within the group, often with the extrusion of members, patients or staff, or by 'acting-out' the unresolved persecution and destructiveness in diverse ways such as violence, suicide attempts and secret sexual relationships. Relief follows the departure of irritant members — but only for a time. The ritual of the 'scapegoat' needs to be repeated.

One, amongst many other less obvious but perhaps more serious effects, is a chronic state: a narrowing of the lives of staff members as well as long-stay patients, who become devoured by the dragon unit. Then, they remain relatively out of touch with the rest of the world in a state of what can be termed an 'exclusive incestuous regression'.

There can be profound effects upon the families of staff, who can either suffer intolerable involvement or, alternatively, envious exclusion. This most important topic deserves close study but it is difficult to elaborate in print for reasons of confidentiality.

Prophylaxis and treatment

I have suggested that the disease can result in the 'death' of the community and serious damage to its members. But it is possible that its more disastrous effects can be mitigated by early recognition of symptoms. The disease might become a 'creative illness'.

I experienced the near-despair of stage 3 after visiting a well-known therapeutic community about seven years after opening Tyson West Two. I did not see what the genuine, dedicated leader honestly saw. Not at all. I returned to Bethlem a sadder, if not wiser, man. If there had been more wisdom the sadness of loss might have led more rapidly to a constructive mourning. The achievement of creative aloneness depends on the acceptance of loss — of an ideal, or of a loved person. The effort to avoid chaos by denying the loss and attempting to bolster up a crumbling idealization resulted in dutiful and yet desperate persistence with increasing isolation. Yet perhaps something was learned. I saw Tyson West Two with new eyes and I decided not to publish my observations. Over the next years in conversations with my colleagues, we explored at least some of the complexities of the disease.

I recalled T. S. Eliot's lines:

Our only health is in the disease
If we obey the dying nurse
Whose constant care is not to please
But to remind of our, and Adam's curse,
And that, to be restored, our sickness must grow worse.

(T. S. Eliot. *East Coker*, IV, 152-6)

How 'grow worse'? To be more aware means to feel more pain more often — as well as more joy. We learn to suffer more. 'Adam's curse' is, I suppose, the original sin of knowledge. We cannot play God or a Divine Hero without a catastrophic Fall. We are faulty. We fail. Eden vanishes. That can be an agonizing loss; but maybe there is the possibility of a creative sickness rather than a debilitating disease.

Explorations, together with colleagues, resulted in many changes and eventually the formation of a new unit in 1971. A 'conversational' approach to psychotherapy emerged and has since been developed with reference to two-person, small-group, large-group and community situations (Hobson, 1974a; Meares and Hobson, 1977). The very broad and somewhat nebulous principles indicated below have provided the basis for a model from which can be derived at least some testable propositions (Hobson, 1977).

Psychotherapy and conversation

Psychotherapy can be conceived as a special sort of conversation which promotes social learning. The word 'conversation' is used in preference to 'interaction' or 'communication' in order to emphasize the central importance of language. Men interact — as do billiard balls. Men communicate — as do bees. But only men use language in which words, looks, gestures and actions are symbols which, as they expand in new and complex combinations, intimate more than is immediately present and known. Language is a peculiarly human mode of being and acting together. Human beings converse. They are 'things' to be inspected, classified and manipulated, and it is proper to study how they interact and communicate. But they are not only things. They are persons who converse by the reciprocal use and creation of new forms of language, fresh ways of living in communion within a community.

In human relationships there is the creation of a new language which is not merely a matter of words. By 'language' I mean a mode of being with people (Wittgenstein, 1968): living together in chats, in games, in the work of a treasurer's office, or in getting together to paint rooms in a hostel. In a 'conversation' there is a mutual reciprocal use and creation of a language between persons. The aim of psychotherapy is the promotion of a situation in which a patient's significant interpersonal problems are revealed, explored, understood, and modified by testing out many possible solutions generated in a dialogue. The problems are directly expressed here and now, not simply talked about. Therapy is designed to promote generalization and/or transfer of learning to varied life-situations. Of paramount importance is the achievement of mutual understanding of experiences and behaviour. Perhaps a central factor is learning how to adjust communication in a significant conversation, i.e., how to correct interpersonal misunderstanding, false perceptions and expectations.

The world 'mutual' suggests an equality, but this is of a special kind. A genuine feeling-response by the therapist does not mean that he talks 'about' the same things as the patient. There is an asymmetry. Patients and staff have different jobs, and it is not for us to burden patients with our intimate problems. It is false to pretend that everyone in a community is or should behave 'alike': to put it at its lowest, our pay-checks are very different. The appellation 'patient' need not be in any way derogatory and, working as a doctor in the National Health Service, it seems that (at least for me) terms such as 'client' or 'resident' can be misleading euphemisms. That is not to say, however, that psychotherapy, in or out of a special community, is best carried out in a medical setting.

The distinction between 'knowing' a person and 'knowing about' him — as in the catalogue of a psychiatric history — is crucial.

Mutuality is to be distinguished from pseudo-mutuality. In the latter there is an investment in maintaining a semblance, an idea, or a sense of relation, an idealization which involves a denial of many perceptions in order to maintain a fantasy of togetherness or fusion which does not permit of anything more than minor differences. All one's expectations must mesh in with those of the other person. Any divergence or independence, including the open affirmation of personal identity, is experienced not only as a painful disruption; it threatens to demolish the entire relation. Mutuality, which involves a recognition and valuation of each other's identity, with its capacities and potentialities for growth, becomes impossible. The pseudo-mutual state becomes more and more empty, stifling and barren. It is a static proximity of two or more isolated people. The 'goodness' of a 'beautiful friendship', an 'ideal marriage' or, not seldom, a 'sympathetic' therapeutic relationship can be a collusive fearful glorification of 'fitting in'. It barely conceals, and helps to create, a resentful loneliness. Although pseudo-mutual 'love' seems to offer much on one level, the 'goodies' are not confirmed on other levels. The uneasy search for security is achieved at the cost of a serious split. What is said in words is contradicted in actions.

The ideal state of a relationship is one of aloneness–togetherness (Hobson, 1974a). The relationship is crucial. 'Growing up' involves the progressive achievement of a capacity to be alone and to be together with others. Aloneness and togetherness are interdependent. I can only be alone in so far as I can be together with others. I can only be together with others if I am able to be alone. That is what it means to become an individual with an identity and to be a member of a community. In the lifelong quest (conscious and unconscious) for a personal identity, I continually seek to make new sense of new inner and outer experience, at the same time maintaining a stable sense of continuity. I have a basic 'need' for relations with others – to maintain the stability of important bonds and yet to remain alone with my own 'middle'.

The state of aloneness–togetherness is not static. It is continually re-created out of verbal and non-verbal conversations between people in a balance of stability and change with a rhythm of intimacy and distance. We need to be in touch, literally and metaphorically; but, just as important, we need space. In promoting a therapeutic living-learning situation, it is most important to distinguish between togetherness and pseudo-mutuality and between loneliness and aloneness. We are faced with the problem of how to 'penetrate to the core of loneliness in each person and speak to that' (Russell, 1967) and yet not to intrude upon the privacy of aloneness.

The great danger is pretence: the promotion of a pretentious pseudo-language. I have in mind the damage done to persons by statistical tables of pseudo-science, by sentimental pseudo-poetry, by pseudo-rational policy-making and (the core of the disease) by the fascinating pseudo-mutual 'equality' in a psychotherapeutic community. With regard to the latter, I have already made a vital distinction between an ideal and an idealization. An idealization involves an admitted or unadmitted clinging to a static belief in a state of perfection in which fantasy is confused with fact. Anything which threatens the 'perfect relationship' must be split off and denied. But, in one way or another, the badness (pain or destructiveness) returns, threatening disorganization and disintegration. An ideal is unattainable. It remains and yet changes. It involves hope – a hope which admits of doubt about the possibility of attaining any particular specified goal. It calls for commitment in the face of a necessary failure. Above all, the ideal of aloneness–togetherness requires mutual trust – a very large and mysterious phrase.

Recovery

In dwelling on the therapeutic community disease, I have given a wrong
impression about Tyson West Two. As far as I can judge, much happened
that was of inestimable value for many patients and for most staff.
Despite many failures, some apparently striking successes urge me on to
pursue the investigation of a possibility: the possibility that a psychotherapy community unit, if suitably developed, could be most suitable
for the resolution of persecutory anxiety which, associated with prolonged hostile dependency, is notoriously difficult to deal with in relatively closed two-person situations. I do not know if this is so.

When the new unit was set up, my colleagues and I hoped to use our
experience of the disease in a constructive way, paying special attention
to the importance of freedom and limits, authority and charisma, and
the judicious selection of patients and staff. It involved a considerable
commitment, but it was a commitment tempered with scepticism. And
hope. The experience is fresh in my mind and, wishing to use the
present tense, I shall quote an extract from an unpublished lecture delivered a year after the opening of the community (Hobson, 1972):

> The characteristics of our new baby are expressions of a considered
> wish for bolder psychotherapeutic friendships between more care-
> fully selected members (patients and staff) in a situation which is
> less of an enclosed hot-house and in which there is an increased res-
> pect for patients as responsible persons who are able to make im-
> portant choices. To assert that patients are persons is in no way to
> suggest a fear of, or guilt about, sometimes studying them (and our-
> selves) as billiard balls and as bees — whilst recognizing the wider
> context of personal relationships. Patients who formerly would have
> been 'looked after' by more or less anxious night nurses live and
> fend for themselves in a hostel with no staff and with minimal super-
> vision. They attend a separate day centre for specialized therapy in
> individual interviews and groups of all sizes. Therapy includes 'inter-
> pretive' psychotherapy, various types of ward meetings of patients
> and staff, art therapy and psychodrama. But the treatment is their
> whole life in the unit — the mutual creation of a language in which,
> it is hoped, distortions are revealed and corrected.
>
> It is not easy to judge when the sonorous phrase 'respect for free-
> dom' becomes a cliché concealing casual irresponsible unconcern, or
> when valuing a person's aloneness drives him into loneliness. The
> 'care' of medical and nursing staff can help to create disturbances,
> yet narcissistic foolhardy risk-taking is wicked. We are scared. Of
> course we are. We stand in 'uncertainties, mysteries and doubts' in
> our efforts to balance on a knife-edge the need for the freedom of

239

aloneness-togetherness, against the need for security provided by a firm structure maintained by definite authority. There is much freedom but there are also some firm rules with clear sanctions. We do not pretend that our odd community is an egalitarian society as we did in the early days of Tyson West Two. The authority is, to a large extent, vested in the whole staff-patient group and it is our aim that important decisions be made by consensus or, occasionally, by majority vote. But there is a curious kind of 'equal asymmetry'. Some are more equal than others.

In certain specified areas, the authority lies with the staff group — especially in the intimate relation between the Senior Registrar, the two nurses in charge, and me. I feel that the most important factor is the authority which arises from a close yet not suffocating, an intimate yet non-exclusive, friendship between two leaders, a man and a woman (the Unit Sister). But, perhaps this view is an expression of my own peculiar needs. Yet, ultimately, there is one boss. That is me. A democracy depends upon power; certainly, the power of love and of respect but, in the last resort, upon coercion. That is a failure. But, to me, it seems to be a fact. In our unit, we attempt to make it explicit, not pretend that it is not so. If need be (but only as a last resort) I decide, as openly as possible, attempting to avoid subtly concealed pressure. But I hope that I listen to everyone. Really listen — deep in my middle. One of the earliest exponents of the therapeutic community concept was St Benedict of Nursia (c. 480–543), and his rule is relevant to such matters as the role of the director, the admission of new members and the ordering of daily activities. He was concerned that all members 'even the most unimportant should have their say' and that no 'just murmuring' should be neglected. Yet he was the boss.

> Whenever matters of importance have to be dealt with in the monastery, let the abbot summon the whole congregation and himself put forward the question that has arisen. Then, after hearing the advice of the brethren, let him think it over by himself and do what he shall judge most advantageous. Now we have said that all should be summoned to take counsel for this reason, that it is often to the younger that the Lord reveals what is best (The Rule of St Benedict, III, 'Of calling the Brethren to Counsel', Benedict, 1943).

But I do not pretend that there is not also a good deal of dimly perceived manipulation.

Just one story. A simple story, but one with many implications.

It is Friday. The Charles Hood Unit has been open for one week only, and the patients are facing the weekend in the hostel, alone and together — or only lonely. I go in to learn that one of them has taken an overdose and cut her wrists. She is returning from a general hospital today and we are faced with the question of what shall be done. On admission, we have told the patients that we do not hold with wrist-cutting nor with suicide attempts. There is a rule forbidding such useless 'language', which can be a reason for discharge. (There is strong evidence to suppose that, for a long time in Tyson West Two, we did great harm by attempting to understand and to analyse — perhaps with some pseudo-mutuality — contagious wrist-cutting.) On this Friday, the staff discuss the situation and the majority are in favour of sending Alice to another hospital. The patients are anxious and non-committal. That evening, I talk to Alice in the lounge with any patients and staff who have chosen to be present. After a short chat with her, I say to three other patients 'You have cut your wrists. You have taken overdoses. As yet, I have done neither. You know how it feels. I hope you have a good weekend.' My weekend was not so good!

On reflection, I consider that, in Tyson West Two, we admitted too many of the most severe personality types with deep-seated paranoid mechanisms. We have our limits, and the situation is particularly toxic for staff with overt or concealed persecutory mechanisms. Maybe the really dangerous leaders are those charismatic personalities who do not seem to be at all paranoid but whose charming facade of honest zeal conceals a deep inner 'split'. A rigid authoritarian personality lies behind the benevolent democrat, maintaining a luxurious 'pseudo-mutuality' which, if it is to be maintained, must create an enemy somewhere. We need more courage to act responsibly, openly and directly, in deciding to exclude or remove some patients and some staff, not waiting for them to be extruded as scapegoats. Ideally, they choose to leave.

I am certainly not suggesting that most emotional disturbances amongst staff (sometimes labelled 'neurotic') are a bad thing. On the contrary, many of those who do not become overtly disturbed at some time during their stay on the unit are either insensitive or do little good or else, by denying their deep dividedness and reinforcing the inevitable persecutory anxiety, they do damage.

There is a need for charisma in the original sense of that word — as a gift for which we give thanks. The use of the Greek word *charisma* is almost entirely confined to the New Testament. It means a divinely conferred endowment being related to *charis* — 'grace', 'savour', 'charm', and *chairo* — 'rejoice'. *Carmen* — 'charm' may contribute to the notion of a charismatic personality. A common source for charity and charisma may lie in the Sanskrit *kar* — 'to be beloved'. The Greek, *kalos* — 'beautiful', 'attractive' is used for 'good' in John 10, 11. (I am grateful to my friend and colleague Dr Stella Ring for drawing my attention to these etymological points.) As there was in

Corinth, so in a psychotherapeutic community, different types of charisma are to be welcomed.

Maybe, then, one answer to the disease is to rejoice in, and be grateful for, the attractive gift or charm which can lead towards the ideal of love. To identify the given with the giver, to play Jesus Christ, is to use pseudo-mutuality coercively on the basis of an idealization. The reference to Corinth draws attention to I Cor. 12, 27-8, in which Paul is stressing the need to recognize the importance of many different gifts in a staff group: prophets, teachers, healers, etc. Student nurses, registrars and even consultants have some charisma. All charismatic persons are not Gandhis or Hitlers. The problem is how to use charisma and not be used by it. Perhaps those community units which attempt to treat long-standing personality disorders, without running a real risk of the disease, are not worthy of the name 'therapeutic'. But we are still a very long way from defining that term.

Formulated 'insight' (the 'Enlightenment?') can be the most effective means of avoiding 'seeing into'. It is a barrier which obscures that new look at the world not only with but also through the eye, which accompanies an emergence from static loneliness into a moving aloneness. This lecture could itself be an example of an elaborate double-bluff, one of the most serious symptoms of the disease. The answer can lie only in taking the risk of explorations in personal relationships, in ongoing conversations in community groups, in staff groups, in personal friendships, in the dialogue of genuine science, and (as patients ourselves) in the curious friendship of psychotherapy.

Following Charles Hood, we are attempting to create situations in which genuine meetings are more likely to occur. Maybe if we can do something about the most damaging taboo we might get somewhere. I do not mean any of the taboos of the Establishment, and certainly not any of those concerning aggression or bodily sex. What I am referring to is the taboo about which an outstanding pioneer, Ian Suttie, wrote forty years ago — the 'taboo on tenderness' (Suttie, 1935). Maybe, if we can become less afraid of tenderness, then we can meet as persons, alone-together — at least, sometimes.

The qualified hope expressed in that lecture seemed to be justified in the succeeding three years, although there were some casualties. But the three years before I left to take up another post was too short a time to make a judgment.

I hope that there is some remedy for the disease. I hope. If there is one, then it lies in knowledge derived from careful but relevant research. A plan of therapy for personality disorders based upon a model of social learning might serve as a guide to future, empirical explorations. But, as yet, we have nothing approaching a psychological theory of language and most of the data that are measurable are trivial. Definition and experiment in social psychology must be directly relevant to such problems as those indicated in this lecture: idealization, persecutory anxiety, loss, loneliness, and the promotion of an openness not only within the community but also between it and the wider societies of the hospital and the local community.

It seems that the disease recurs in cycles and that, if recognized with intellect and passion, it can be modified, becoming a 'creative illness'. The duration of the cycles can be shortened, the damage lessened, and a state of 'relative disintegration' can result in new patterns of differentiation and integration of individuals and the whole group (Hobson, 1964). It can, but often does not. The various phases, which often interpenetrate, can sometimes be 'lived through' within one group session. My hunch is that the important problem is the understanding of the mysterious term 'persecutory anxiety' and how its escalation is promoted, not only by certain social structures but also by certain types of person, whether patients or members of staff (Meares and Hobson, 1977). But, I suppose, the Messiah will continue to creep in somewhere.

We need to be explorers, not bound by an elitist fashion of what is a proper or real therapeutic community. If not as the 'old men' referred to in the epigraph of this essay, at least in late middle age — Eliot's 'middle way'. I do not expect a quick cure, if indeed there is one. My speculation is that a community such as Tyson West Two attracts people who express a partially concealed sickness rooted in the values of our modern competitive-acquisitive society. Perhaps the structure of the unit makes this disturbance more evident. It can reinforce the splitting but, in the failure to achieve an ideal, there lies a possibility of a different sort of success. It is often in grappling with a failure to communicate that a new mode of togetherness emerges. The disease can result in a cynical disillusionment and self-destruction which I have experienced, but it can lead to an exploration of exciting possibilities. So we start again and again in the quest for an impossible ideal, expecting to fail in our efforts to create a therapeutic language. Perhaps we can hope to do a little less damage than before. And that is important. But, as yet, we do not have a vocabulary, let alone a language.

> So here I am, in the middle way, having had twenty years —
> Twenty years largely wasted....
> Trying to learn to use words, and every attempt
> Is a wholly new start, and a different kind of failure
> Because one has only learnt to get the better of words
> For the thing one no longer has to say, or the way in which
> One is no longer disposed to say it. And so each venture

Is a new beginning, a raid on the inarticulate
With shabby equipment always deteriorating
In the general mess of imprecision of feeling....
There is only the fight to recover what has been lost
And found and lost again and again: and now, under conditions
That seem unpropitious. But perhaps neither gain nor loss.
For us, there is only the trying. The rest is not our business.

(T. S. Eliot. *East Coker*, V, 160–80)

'The wounded surgeon plies the steel.'

Acknowledgments

I am deeply grateful to many patients and colleagues, especially to Miss Eileen Skellern for sage advice derived from her long experience of therapeutic communities, for her unfailing support during difficult periods at Bethlem Royal Hospital, and especially for the aloneness-togetherness of an expanding friendship.

23
The large-group syndrome[*]

R. D. Hinshelwood and Sheena Grunberg

The main debate at every conference of the Association of Therapeutic Communities that we have attended has centred around the issue of structure and organization. It has been the flashpoint of many heated exchanges; and at a previous conference such division was reached over the simple structuring involved in the appointing of a secretariat that many members abandoned the conference. Within this large group of the ATC there is the widely held belief that this is a structureless group; but we believe that, whether structure is recognized or not, there is an elaborate structuring that, if it were explored, would lead to a creative development in the ATC.

Also, within the various therapeutic communities themselves there is wide variation in organization and structure, from the Henderson with its elaborate structure and organization to the Paddington which has abandoned all formality, allowing the patients to organize their own structures. It is to this tetchy subject of structure, its development and uses that we address ourselves.

In an earlier paper (Grunberg and Hinshelwood, 1973), we discussed the way in which we conceptualized problems at the Marlborough Day Hospital using the formula of structure, process and content; and today we would like to develop one aspect of this theme, which is looking at structure as content.

Structure means the act of putting together, the relationship between the parts; and the actual subject matter of this chapter is an examination of the ways in which structures articulate; for it is the idea of articulating structures that distinguishes us as therapeutic communities from traditional psychiatric practice.

We use the word 'articulating' advisedly, for the verb 'to articulate' has a double meaning. The Chambers Dictionary defines it as 'to join,

[*] Read at the conference of the Association of Therapeutic Communities, October 1974; published in *Group Analysis*, VII/2, May 1975.

to connect as by joint, to form into distinct sounds or words' and the Shakespearean usage was 'to come to terms, to speak distinctly'. It therefore expresses concisely the idea of parts brought together by words and speech. This is not a new idea, for it was Einstein who changed scientific thought by his startling idea that it was not the charges nor the particles but the field in the space between which is essential for the description of physical phenomena. In Pat de Maré's book (1972), he says: 'Marxism, Gestalt psychology, field theory, communication theory all have in common that it is neither the individual nor the group, neither the part nor the whole which is primary but it is the interstices of intercommunication, interaction and interrelation which play the primary part.'

We feel that it is through this line of thinking that we will be able to make advances in the treatment of our patients, especially in the following areas: (1) integration; (2) feeling of relatedness; and (3) identity; and we will pause for a moment to define identity as having a boundary and a focus, and this again is a structural concept.

We would like to illustrate the kind of problem we mean by demonstrating the events that emerged a few months ago at the Marlborough. We have since evolved a new system, but prior to this the sequence of events was as follows: Staff Meeting/Large Groups plus on different days Small Group/Patients' meeting/Work Group/Gestalt/Encounter/ Dream/Projective Art/Sanctions/Leavers' Group/Staff Groups. During this time there was growing discontent on the part of the staff and patients concerning two aspects of the hospital. One aspect was the large group functioning with what might be described as the large-group syndrome, i.e. long silences, staring out of the window, no proper exchanges. This was becoming so depleted that it was even mooted that perhaps we should abandon using the large group since so few of us felt there was any therapeutic value attached to it. It seemed that we were only holding on to this structure because it typified therapeutic communities. Hand in hand with this large-group syndrome came the awareness of the proliferation of small specialized groups. These groups appeared to have an autonomy from the main life of the community and seemed to detract from it. The connection between these two aspects, that of the large-group syndrome and the peripheral splintering was quite remarkable, and in fact leads us to propose a direct correlation between the two.

This state of affairs we knew to be serious, but it was only when the alarm was raised by fire-setting that we were able to appreciate the extent of it. Every Tuesday for several weeks mysterious fires broke out, and we were left helplessly at the mercy of this patient or patients, who continued to remain anonymous. Nowhere in any of the many therapeutic groups in the hospital was there a clue as to who had set the fires.

It seemed that the particular use of structure had facilitated splitting. The explosiveness that should have emerged and been contained, if not in the large group then in some other part of the programme, had been split off to such an extent that none of the therapeutic potential could get at the problem. We did, however, feel that there was some connection between the fire-raising and our difficulties in running the large group. In our opinion, the large group is something in which the general condition of the community is reflected, so that clues leading up to the fire-raising should have been available. However, in this case we could detect clues neither from the large group nor indeed from any of the smaller subsidiary ones. But it was particularly in the large group that we hoped to see the projections that could lead us out of this disorganization. The combination of the sub-groups functioning autonomously and the depleted large group is an example of what we mean by a structure which is not articulating.

It was not then surprising to find that our fire-raiser, a girl with a potentiality for psychosis, should be the person to act-out. We were in fact allowing a psychotic structure to develop. It was Comte, the French philosopher, who said that the structure of society itself is the human mind, and it was only too clear how our structure was analogous to psychotic functioning. The parallel between the patient's mind and the level of articulation between the structures is actually more than an analogy; for we believe that the integration, relatedness and sense of identity of the individual patients is mutually interdependent on the efficiency of the articulating structures. We therefore concluded that our fire-raiser in her psychotic acting-out had demonstrated clearly that we, as a community, were out of touch with reality.

The first essential was to institute proceedings to get back to reality and remind ourselves of the most important development in the elaboration of the concept of reality, which has been to give to the term reality a real meaning by substituting the description of maternal personality for that of primary object. What does this mean? Using the model of the baby's emerging sense of reality, we see that the first organization of his emotional life is made by splitting the good and bad aspects of mother. Translating this idea back to the community, the logical development in terms of organization would be from a split-up community with a depleted large group to an organization where the large group would be replenished with all of these projected parts so that the community personality could be explored as a whole.

So we made minor modifications to our structure; these consisted of introducing a feedback session into the first quarter of an hour of the large-group time where literally anything that happened the day before, from the Work-out in Gestalt/Small Group/Working Groups, etc. to teatime chat, would constitute material. The remaining three-quarters of an hour of the group is then open, 'free-floating' as we call it, and it is during this time that we hope to see the projections onto the 'community personality' which is the focus.

We feel that it is important that there is a spelt-out focus, however loosely described, as a kind of guideline and idea against which we can assess the fantasies and realities expressed about the community. Otherwise it would only be too easy to get bogged down into the kinds of difficulty that we have called the large-group syndrome, which Tom Main (1975) so ably describes in his paper 'Some Psychodynamics of Large Groups'. With such clarity of perception he describes how projective processes can degenerate to such a degree that staff get hardened into set roles, to the point where they scarcely recognize themselves and need time after the group to get back their projected parts. He feels that one of the characteristic features and faults of such a large group is that staff make interpretations about 'the group' which he feels can only lead to alienation and depersonalization, and advocates comments of a simple kind like 'You are looking upset, John.' Main feels that such interventions confirm the self rather than depersonalize, and we would agree. However, we feel that such simple interventions are not sufficient to pinpoint the state of the community personality on which we feel will depend the increasing integration and sense of identity among our patients.

Let us demonstrate to you how we feel this could work, by going back to the fire-raiser and the large group using psychodrama techniques in which the confession was made. At the beginning of the group the structuring and configurations within the community were examined and developed to the stage where an emotional point was reached when the fire-raiser owned up, in the backdrop of a group who felt that any one of them had the potentiality to set the fires; i.e., the fire-raiser could take back her ability to verbalize and the others could take back their fire-raising parts. We feel this could only have happened in a setting in which the community personality was made the focus.

What we are saying is that the large group at the outset is structureless but thereafter becomes highly organized, expressing, through structure and personality, ideas about the community personality. In changing our programme we hope that we will be able to replenish the large group by (1) confronting the community with the split-off parts; and (2) giving to the large group a real identity with a boundary and a focus and calling it the community personality.

24
Thinking and the development of structure in a community group

Sheena Grunberg

One of the crucial issues that therapeutic communities have to deal with is the problem of structuring the day. There seems to be no set pattern or meaning in the particular method of structuring that exists, with little emphasis placed on the study of structure. However, there does seem to be a general belief that the community meeting is an important arrangement which helps in the management and integration of the therapeutic community. But perhaps most importantly it has been the tenacity of the anti-authority belief systems which have impeded the study of structure, resulting in the idea that structuring undermines the ideology behind the therapeutic community system. My belief is that, on the contrary, structuring and the study of it promote the therapeutic community ideal.

Whilst this anti-structure lobby has impeded the development of structure, there is indeed a profound truth about structuring and institutionalization. Much has been written on the topic of the development of the structure as a defensive operation. For example, Rosenberg (1970) writes:

> The hospital sub-culture provides a setting in which a number of people can share in a common system of ego defences, in a way that simultaneously helps to reduce intra-psychic tension while permitting the maintenance of a stable institutional structure.

It is this stable institutional structure, usually fossilizing into traditional hierarchical patterns unhelpful to the patients, which has been anathema to the therapeutic community movement.

Despite acknowledging all the very important literature laying emphasis on social structure as a defensive operation, my perspective is of a social system seen as a constructive operation. Whilst the process of structuring is defensive, it is also developmental and differentiating, and it seems to me important to expound the full meaning of structural expansion.

My viewpoint derives from Ward (de Maré, 1972), who described evolution as a struggle for structure, rather than the survival of the individual organism; and, by this statement, I take him to mean the evolution of both external and internal structure. The assumption in the paper is of there being a harmony between the structures of the mind (internal structuring) and the order of the outside world (external structuring), and my aim is to trace the nature of this harmony. But, more specifically, it is the correspondence between the development of external and internal structure and their relationship to man's greatest potentiality for evolution (i.e. his thought) that I want to pinpoint.

In Chapter 23 we (Hinshelwood and Grunberg) suggest that, in order to make sense of the working of a therapeutic community, one has to conceptualize the large group (as the main vehicle of expression of the community) as having a real identity and focus, called the community personality. The assumption is of a community mentality that thinks, and the state of which can be assessed. Bion showed that the process of personality development and the process of thought development are not only emotionally but also structurally related. More importantly, they are structurally linked at a particular point in the development, which Klein (1975) describes as the depressive position, that point in the development of the infant where the mother is, for the first time, conceived of as a whole parent. To put it more clearly, in the emotional climate of the depressive position, the structural step is to see the whole person. This structural step is worth tracking down in the therapeutic community.

The philosophic background of this chapter comes from ideas about structure and thought propounded by Marx, whose vision of structure effected monumental changes in our society and attitude. Marxist views are in striking contrast to those of Hegel:

> To Hegel, the life process of the human brain, i.e. the process of thinking which, under the name of 'the Idea', he even transforms into an independent subject, is the demiurgos of the real world and the real world is only the external phenomenal form of 'the Idea'. With me, on the contrary, the ideal is nothing else than the material world reflected by the human mind and translated into forms of thought (Marx, 1889).

The Hegelian viewpoint broke all links between thinking and the external environment, incarcerating thinking in the realm of 'the thinkers'. The real world was secondary and dependent on the thinker's thoughts. The Marxist viewpoint, disgusted with such an elitist approach, propounds that the environment profoundly influences our thought and that everyone contributes to it, whatever his place in the social structure.

Marx's *tour de force* spells out a major shift in attitude in the twentieth century, and our developments in thinking rest on its understanding and implications. Thought as a process of a social group must, therefore, significantly alter our approach to treatment in the therapeutic community in terms of the way in which we use structure.

A case study

These ideas can be explored in some major changes in the structure of a large community group over a three-year period. Changes have been made in the group immediately after the large group, with the rest of the programme altering in consequence.

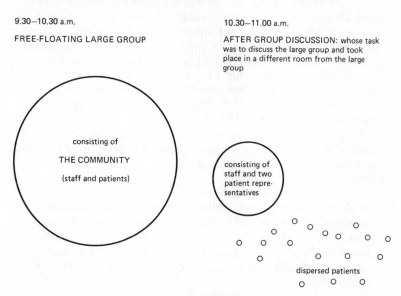

9.30–10.30 a.m.

FREE-FLOATING LARGE GROUP

10.30–11.00 a.m.

AFTER GROUP DISCUSSION: whose task was to discuss the large group and took place in a different room from the large group

consisting of

THE COMMUNITY

(staff and patients)

consisting of staff and two patient representatives

dispersed patients

Figure 24.1 Spatial arrangements in the daily programme

The community meeting in Figure 24.1 was characterized by a heavy atmosphere with the main communication coming from staff, or from 'leading' patients imitating their small-group leader's approach. Interpretations about the group often either fell flat, or were received with sullen silence or even actively resisted, individual interpretations being found much more acceptable. In retrospect, it seemed that any feeling of a real community was often at a low ebb.

It was a great relief to get into the staff meeting afterwards where one could let go of one's feelings, and at the beginning of this meeting there was the release of tension by laughter, heated discussions, smoking and the hugging of coffee cups. This was the place where Tom Main (1975) suggested that the staff were able to get back their projected parts and assume their own identity after the emotional draining of the large group and perhaps begin to make sense of it, i.e., an attempt was made to think about the large group. The dispersed patients met in the kitchen and obviously had the need to do the same, but were deprived of the opportunity to recover their projected thinking parts.

A clear picture of structuring emerged at that time with a depleted large group and many lively and autonomous small groups running concurrently, whose work we heard nothing about in the large group. Elliot Jaques (1953) writes that 'All institutions are unconsciously used by their members as mechanisms of defence against psychotic anxiety', and we felt that our particular structure supported a psychotic state of mind in that more and more of the community personality was being split off from the community meetings, making them lifeless; and the energy was being used up in an endless proliferation of small groups, none of which bore any relation to the other. It seemed that treatment was being done in these small groups in a piecemeal fashion, and it was hard to justify the community meetings and this expensive form of treatment if that were the case.

This splitting seemed to correspond to the sort of projective identification of the psychotic personality documented by Klein (1975), the purpose of which is to deny consciousness of reality. Bion (1957) writes:

> It is to be expected that the deployment of projective identification would be particularly severe against the thought of whatever kind that turned to the relations between object impressions for, if this link could be severed or, better still, never forged, then at least consciousness of reality would be destroyed even though reality itself could not.

These broken links or fragmentation of the community personality seemed to have their internal counterpart in the staff. After the initial relief of tension, a different tone came upon the staff group, as one version of reality conflicted with another and strife emerged. The pervading ethos of this staff group was of theirs being the 'right' interpretation, and conflicting reports of feeling from the large group were almost entirely considered to rest with the idiosyncrasies of the individual, if they did not concur with the majority opinion. This led to power alignments with the winning faction controlling events, and this was destructive to any therapeutic progress. The richness of the differing points of view, containing as they did different aspects of feeling from the large group, projected into staff members, was thrown to the winds. We seemed to be trapped in this unbalanced state of mind, only seeming to emerge when visitors brought us back some awareness of the kind of reality denied us within the framework of our structure. The structure was designed to avoid thinking and linking from taking place.

Pat de Maré (1974) in 'The Politics of the Large Group' says that the large group's equivalent to thinking or mentation is by controlling and structuring. He suggests that it becomes organized as a result of the frustration, hate and aggression brought about by the situation in the large group. For example, the large group may have to resort to an overly developed control by hierarchy, which can easily result in an abuse of hierarchy, resulting in mindless and dehumanizing organization.

I am assuming that the same type of organization can also be seen in a therapeutic community in a modified form, because of the closed nature of the community. We consider that the large group is the most significant event in the therapeutic community, all the other groups and activities being seen only as lateral outcroppings of the large group. Their functioning has to be constantly under observation, because they contain and control important operations which are at the centre of the process of mentation. So, what I am saying is that what is reflected in the control and structuring of the whole community with its large group and lateral outcroppings, constitutes the mentality of the community.

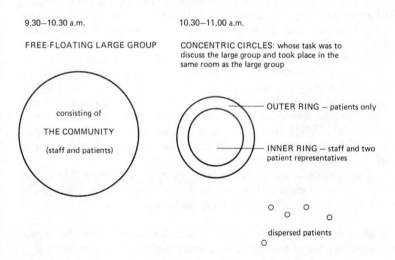

9.30—10.30 a.m.

FREE-FLOATING LARGE GROUP

consisting of

THE COMMUNITY

(staff and patients)

10.30—11.00 a.m.

CONCENTRIC CIRCLES: whose task was to discuss the large group and took place in the same room as the large group

OUTER RING — patients only

INNER RING — staff and two patient representatives

dispersed patients

Figure 24.2 Spatial arrangements in the daily programme

Concentric circles (Figure 24.2) as a structure were developed after this difficult time when the particular structuring had made it difficult to think about the community as a whole. It evolved ostensibly because of a need to include more patients in the staff meeting because of the undue pressure on the two patient representatives to report back accurately to the patients not included in the staff discussion. What seemed to be a sort of galloping persecution of the patients about the staff group was really their only way of exerting pressure on the staff to change the system. However, because it was felt that it was easier to think in the smaller group, this 'fishbowl' technique was used. At first, it was decided that no one in the outer group was obliged to attend and they were not allowed to speak. This was later modified to the point where the outer ring was allowed to speak after a quarter of an hour and then, finally, no time limit was imposed. Here was a fine example of control by hierarchy! Although the decision to institute concentric circles was ostensibly taken by the community, it was, nevertheless, controlled in effect by the staff who held the thinking and deciding function in the organization at that time.

The atmosphere at the concentric circles was of a tense inner circle thinking very intense thoughts; gone were the laughs and jokes of the previous staff meeting as we set about the task of analysing the community. Here were 'the Dons' of the community, putting before the community what Tom Main described so aptly as the Nobel Prize-winning interpretations. The outer circle of patients was poorly attended and supine. Clandestine conversations took place behind hands, reading of newspapers and an occasional vigilante sitting bolt upright listening to the endless intellectualization. Let me reconstruct the atmosphere for you with this example. One particular morning the inner circle was debating about two significant events which had been raised in the large meeting, and inevitably, an erudite discussion about the relation to the two breasts resulted. This revelation met with nodded approval by the inner circle, but was blasted by an illegal and outraged voice from that lone vigilante, who cried out: 'two ears – two eyes – two hands – two legs – TWO FEET!' Here was a plea for the community feet to be firmly placed on the communal floor. This was the beginning of a new upsurge of the demand for participation.

This gagging of the patient group was, not surprisingly, felt as that kind of controlling reminiscent of political repression. In relation to this behaviour, David Cooper (1967) has this to say of Villa 21:

Perhaps the most central characteristic of authentic leadership is the relinquishing of the impulse to dominate others. Domination here means controlling the behaviour of the others, where the behaviour represents for the leader projected aspects of his experience. By

domination of the other, the leader produces for himself the illusion that his own internal organization is more and more perfectly
ordered.

Intellectual activity came to appear separate from man's practical
activity only when the division of labour progressed sufficiently for
some men to become thinkers. We can see how a thinking class developed in the hospital, not only from this example, but in other areas of
the hospital where patients were put in the role of 'the mindless workers'.
One of the severe criticisms by the patients at this time was of being
asked to play out empty roles in the community, and in the work groups
particularly. The development of concentric circles is a fine example of
the way in which distorted solutions can be reached when the thinking
involved included only a section of the community. At the time, it was
done in all good faith, but it clearly served the staff's need to control.
However, it also represented the giving up of some control by the staff,
which must also be recognized.

As the concentric circle function became redundant due to the thinking function being given back and, therefore, more equally distributed,
ten half-hour sessions were allocated solely to the discussion of the
present structure, and this was the first time that such an occurrence
had taken place. Throwing open these ongoing discussions to the community as a whole was a radically different procedure from those which
took place in moving from Figure 24.1 to Figure 24.2. The task of
these sessions was to examine the concentric circles arrangement with a
view to reorganization to a structure which would facilitate greater integration within the community. The most salient difference was the
openness on the part of the staff to entirely new ideas about structural
rearrangement thrown up by these many discussions whereas, before,
the concentric circles arrangement had been the only structural change
on offer and somewhat predestined. At the end of these ongoing studies
of the structure, a final decision was reached jointly to establish the
situation as envisaged in Figure 24.3.

Simultaneously with these changes, there took place full patient participation in the policy and assessment groups which, prior to this time,
had consisted of staff alone with patient representatives. The inclusion
of the patients in the assessment group, which goes through the case
history of possible new patients and where it is decided jointly whether
to admit or not, presented us with some ethical problems which we
have surmounted, and the details of which are not relevant to this discussion. The inclusion of the patients in the policy meeting gave to
some patients a real say in the making of their own destiny. There was
also the collapse of the work groups, which were those groups which
did such tasks as gardening, repairing toys, painting old people's houses,

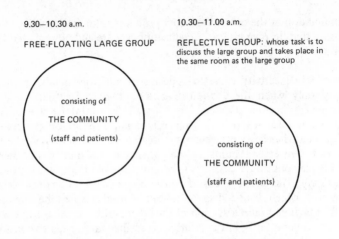

9.30—10.30 a.m.

FREE-FLOATING LARGE GROUP

10.30—11.00 a.m.

REFLECTIVE GROUP: whose task is to discuss the large group and takes place in the same room as the large group

consisting of

THE COMMUNITY

(staff and patients)

consisting of

THE COMMUNITY

(staff and patients)

Figure 24.3 Spatial arrangements in the daily programme

etc. Work was considered empty and peripheral to what was considered to be the actual work task of the community.

A different quality of interaction accompanied this total participation; and it became possible to put forward interpretations about the community without being given the rasp, and for them even to be welcome. Patients themselves learned to make real group interpretations with considerable skill rather than by imitation. An apt interpretation brought about considerable closeness of the community and there was also a greater capacity for acknowledging the experience of others, which was no longer embarrassing. There was also a change in the character of decision-making in the community, from the imitating of staff members in Figure 24.1 to the development of the capacity of the patients to deliberate on issues and wait for a decision to come to fruition. Sometimes a patient would be asked to wait until the next community meeting for a further discussion of the problem before a decision could be reached. However, it was interesting that a special staff meeting of three quarters of an hour was instituted immediately after the change to Figure 24.3 was brought about, which seemed to be the result of residual staff anxiety and, possibly, the need to hang on to some control over policy-making. The staff were quickly able to realize the new function of this staff group, and its role is now severely circumscribed.

Our therapeutic community working party demonstrates the kind of thinking now taking place amongst the patients as a reflection of the level of organization and capacity for thought now possible. This working party consists of three patients and one junior member of staff. The openness to new ideas and eagerness to learn is outstanding. The working party, however, reflects dissatisfaction; it is searching for ways of developing the present system, and here is the struggle for structure rolling on.

We have reached the point of a thinking community, where the structure supports the whole group reflecting upon itself — a state of affairs that Marx would have applauded. Let us return to our Hegel-Marx statement and note how the development of the large group recapitulates the evolution of a society from a point where thinking belonged to 'the thinkers', where thought was reified in the concentric circle structure, to a point where the structures support a system allowing the thinking function to be redistributed and belong to everyone. Here, the whole group reflects upon the community, translating internal structure in the form of the content of the large group into forms of thought useful to the community. In my view, the structuring involved in each stage constitutes important developments in thinking, particularly the complicated and convoluted structure of concentric circles which can be considered as a piece of mentation of the group, which enabled the final structuring in Figure 24.3 to become possible.

It is relevant here to return to the previously illustrated separation of staff and patient groups which seemed so rigid and laughable, and to note that it appeared to be a necessary stage of development. The inequality of Figure 24.1 that seemed to be so flagrantly uncharacteristic of the therapeutic community ideal does seem, in fact, to be a necessary prologue to the development of important mental mechanisms and to the development of integration. This sharply contrasts with one of the aims of the therapeutic community movements: that of role blurring, as stated by Maxwell Jones. If, in fact, role blurring had taken place to any great extent during this time, I doubt whether the kind of progress reported here would have been possible. It was vital to know exactly who was playing the thinking role so that the role function could be reclaimed by the group, and I shall be returning to this topic later in the chapter.

What did these structural changes mean in terms of the development of thought? What are the processes involved in their transition? Here I must return to the breast at the risk of being hoist by my own petard! To have thoughts and then to think originates in the experience of feeding. The development of thought has a great deal to do with the development of the mother and baby relationship. At the beginning of this relationship, the mother has simply to try to feel and understand what the baby wants and needs. A mother with a new baby cannot understand initially what the baby's cry means, but she knows that the cry is the baby's only means of expressing that something is wrong and, in thinking about what that might be, goes through the various routines of feeding, changing and checking the baby, in order to satisfy him.

Soon enough, her own feelings guide her and she learns to pick up the baby's projections and differentiate between the hungry, windy, discomforting and desperate cries. This capacity of the mother to think and understand the needs of the baby is the containing function. With the satisfaction of mothering (i.e. containment and maturation), the baby learns to wait (if there is a sufficient toleration of frustration) and to take on the capacity to contain and understand his anxieties himself, and this process involves introjection (Bion, 1962). So the two significant processes which have to occur before the infant can begin to think are: (1) the satisfactory development of the mother and baby relationship through the process of projective identification; and (2) the introjection of this mechanism.

Let us return to our examples.

The transition from Figure 24.1 to Figure 24.2

Characteristic of this stage was the extensive projective identification, with the staff and patients having clear demarcation lines in terms of roles, with the staff taking the role of parents and the patients as children. Here was the mother–baby relationship in its inception. The way in which the projective identification was contained and converted into useful thoughts was by a renewed interest on the part of the staff to try to contain these orbital projections into staff and small groups, by the introduction into the large group of a feedback section (lasting a quarter of an hour). This meant that important happenings, impressions and experiences about the previous day's events were fed into the large group. Staff slowly became able to communicate some of their own feelings of the day before, and a picture started to build up of the experience of the community against the background of the present group; i.e., we began to understand the needs of the patients and community.

This feedback section no longer operates as such, because feedback itself has now become a part of the culture of the group. At the time, it had to be propagated by the staff and, for about a year, we struggled with the problem of only staff feeding back and making the links. Little did we realize at that point that it could not have been otherwise. We were, in this operation, seemingly reversing the process of projective identification which Bion stresses as one of the essential aspects in the treatment of the psychotic elements of the personality and an essential step in the process of thought development.

The transition from Figure 24.2 to Figure 24.3

The development through concentric circles seems to have some correspondence with the second significant process which has to occur before thinking can take place. Let us now focus on the concentric circle arrangement, and conceptualize the inner ring as the containers, those people who are in the role of containing anxieties, i.e. mother, or, in our case, the staff and two representatives; and the outer ring as those who require their anxieties to be contained, i.e. the baby, or the patients. Then the whole concentric circles transaction can be seen as the large group's equivalent to the process of mentation involved in introjection, i.e. the containers becoming contained within the large group in a very concrete way. Esther Bick (1968) writes about this process thus:

> Until the containing functions have been introjected the concept of a space within the self cannot arise. Introjection, i.e. construction of an object in an internal space, is impaired. In its absence, the function of projective identification will necessarily continue unabated and all the confusions of identity attending it will be manifest.

The clearing of the inner ring, creating a space in the centre of the large group, seems to me to be symbolic of the development of a community internal space in which the internal constructions of the community personality can be made and understood. The ramifications of external structuring here demonstrated seem to have been a necessary antecedent to the development of the capacity for internal structuring. In fact, one could hypothesize tentatively that external structuring bears an inverse relation to internal structuring as a community develops.

Whilst I respect highly Maxwell Jones's attempts to change a ghastly system, I feel that rapid role blurring can really blur vital areas of conflict in a therapeutic community which contains the kinds of relationship between the staff and patients essential to the progress both of the therapeutic community and the individual. What I think he must have meant was role redistribution.

So we see that the structure of Figure 24.1 was a psychotic structure untenable and extended and inevitably producing psychotic thinking or, in a different metaphor, a mother preoccupied and therefore out of touch with a new baby. The structure of Figure 24.2 seems to represent the turning point from external to internal structuring and supported the mechanism of projective identification and introjection and the laying of the ground necessary for the beginnings of a relationship where thought can develop, or the start of a mother and baby relationship. The structure of Figure 24.3 seems to show the external and internal structuring supporting wholeness with the capacity for reflective thought:

a mother able to develop her baby to a significant stage of development.

Bion's distinctive contribution is to suggest that an essential element in thinking lies in the interplay between seeing the object — in our case the community as a whole — and seeing the part-objects which are all the various relationships making up the whole. This interplay is the daily routine of the large group and reflective group; this is the internal structuring which leads to the development of mature thinking and is the structural step that we hoped to track down earlier, where the structure supports the linking between intellectual and emotional development. Every morning we start with a new selection of events which then gets built up into an attempted whole view of the community. Each day we reconstruct the image of the whole, which is the internal structuring of the community and this process is thinking. Let me just add here that we are far from believing that we have found Utopia, but Figure 24.3 does seem to be the best structural system that we have developed to date, in its capacity to promote reflective thought and to support wholeness. In the following example, you will note that some of the difficulties earlier cited as belonging to Figure 24.1 emerge again, but my point is that the system as seen in Figure 24.3 does give more support in its structuring to a more satisfactory outcome.

Let me illustrate what I mean. At the end of September, there was to be a break-up of the community. Eight students from the Student Scheme together with twelve of the patients from the regular programme were to leave; also the head occupational therapist, the doctor and psychologist involved in the Student Scheme and the two student occupational therapists — twenty-five people in all. The loss to the community is obvious, and one would expect this to be reflected in the community meetings. This particular large group meeting was preoccupied with what seemed to be the persecution of one patient who was being grilled as to why she wanted to join the Gestalt Group. It seemed that demands to answer for herself were excessive and the patient broke down into sobs. Eventually, the girl got up and walked out, and there was further quarrelling and blaming amongst the patients and staff. Interpretations about the loss to the community of the leavers fell on stony ground and only seemed to exacerbate irritation, resulting in bickering between staff members. The large group ended on that uncomfortable note. We all knew that feelings of loss were there, but could not get at them.

The discussion afterwards began with some sort of ill-humour, until it was suggested that the group could not mourn because the community, although present physically in the large group, was not perceived as a whole. The recent long holiday break had involved closure of the hospital for two weeks. The build-up to the perception of the whole acts as the fulcrum on which the balance of the community health depends. This significant perception of internal structure reflecting the community fragmentation galvanized the group, and the patient's crying was seen less as a result of persecution and more as a split-off piece of mourning of the community. It was a moving experience to see this process in action, and felt as if the engine of the community had started up again.

It is interesting to track down one significant event that helped us on our way from Figure 24.1 to Figure 24.3. As a result of continuous anonymous fire-raising, about which we were helpless, we, in desperation, asked a member of another department if he could use psychodrama techniques to elicit information about the fire-raising. This was a one-off event, but what actually happened on that occasion was an examination of the structuring and controlling within the community, tapping the patients' thoughts by the use of sculpting techniques; i.e., giving an ear to the lost thinking of the community. It was after this event that we were able to get back on to a saner path. It is interesting to note that sculpting techniques have been introduced into the programme very recently and only after the structuring of Figure 24.3 was realized. This provides us with some proof of the stage the community has reached.

Looking back to the days of Figure 24.1, what can be remembered is the sweat and blood that went into the restructuring of the community: whether the large group should be at the beginning or end of the day, or both; what work groups should do; whether the small groups should be once or five times a week. We even, on one occasion, closed the community for one morning in order that the staff could have a think-in. We struggled after structure in an effort to sort out our relationship difficulties because we knew that our survival and development lay in the structuring. But we were only tinkering with the system, playing the Hegelian demiurgos, out of touch with the community reality. We denied the community's capacity to create by its own structuring and controlling, because of our own need to control. Being in touch with reality in a therapeutic community has to do with conceding to the community its own capacity to think and create, through its capacity to structure. The real work is then for all members of the community to bring together associations, dreams, experience and interactions of the members, whether staff or patients, and translate them into thoughts and ideas about the whole community and not allow them to be dissipated. Inevitably, there must always be some dissipation for a multitude of reasons, including the difficulties intrinsic to the large group, so that the threat of a Figure 24.1 situation emerging must be an ever-constant danger. But, in general, in Figure 24.1 the staff used to think and structure later, where now our aim is to note the structuring and begin to think again.

261

Current issues

The authentic consultancy

I want to conclude on a point of contention but of great relevance in therapeutic communities, and especially those in the Health Service, by introducing the concept of the authentic consultancy. The arrangement as visualized in Figure 24.3 represents that kind of structuring which is more supportive of the capacity for development of a mentality consistent with mature thought, and here is the authentic consultancy of the therapeutic community. The authentic consultancy must be distinguished from the person of the actual consultant; the former is not about clinical responsibility.

The authentic consultancy is the abode of the thinking and consulting function of the therapeutic community and everyone contributes to it. The functioning of this consultancy depends on everyone consulting everyone else about the community affairs and out of these consultations creating thoughts and ideas about the community which will facilitate growth. The change from Figure 24.1 to 24.3 constitutes the move of the consultancy and thinking function from the consultant and staff and two patient representatives in Figure 24.1 to the community as a whole in Figure 24.3.

The consultant plays a special role in this transfer as he initially carries a full complement of projective investment of the consultancy and thinking function. His role must be to see to the re-investment of these functions.

The authentic consultancy and its effectiveness are expressed through that structural arrangement whereby the world of the community can be reflected by its members both staff and patient, and translated into thoughts about the community as a whole; development and management of the community rest on these important thoughts; executive action submits to the exigencies of authentic consultancy. The function of the actual consultant must be to ensure that this work is done.

Lest I fall into my own trap of becoming the Hegelian demiurgos, I would like to add that, although these are my interpretations of events, they also constitute part of the thinking of the community. This thinking has been fed back to staff and patients of the therapeutic community; it is part of the community mentality and I gratefully acknowledge the part played by the staff and patients of the Marlborough therapeutic community in the creation of these thoughts.

Acknowledgments

To Bob Hinshelwood for his encouragement and useful suggestions in the writing of this chapter.

262

25
Attempts at democracy

Anne Crozier

A person first entering a therapeutic community must be impressed by the novelty and strangeness of what goes on. In fact, for most people the experience is of overwhelming confusion, about where they fit in, and how it can possibly help to be there. Things take place as if on a stage, and it is hard to be involved in what often seems like petty bickering over trivialities, and fruitless arguments. But people find out about themselves and their place in the community by experimentation and expression, and democracy works rather as the little girl meant, who said, 'How can I know what I think until I see what I say?'

It is often very difficult for patients to say how they feel about community issues, especially in the large group. Many people are chary of becoming involved in a situation that binds them to accepting the will of the majority, especially where they disagree with it, as it seems like an infringement on personal liberty or even as an attack on their identity. Sometimes people do not feel that they 'belong' sufficiently to the community to take an active part, or they feel that it is threatening to do so. There is always a waxing and waning of interest and involvement in general community matters; people feel that certain issues do not interest or concern them. On the other hand, people sometimes become intensely emotional about otherwise objective or trivial issues. Democracy may seem to be the expression of the most powerful characters, and patients fear the domination of those who have more expertise in expression than they have. The staff are thus often seen ambivalently, as having more power in this respect; but also patients appreciate their ability to see more clearly what is going on. As the final vote which decides the outcome of an issue seems such a rough-shod, haphazard justice, it is often difficult to feel that the many aspects of the subject discussed have been taken into account. But if an issue has not been resolved by the discussion, it usually appears again in the agenda after a while, as in the case of the staff meeting (see below), which came up many times, over about a year and a half.

In this chapter I follow the evolution and development of certain changes which took place at the Marlborough Day Hospital between June 1975 and January 1977, as a result of discussion and democratic decision by the whole community, everyone having an equal vote. As a comparison I refer very briefly to the Paddington Day Hospital, and some events that took place there.

The staff meeting

When I first came to the Marlborough, the staff meeting was held in an upstairs room directly after the community meeting to discuss what had happened there. Two patient representatives were allowed to attend, and they related to the rest of us at lunch what had been discussed.

Patients were dissatisfied with this. We wanted to be able to attend the meeting itself. We were concerned about what the staff might be saying about us, and felt that either we were being torn apart, or that perhaps we were not important enough to be discussed at all. The presence of the two representatives did not alleviate these fears, as patients still did not know what 'really' happened.

There was a lot of discussion about it, and some of it was quite heated. We were challenged about our curiosity to know what was going on upstairs. Didn't the two representatives provide a safeguard against malice and slander? Did we not believe that the staff were only concerned for our welfare? The staff saw a proposal to open the meeting to all patients as bound to make their task almost impossible, and therefore bound to increase tension.

A vote was taken, and the majority was in favour of an open meeting that patients could attend. It was to be held within the large group, but with the staff drawn together into an 'inner circle' and the patients sitting outside in a wider concentric circle, although they were not allowed to speak. This form of meeting was introduced for a trial period of three months, after which it was to be discussed again. In the event the final decision on its adoption was postponed for several months more before it was accepted as a permanent change.

Many of the staff felt threatened by this arrangement. They thought that it greatly hampered their ability to be open with each other in that meeting, especially when there were difficult matters to discuss or when there were disagreements between members of staff. Some reacted by speaking philosophically or by using technical terms, as if to obscure and mystify what they were saying. One staff member even protested: 'I can't understand all that jargon!' Somebody remarked that now they were to be observed working, they must be seen to be working, and the open meeting prevented them from being too sloppy.

About six months after this form of meeting had been accepted as a permanent change, it was discussed again. The staff still found the situation difficult and felt ill at ease. One said she felt as exposed as in a 'shop window', with people sitting behind whom she could not see. They were resentful that what they said seemed to fall on empty ground: there was very little feedback from the patients as to how they felt about staff comments. Some complained bitterly about the frustration and difficulty they experienced, and wanted the meeting to go back upstairs.

Patients were certainly against a return to the old style. Many said it was tedious to discuss again something which had been accepted long ago. We appreciated the closer contact with the staff and the greater understanding of what they thought and how they worked. There was a sense of relief in realizing that what was discussed was the general issues of the community meeting and not the idiosyncrasies of individual patients. Although not everyone came, we valued being able to attend if we wished.

As patients were not allowed to speak at the meeting itself, any comments had to wait till the next day's community meeting, and by that time the issue had gone cold; there was fresh matter to be discussed and nobody liked digging over dead bones. To try to lessen staff paranoia, the community decided to let patients speak in the last ten minutes of the meeting.

This proved to be very restrictive of the natural flow of discussion, as a patient had to wait till the appointed time to speak on an issue that had already been discussed and passed over; or someone would forget about the time factor and interrupt anyway. It seemed stupid to restrict the meeting in this way, and after a while the time limit on patients' comments was dropped, at first tacitly and later by formal vote. From there it was a simple step to acknowledging that there was no point in having a special form for the meeting (i.e., staff withdrawing their chairs into an exclusive inner circle), and so the system of concentric circles was abandoned and the staff meeting became an open discussion for all present.

There were still many difficulties about this form of the meeting. There were always problems about differentiation in the content of the discussion. Often it seemed difficult to break away from the form of the community meeting, especially when things seemed only to have warmed up a bit towards the end, or when there was a great deal of urgent material to discuss that was hard to leave over to the next day. Some people said that patients dominated the discussion with irrelevant comments and did not give staff sufficient space to have their say. The staff constantly wanted to be able to get away from the patients for a time, to relax and be on their own. They said that the staff meeting should be their time, and it was a special privilege for patients to attend. Some proposals had been put forward which in retrospect seem ridiculous; e.g., to have two separate meetings in the same room, for patients and staff, or to have patients in the inner circle with staff outside, not speaking. (Other proposals were for staff to go upstairs as before, with patients 'having the opportunity' to go away and discuss the meeting on their own; or to open the meeting entirely to all present.)

In spite of the obvious wish and need of the staff, the patients almost unanimously voted to keep the meeting open, although they were not able to put forward many arguments in its favour (other than that they wanted to know what went on, or that it lessened feelings of paranoia), which further dissatisfied many of the staff, who had presented their case so much more forcefully. However, it is an 'injustice' of democracy that the community has to abide by the will of the majority and not necessarily follow the course which has most arguments in its favour. Thus the patients have more power in that they usually have more votes; but also they are not as well organized as the staff, who have greater experience and training in group therapy, and are able to exert considerable influence on the course of events. Patients are aware of needing a different way of seeing things, and although in this matter we wanted the open meeting in spite of staff opposition, nevertheless we tried to alleviate the stresses of the situation. Was it better to have everyone in the same circle so that we could be eye to eye with each other? Should we allow everyone to make comments at any time if they wished? Maybe the staff needed extra time alone upstairs to discuss the problems in the operation of the meetings.

Involvement of medical staff

One of the doctors was fond of remarking that therapeutic communities are often dominated by a 'charismatic medical figure' who, by influence or direct leadership, affects the way the community is run. Perhaps it is an ideal to hope that in any democracy everyone should have a voice as well as a vote: and in a community such as ours the difficulty is to find a public voice for a private disaster. Everyone seems to be so concerned with his own affairs that you feel that your voice is ignored in the ferocious chorus.

As a contrast to the struggles and developments described here, the changes that took place at the Paddington Day Hospital (*Guardian*, 25 June 1976; see note p. 271) were brought in by the consultant against the opposition of both patients and staff, as part of a policy to eliminate everything which he thought interfered with the practice of psychotherapy (including small groups, and other therapy and activity groups, also material facilities such as telephones). He tried to withdraw the provision of lunches and medical certificates and reimbursement of fares. All that was left was one large meeting a day where everything, even a request for medical certificates, was treated as a symptom to be analysed. I visited this institution in August 1976, and was appalled by the chaos of bitterness and frustration, and the resulting intolerance and indifference between staff and patients. Nobody listened to others' complaints or comments, or offered any interest or constructive suggestions. The large meeting was constantly interrupted by shouting and noise from outside, which was analysed and not dealt with, and by people wandering in and out as they pleased. Instead of feeling that the structure gave them support to take control of their own lives, and gain for themselves what they needed (a sense of being able to influence the course of events in the community by discussion and democratic vote), the patients felt that they were being used as 'guinea-pigs in some bizarre experiment,' (*Guardian*, 1976) 'to see how much suffering and frustration it was possible for anyone to bear', as one patient said. Their experience of community life there was the opposite of therapeutic: they were continually confronted with a state of absolute chaos they had no way of dealing with. I spent only one day at this community, and was too horrified by the experience to wish to repeat it. Dr Goodburn said in defence of his policy of withdrawal of facilities, 'Depressed people cannot take what really matters, i.e. psychotherapeutic help — when they are proffered things that are irrelevant and unnecessary.' (*Guardian*, 1976). But surely one needs to be treated as a whole person, with physical as well as psychological needs, and to treat only one aspect, in a community supposedly offering full-time day treatment, seems insulting to patients and contemptuous of their needs as human beings.

In a democratic community you don't expect the medical staff to dominate in this way. At the Marlborough, when the consultant was withdrawing from the Day Hospital, we discussed which meetings he was to attend. He decided that he wanted to go to business, admissions and policy meetings, and also to the patients' individual three-monthly reviews. We said he should stay out of the community altogether, rather than come irregularly and only to some meetings, and we objected particularly to his going to reviews, as he would not be able to keep effectively in touch with patients' progress, on account of the esoteric nature of the reviews. His appearance only at reviews could be extremely stressful to some patients, or else encourage fantasies that someone could come in from outside and sort everything out. He could much better be briefed by the small-group therapists as to the patients' progress. He then said that as consultant he had the right to attend what meetings he chose. We said that if he asserted his authority in that way there was obviously nothing we could do, except make it plain that we did not approve of his appearing in a part-time supervisory capacity. 'We're just keeping your job open for you,' someone remarked. However, he withdrew and agreed to attend only admissions and policy meetings.

Recently the consultant again wished to be part of the day community, but he had accepted much more readily the community's decisions about which meetings he should attend, and how often.

The patients' committee, Marlborough

An important development which took place was in the working of the patients' committee. It consisted of a representative from each small group, and one other person, who met each week to discuss the state of the community, and to compile a list of patients who needed special care or attention. This was discussed in the community meeting the next day. There were always problems with the committee: many patients found it difficult to commit themselves to it for a three-month period. Some people found it hard to discuss others when perhaps they felt themselves to be in so much need of help, or found it easy to talk about others but very difficult to mention themselves. The committee resented being put in the role of caring for others, writing to absentees, or recommending some strong action, when they did not get much support from the rest of the community. Also some patients resented being discussed by the committee behind closed doors. It is always easier to talk about people who are not present, and more difficult to say those things directly to them. The committee was hampered in its working especially when all members did not turn up for the meeting, leaving the rest to bear all the responsibility.

Why should they? The whole community should be responsible for those who needed special concern, or for making contact with errant members. The committee felt that the community made them do all the work, while at the same time often disagreeing with what they had done, or criticizing them for not mentioning a 'self-evident' case. Much of their concern was seen to be threatening or persecuting: 'What have I done to be brought up? You only want to have a go at me.'

It was proposed that the committee should be an open meeting in which all patients should participate, and they should all be responsible for suggesting those who needed special attention.

Some patients felt that this proposal merely demonstrated the ineffectiveness of the members of the committee, and thought that we should rather look for other representatives who would be willing to take the responsibility of caring and would be prepared to take strong action against lax attenders. The committee must be a strong backbone for the rest of the community.

It was very difficult to discuss this issue with the patients. There were several weeks of violent arguments with nobody seeing anyone else's point of view, and some people disrupting the meetings by walking out, feeling that the decision would be taken against them anyway, without their views being taken into account. Finally, the dissenters did not come at all, and although the handful of people who did come all agreed with the motion, we felt we could not push it through without more support from the community.

In the event, the change came about of necessity. The committee was much weakened by lack of attendance, and one or two small groups did not even have representatives. As only two members came to the committee meeting one evening, it was not held, and next day the concern meeting was open to all the community to discuss.

The programme

There had for a long time been arguments about the programme. Staff felt that there were too many therapy groups, the work was too intensive, and there was too little emphasis on the practical or creative side of people's lives. The occupational therapy staff were not using their practical skills and felt we ought to be doing regular work groups in pottery, sewing, woodwork, etc. There was too much sitting around talking, not enough doing, especially of practical things in groups, co-operating with other people. Patients, on the other hand, never attended work groups regularly: only when there was a specific project, e.g. making stuffed dolls for a bazaar, producing a magazine, etc., was anything done. We felt that it was 'useless work', doing something for the sake of it only, doing meaningless repetitive things which did not even constitute learning a skill (someone once asked that we should have classes in, for instance, German, and was told to go to an evening class). Work groups seemed only to emphasize the difference between ourselves and the staff, who had real work to do, were so busy they did not even have a proper lunch break, and patients who had nothing real to do, and were unable to get on with their lives.

So when the staff arrived with a large blackboard with a new programme written out, mostly worked out to suit availability of staff, but also including a great deal more occupational therapy, as well as two community lunches a week, there was an outcry. Most of the objections were about the community lunch: it was quite fun to produce a lunch every few months, but twice a week seemed too much like an attempt to make work for patients.

269

Staff gave as reasons for the lunches that we would be doing something useful for the whole community, that it would be an opportunity for staff and patients to meet socially, and it would provide staff with an excuse for a lunch break. We were not convinced. As it was, staff had no time for lunch; how many would really come, or do more than snatch a bite to eat? How much socializing can really take place between staff and patients, considering the difference in our social positions? It seemed artificial and patronizing.

Perhaps the main objection was to staff coming in with a prearranged scheme of 'what was good for us', which left us no room to say what we wanted. We could only say what we disliked about the proposed programme, instead of being able to discuss it from the beginning and make suggestions from our side. We were only able to be negative about it; the prepared timetable seemed to prevent any kind of discussion, and separated staff and patients into two opposing blocks. After a week or two of violent objections by patients and surprise and bewilderment on the part of staff, we realized that we would have to scrap the timetable and start from the beginning with a discussion of why they were dissatisfied with things as they were, why certain changes were needed, and how patients and staff felt about the proposed changes.

As this incident shows, any change which is brought in by one section of the community, without a discussion of how the other half feels about it, even if the form of the change is limited by practical considerations (such as hours that staff work and their availability), seems doomed to failure. One cannot help casting a glance at events at the Paddington, where the changes were brought in by the consultant without any discussion, and the staff as well as the patients had simply to accept many of his decisions, even where they disagreed, and no democratic vote was taken to indicate the wishes of the majority. The staff seemed to be reduced to merely 'doing their jobs', without being involved, and patients felt that they were being treated without consideration of their status as human beings. What seems ultimately so cruel in their position is that it is by having a say in how our lives are run, and particularly by being able to take some action to get what we want and need, to make our lives more tolerable, that we can take responsibility for ourselves and change our status from that of dependent mental patients to that of independent people able to run our own lives. Precisely this right was denied to the patients at the Paddington. They were made to feel like pawns in a game, becoming increasingly helpless to control their own lives, and unable to influence events or even have any relationships with others in the community. There were no 'common causes' that could link people together. Where one is denied the sense of being a real person with human needs, or where these needs are not recognized as real requests but as psychological requests only, one is continually thrown back into a state of chaos more extreme than any one could meet in the outside world. It becomes impossible to distinguish between realistic need and wants that others agree are reasonable, and the unreasonable or impossible ones no one can accept. It is never possible to go back to the beginning: one can only ever try to go forward, and that using what one has as given.

Conclusion

There are all sorts of difficulties in the operation of a community supposedly run on democratic lines. There are certain external limits that obviously have to be observed, things that are not practicable. It is impossible in a vote to take account of the feelings and points of view of everyone in the community, and therefore the solution often seems very unfair to some, who feel ignored and neglected. The discussion and decisions are a way in which people are involved in community life, and a means of expression through which we find out what we do think, and how it affects other people, and so an important way of achieving some personal development, and achieving an individual and independent way of being. It is necessary to take into account that other people feel differently, or see a situation differently, or want different things from it; and this increases awareness of other people as individuals, and the social responsibility one has towards them as members of the community. One has the opportunity of assessing what one can realistically and humanly expect of others, and what one has to concede to them. But there is all the difference in the world between the conflicts of discussion and sometimes violent arguments which we were involved in, and what was happening at the Paddington, where every attempt to deal with practical issues was frustrated by not seeing them as events in a real environment, but merely as symptoms of their own neurotic state, to be analysed without ever being dealt with practically.

Note: The unfortunate conditions at the Paddington Day Hospital, referred to above, ceased in 1976 (eds).

271

26

The management of boundary crossing

Angela Foster

Introduction

The aim of this chapter is to describe how two therapeutic communities have tackled the management of boundary crossing with special reference to the admission and discharge of their members. I shall draw from both sociological and psychological theories in an attempt to explain the process of management. Only by doing this is it possible to represent adequately the nature of the thought that members of therapeutic communities invest in the work of (a) providing treatment for patient members, and (b) creating and maintaining a social system that facilitates the psychotherapeutic process. The latter implies that the social system must be flexible if changing needs are to be met.

Boundary issues

The term boundary crossing is used sociologically to refer to an individual's transition from one social system to another. This process places a person in a crisis situation, which 'requires the learning of new sets and their integration into the ego, or the reorganization of the ego following the loss of old sets' (Cumming and Cumming, 1962). For patients in therapeutic communities the times of admission to the community and discharge from it are the most significant transition periods.

However, there are many other aspects of boundary crossing in therapeutic communities which need comment in order to give a more complete picture of the context in which discussions about admissions and discharge take place and the process by which management functions are carried out. Therapeutic communities vary according to their clientele, and this has a bearing on their approach to boundary issues. Some residential communities cater for people with delinquent or psychopathic tendencies, offering security and containment for their members;

this, in turn, means that strong group pressure can be exerted on members to change their behaviour. It usually follows that the social system in such communities is considerably different from that in the wider community; and that admission and discharge are traumatic periods when a person has to make large adjustments in his way of life. In contrast, members of day hospital or day centre therapeutic communities are expected to cross the boundary between the therapeutic community and the wider community daily, and to cope independently at weekends and public holidays. They may, or may not, have easy access to a hospital bed in times of crisis in a setting with which they are familiar. In these communities the difference between life inside and life outside is usually less striking, but problems surrounding the crossing of the boundary from one to the other are frequently brought to the community's attention.

More psychologically, the treatment process requires people to cross or not cross boundaries within themselves. People may be expected to express themselves in a way which they would not normally use, or even in ways that would be unacceptable outside the therapeutic setting; for example, to express previously repressed feelings in a cathartic exercise, thus breaking through psychological boundaries or defences. People may also be expected to develop tighter psychological boundaries; to contain their feelings more and not resort to manipulation or acting-out. They are required to adjust to these new wider or narrower boundaries of the community without overstepping them; to express themselves freely but refrain from physical violence.

One of the aims of therapeutic communities is to avoid through their social system the anti-therapeutic effects of institutionalization, the dehumanizing and de-skilling processes described by Goffman (1968) which reduce a person's ability to cope with life outside the institution. The four main characteristics of this social system are described by Rapoport (1960) as democratization, permissiveness, communalism and reality confrontation. A fifth, implicit in the other four, is the large group, the setting where all members of a community (staff and patients) come together and freely discuss issues that concern them. These measures encourage patients to maintain and develop their social skills and to exercise responsibility both for themselves and for the management of the community as a whole.

The large group is a concrete manifestation of the boundary of the community, open to all members, and closed (except on visitors' days) to non-members. It is in the large group setting that discussions about management issues concerning the community take place. Here thoughts and feelings can be shared by everyone concerned, discussed and, it is hoped, understood. Having reached this point, in relation to a specific issue, the community is in a position to act. I shall give examples from large-group discussions at the Marlborough therapeutic community.

The community can decide to maintain existing boundaries, perhaps by imposing these on an individual; e.g., by insisting that a person leave on his discharge date, though he may wish to stay; or by imposing sanctions on someone who has overstepped the boundaries; e.g., by suspending or discharging a person for physical violence. Alternatively, the community can initiate discussions to widen or tighten its boundaries; for example, by recognizing that there could be therapeutic reasons in a person's request to change small group – something previously unrecognized, or in deciding to impose new sanctions for bad attendance.

The discussion and clarification of boundary issues is such a common feature of large groups that members become skilled at working with them. Despite this, it is those boundary issues surrounding admission and discharge that often require more attention than they are given. It is regrettable that members can be expected to cross these boundaries with the minimum of support. Therapeutic communities can appear unconcerned about a newcomer or leaver, and yet be aware of a high drop-out rate among new members and a regression in those recently left after completing treatment. This 'blindness' is a defence against the insecurity experienced when a community's boundaries are stretched to let in new (unknown) people and to let out familiar people with whom one feels safe. Anger about this process can lead to denial of issues surrounding admission and discharge and a collusion in the fantasy that the community will go on indefinitely with the same population. It is not surprising that without support from the community individuals suffer; and in the long run the community itself suffers because, having lost sight of its purpose it becomes out of touch with reality, thus demonstrating a form of madness.

The residential community

When I was first appointed on the staff of a therapeutic community, I was asked to tackle this type of problem. It was a community for ex-drug addicts, and the issue was highlighted for me by one resident who had been in the community for over two years. He was respected by the community for his high level of competence in management and therapeutic situations within the community and was extremely well liked for his personal qualities. In spite of this, he suffered from intense fear and anxiety of going outside the community, even for an evening. The community appeared to be helping him with this but failed because of its investment in seeing him as a success on the one hand, and keeping him there on the other. This man was in a trap and the community had lost sight of one of its stated purposes, that of rehabilitation. It was sad that a community which could obviously do so much for people should fail to enable its members to live independently of it. While the social system in this therapeutic community was vastly different from that of a traditional mental hospital, the residents were becoming institutionalized; and crossing the boundary from the community to the outside world was confusing, disorientating, and as bizarre an experience for the individual as those Goffman describes.

I now want to describe some of the ways the therapeutic communities in which I have worked have used the community process in attempts to overcome difficulties relating to the periods of admission and discharge. In the community for ex-drug addicts, the dependence of long-stay residents was seen as the chief problem, but there was also a high drop-out rate among new residents. The culture of the community was so different from that of its surrounding community, that its members tended to split the two, idealizing the therapeutic community at the expense of the 'bad' outside world. In fact, the amount of effort and care that residents put into their community did tempt one to feel that life outside could never be so good.

At the time I joined, the management committee had just made several staff changes, prompting most of the residents to leave (although many re-applied and later returned). We were, therefore, in a position to build up the community, modifying admission procedures and treatment. Our task was to work out which policies were therapeutic in that they provided an extremely vulnerable group of people with the security and sanctuary they needed in order to cope with psychotherapeutic treatment, and which policies hindered both their treatment and rehabilitation.

Boundary crossing was described earlier in terms of learning new sets, or losing old sets of behaviour. Treatment and rehabilitation for ex-addicts involves an enormous amount of change at these points. A person newly off drugs coming into a therapeutic community is required to leave his whole way of life, and many changes have to be made immediately if the community is to remain a safe, drug-free place.

Thus, a certain amount of ritual about admission is useful, marking an intended change in life-style; but some of the existing policies seemed excessive, making admission more of a crisis than was necessary. Through discussion we discarded those policies, deciding that new residents should no longer automatically have their hair cut, give up personal possessions, or break contact with their families, girlfriends or boyfriends. We had special groups for new people when it was felt to be appropriate, and more senior residents spent time explaining and re-explaining the therapeutic community process to them. People were still searched to make sure they did not bring drugs into the house, and we maintained restrictions on their personal freedom in an effort to prevent them having access to drugs. People who have just stopped using drugs are strongly tempted to use them again in order to avoid painful emotional feelings; and the sense of failure and guilt, if this happens, becomes an added burden. For the same reason, prospective residents who were still using drugs could not visit the community before deciding whether they wished to come or not, so we took the community to them in the form of groups in hospitals and clinics run by staff and residents. We developed the same approach in prisons, and women from Holloway were allowed to visit the community before they were released.

The assessment of new residents included discussions about the appropriateness of admitting people in relation to the culture of the community at any given time. We found that despite having room for thirty residents, we were rarely able to keep more than twenty. It seemed that people felt crowded emotionally as well as physically if we were larger, so we lowered our quota. We noted, as did Rapoport, that in times of stress the community could not cope with new people, as they would tend to be the most vulnerable and therefore leave. We could contain only one or two borderline psychotic people at a time, and it was best to keep the sex ratio as equal as possible (this was difficult because we had fewer women referred and they tended to be more difficult to treat than the men).

Treatment policies included some degrading disciplinary methods. Communication at all levels often resembled indoctrination rather than open discussion, and personal freedom was more limited than seemed necessary. This situation made it difficult for some people to stay, and tended to promote the institutionalization of those who did. We attempted to become more flexible in approach, recognizing different individual needs with treatment plans and reviews, and we discussed and used a greater variety of therapeutic methods. One no longer had the impression that the community was forcing its members into a mould. In making these modifications we were constantly aware of the danger of becoming lax under the guise of being flexible. If the degree of sanctuary was high, and social demand low in terms of pressure to change, it was likely that the community would be considered a soft option and illegal drugs would be brought in. If this happened people would revert to their 'street' personalities, destroying the trust and honesty in the community which was highly valued and essential for the therapeutic process. Considerable authority was vested in the ex-addict staff members and senior residents as they were most in touch with this anxiety. It was significant that the impetus for change usually came from the staff, and the residents were often initially resistant to the suggestions. For these reasons the more harsh disciplinary policies were kept although rarely used.

Rapoport (1960) states that, 'A relevant distinction in differentiating aspects of the therapy programme would be between groups or activities that are primarily orientated to treatment goals, and groups that are primarily orientated to rehabilitation goals.' He is differentiating between goals of personality change and goals of social adaptation. This is something that it seemed important for our community to do, as previously it had lost sight of the rehabilitation goals and aspects of the therapy programme which would promote these. The community reduced the length of stay and treatment to nine months. This was not because ex-addicts only require nine months of psychotherapeutic help, but because to offer a longer time in residential treatment hinders their rehabilitation. We encouraged people to go out more throughout their periods of treatment; so they gradually became more independent of the community.

We planned a further three months in the community following the treatment period, where residents could live in a flat at the top of the house and make arrangements for future work or study. This period of their stay was called re-entry. We also set up a weekly evening group which people joined whilst in the re-entry stage and continued with for a while after they had left the community. It was described in this way:

> The group operates in three main areas. It can be supportive, enquiring or directive, depending on the needs at any one time. Moreover, its main function is to encourage the development of a cohesive re-entry peer group where mutual support and concern for each other is always present. To take a simple example, going out alone can be extremely threatening or depressing. Whereas to be part of a small group is not only more fun but also more relaxing, and so it becomes easier to make social contacts. There is considerable advantage in mixing pre-re-entry residents with re-entry in these groups. Those already in re-entry help others to be aware of the type of problems they'll be facing and ways of coping with these; whilst people in treatment can often remind those re-entering of parts of the Phoenix concept which they have overlooked, and which can be very helpful in the struggle to clarify problems or difficulties (Foster, 1973).

In spite of these changes, the leaving period was still the most difficult hurdle for the residents in this community, not least because of the specific problems facing ex-drug addicts. On leaving the therapeutic community, they are not going back to the world they left and, therefore, face a crisis situation where they have to build, often from scratch, their work life and social life. Going into the West End of London can be a frightening experience because they know exactly where they can find drugs, and old friends may even come up and offer them. Even

277

going to a party or a pub can give rise to difficulties, because of anxieties about replacing heroin with alcohol and becoming alcoholic.

In general, it did seem possible to modify the trauma of admission to the community, thus enabling people to settle in more easily, and to modify treatment in order to promote the aims of rehabilitation. It was also possible to make the rehabilitation process a more gradual one as, throughout their stay, people were working towards a time when they would be leaving. Nevertheless, this was a true crisis situation for every resident who left, and the most important thing we could do was to support them over this period.

The day community

A similar situation to that described at Phoenix House was experienced by the Marlborough therapeutic community a few years ago. Members were concerned about the difficulties patients had over leaving. This concern was especially centred on a group of patients who had recently been discharged, having spent up to three years in treatment. These ex-patients were spending a great deal of time on the premises of the therapeutic community and were seemingly unable to organize their lives in any other way. As patients leave the community to go home in the evenings and at weekends (except in times of crisis when they may be admitted to a bed in the hospital), such problems had not been anticipated. John and Elaine Cumming (1962) describe the stages of transition crisis in this way:

> The first reaction is a psychological and physical turmoil, including aimless activity or immobilization and disturbances of bodily mood, mental contact and intellectual functions. The second stage is characterized by a painful preoccupation with the past; and the third is a period of re-mobilization, security and adjustment.... All stages of response seem necessary for recovery or ego reorganization. If any stage is omitted the prognosis must be guarded.

These stages are those of a mourning process, and in this case it is the loss of the therapeutic community that is being mourned. It appeared that the people in question were stuck in the second phase and unable to progress into the third.

In an attempt to facilitate this progression I started a club one evening a week in a local community centre. The choice of location for any social group work is significant and in this case the physical movement from the hospital community to an outside community symbolized a future psychological movement. These ex-patients were depressed by their dependence on the hospital, and showed interest in the project. At the same time the current community patients, knowing that this group had an alternative venue for meetings, felt less guilty about their plight and were able to be firm about banning them from hospital premises. Thus the club was seen as a potential way out of a difficult situation both for the ex-patients and the therapeutic community, although it was not clear at this point why the club should succeed where years of psychotherapy had failed.

I undertook to be at the club each week but took no direct responsibility for its management or organization. The club went through three stages, the first being typical of the formation of any social group. Gradually the ex-patients organized themselves, negotiating with the people at the community centre, planning membership, ensuring that sufficient people were there each week to cover the required payments. The middle stage was when the club was most effective as a club with a consistent group of people attending weekly. They worked to make the room more comfortable, assessing their needs and organizing themselves to meet these. Some members helped to run the centre by undertaking voluntary office work in the evenings. Through developing the club many members began to recognize that they had abilities which could enable them to be more independent of the hospital. In contrast, we all became increasingly aware of those members with chronic dependence problems. This was most obvious through dependence on alcohol; and when the group restricted the amount of drinking in the community centre because of anxiety about this leading to violent outbursts, one member in particular began to spend most of his time in the pub over the road. This stage was, therefore, characterized by the emergence of social skills and social problems.

The third stage was when those who felt able to get work and plan their social lives became increasingly independent of the group, while those whose difficulties had become more apparent began to discuss these, sometimes seeking me out individually for this purpose. Much of the concern was focused on a core group of three, two of whom felt able to do some part-time work but were anxious that if they did this the third person (the man with the greatest drink problem) would feel abandoned and might kill himself. This anxiety was an illustration of the amount of pressure these three put on each other to conform to the norms of their sub-group. The destructiveness in this situation was recognized by the group and by other friends in the club.

Originally all these people had been on my case load for supportive social work, but as the club became a setting for mutual support and individual needs of its members became clearer I was able to redefine my contracts with them. I discharged most people. This gave me time at the hospital to see a few individually for further therapeutic help; for example, I saw the man with the drink problem weekly for a limited period of time. This provided him with extra help and attention which he felt he needed, and relieved the others of some of the burden they felt they had been carrying.

Although initially no time limit had been imposed on the duration of this club it finished after a year, indicating, I think, not its failure but its success. The club had served its function, which had been to enable this group of people to complete the mourning process involved in leaving the hospital and to organize their own lives. Necessary changes in attitude had occurred both in the hospital and within the club group, making this development possible. The hospital no longer offered in-definite support, either in the form of a place to 'hang out' or in un-limited social work time. We realized that these had not been supports at all, but part of a collusion with the patients in the assumption that life without the possibility of coming to hospital at any time was too difficult for them to cope with. The community had both been over-protective of its members and doubting of its ability to treat and re-habilitate people effectively. The club members, on the other hand, recognized through the club that they had skills which could be put to use in improving their lives. Despite the fact that many of these people still felt unlimited in what they were able to do, and continued to live rather impoverished lives, their self-respect had increased.

During this time members of the therapeutic community had been concerned that future leavers should not face similar difficulties. It was decided that the average length of stay should be about a year, and that patients would be made aware of this when they came for their assess-ment interview. Each patient is expected to name his leaving date, which he does well in advance, providing himself and the community with a boundary to work towards that can be altered nearer the time if there is good reason for doing this. The community also decided to have a leavers' group. This was poorly supported in its early stages, indicating the reluctance of the community to face leaving. However, as leaving became recognized as an integral part of treatment, through the discussion of leaving dates and feedback from the leavers' group into the community meetings, this group became well-supported and effec-tive. Later the group continued well but feedback and discussion about leaving decreased in the community. When members of small groups (which meet three times a week) became concerned that individuals about to leave were not discussing their feelings we realized we had again been denying issues surrounding leaving, this time by splitting them off into the leavers' group. We wondered whether the existence of a leavers' group encouraged this sort of split to develop, and considered closing the group. In fact, we have continued with the group for two reasons: it is useful to have a separate setting to discuss the practical aspects of leaving such as plans for jobs, or courses of study or training; and it is important to support people through the mourning process for a short period after leaving. However, considerable discussion now takes place in the community about the feelings of members who are leaving and the feelings of those who are being left. In addition to these discussions, someone's leaving day is recognized by the preparation of a special tea and the giving of cards. More formally, discharge forms are made out summarizing a patient's treatment in the community, and copies of these go to the patient, his referrer and GP. These are prepared by staff, ideally before patients leave, so that they are encouraged to arrive at personal assessments of their time in the therapeutic community and to sort out any discrepancies between their views and those of their therapists.

The relationship between the leavers' group and the community is an interesting one, which can be explained in terms of Gestalt psychology. If healthy development is to occur an individual must identify his current need, act on it, and then assimilate this process back into his whole personality. The assimilation phase is perhaps the most important one, as without this process one tends to create rather than heal splits. If we take the community as the whole one can see that the need to help people over leaving was thrown into the foreground and recognized (initially by the dependent group of ex-patients), and measures were taken to cope with the need in terms of the club and the leavers' group. But it was only when the leavers' group was assimilated into the community and not split off that the problems were really being dealt with and the community could develop healthily in this area, enabling individual members to do the same.

The management of admissions, unlike that of discharge, has interested the Marlborough patients only recently. This seems strange as all patients (unlike staff) have first-hand experience of the procedures involved: indeed, when attendance is poor, the whole community discusses problems of crossing the boundary in. One of the assumptions of Gestalt psychology is that the 'whole determines the parts' (Perls *et al.*, 1973), indicating the importance of examining the relationship between community meetings and sub-groups within the structure. For further discussion of this see Hinshelwood and Grunberg, Chapter 23 of this book. It is useful to comment briefly on developments that have taken place in the relationship between the staff and patient groups within the community, as patients' involvement in the admissions meetings arose out of these developments.

Community meetings are held for one hour at the beginning of each day. After this there used to be a staff meeting with two patient representatives where the community meeting was discussed. The structure was such that the patient representatives had no time to assess the opinions of those they were representing or to feed back to them. Consequently, most patients found this role difficult. Moreover, it seemed that we had created a split between the community meeting itself and the understanding of the community meeting, the latter being the task of the staff and two role-confused patients. We discussed this situation at length in business meetings and eventually arrived at a structure where the community meeting is discussed in the following half hour by the large group as a whole. In breaking down the false and anti-therapeutic aspects of the boundary between staff and patients (which split off understanding from feelings, investing the former in staff and the latter in patients) we have begun to share our experiences and skills more openly (Grunberg, Chapter 24). We are working on real boundary issues between the two groups as they arise, clarifying roles and defining areas of responsibility. It is significant that as soon as this change occurred patients wanted to take on more tasks concerned with management of the community; and the admissions meeting was made open to everyone.

This inevitably led to further changes. The admission procedure had involved an individual interview for assessment with a member of staff and an informal visit to the community. The applicant was discussed and a decision regarding admission reached in the admission meeting where, it was hoped, the patients' representative was someone who had met the applicant. The new member was introduced into the community meeting on his first day and would start his small group the following week, or possibly later if he had difficulties in attending other meetings.

Through the open admissions meeting problems in this procedure have emerged, and been discussed. Our first problem was that of confidentiality. We developed the following system, which enables us to work in the way we have decided is best for us without undermining the prospective patients' rights or upsetting referrers. Referral letters go only to staff members, who still do the initial assessments. If considered suitable, applicants are asked if they want to continue with their applications after this interview. If they do, they are told (a) that their names will be given to the community in order that a visit can be arranged, and (b) if after this second visit they wish to join the community then the content of their interview (not the referral letter) will be shared with the community, in the admissions meeting along with the opinions formed by others who met them. This community group then decides whether or not this person may join. It is useful to consider new members in the light of the existing state of the community. We may decide not to admit very disturbed people if the general feeling is one of insecurity; or we may ask people to wait, sometimes deciding that it is better both for new people and the community if they start in twos or threes.

Most change has occurred over admission to small groups. When patients became involved in the allocation of prospective patients to small groups they asked what criteria the staff had formerly used. This led into a discussion about what criteria should be used. We decided that if we were aiming to select on personality grounds we should do this when the new person had already started, so that we would know this person better and he would have the benefit of the discussion. This proved to be an uneasy experience, where the disadvantages seemed to outweigh the advantages; so this policy was quickly changed. Instead, we decided that our main consideration would be which groups needed new members and whether they needed men or women, as we aim to keep the sex ratios as equal as possible. In addition to this, if any people in the community felt that they would like this person in their group then this was noted.

New patients began questioning why they were not allowed to join their small groups immediately. Our superficial reason was that they should settle into other groups first, but this did not stand up to scrutiny. It seemed that staff and patients had been colluding to keep new people out of these rather 'sacred' groups. New patients had sensed this and felt excluded. We, therefore, decided that people should join their small groups on their first day. Later people began to say how difficult it was to come straight into the community meeting on one's first morning, and it was proposed that people should start with their small group. We wondered if by allowing new patients to identify first with their small group we would be hindering the development of their identification with the community as a whole. We could not answer this question, so decided to accept the proposal for a trial period and assess the effect of it on the community. Thus, problems surrounding the crossing of the boundary from the outside community to the therapeutic community on admission were left unexplored until the community as a whole was sufficiently integrated to allow these to emerge, and within the present structure problems continue to emerge: 'In health the figure and ground is in process of permanent but meaningful emerging and receding' (Perls *et al.*, 1973).

A further development between groups in the community which has influenced our work on crossing the boundaries of admission and discharge has been the annual introduction of a group of patients just for the summer months (Hinshelwood and Foster, 1978; Foster, 1976). Each year the community is involved in the assessment of people for this group and the planning of their treatment programme. The advantage of having a complete small group start at the same time is that issues surrounding admission are highlighted. Similarly, issues surrounding discharge are central in community meetings around the time the student group leaves. The relationship between this group of short-term patients and the longer-staying members of the community is often intense. The time boundary on the short-term group creates in them a sense of urgency, which is transmitted into community meetings where problems between this group and the community are brought to the fore and worked on. Consequently, by the end of their stay, this group of people are usually well integrated into the community as a whole. This type of interaction, facilitating as it does the identification of conflicts, their resolution and assimilation, promotes healthy development of the community in many ways. These annual student groups, through their eagerness to take from the community, have given a lot.

It is difficult to conclude a chapter that is essentially about ongoing experiences, but I hope the description of changes made by these two communities may be of help to others struggling with problems of boundary crossing in the areas of admission and discharge. I also want to stress that the essence of a therapeutic community is the process by which management functions are carried out, not the specific structures or policies that are created. Participation in this process, which encourages members to take responsibility for problem-solving within the community, also helps them in coping with personal crises such as those of transition from one social system to another which are experienced throughout life, not just during periods of admission to, or discharge from, a therapeutic community.

Section G
Research

In this final section we consider the difficulties of setting about systematic reflection on the processes within and effectiveness of therapeutic community work. The therapeutic community movement began as an experiment. In the early years research was a fundamental part of the whole approach. With the passing of time, despite a commitment to careful self-reflection, therapeutic communities have tended to become both defensive of their new 'faith' and perhaps self-satisfied that their ideas are sufficiently developed.

The three chapters in this section argue initially the case for doing research (Chapter 27), and then discuss some of the simpler questions which can usefully be posed and answered (Chapter 28). Finally, Chapter 29 tackles the more fundamental methodological difficulties which need to be confronted before any adequate evaluation of the effectiveness of therapeutic community work can be gained.

Research was not split off as a separate activity in the early years. Today, with the growing specialization of such activity, the research worker is all too often an outsider, a stranger, a threat. However, therapeutic communities offer a good opportunity to repair this split; the opportunity for practitioners to think about their work, and for research workers to help to meet the needs of the community rather than their own career and publishing expectations.

27

The politics of survival: the role of research in the therapeutic community*

Nick Manning

This chapter is concerned with the processes surrounding the survival of therapeutic communities, and in particular with the role of research in those processes. I have discussed at length elsewhere (Manning, 1976a) some of the characteristics that the development of therapeutic communities has shared with scientific innovations and social movements. In the course of my investigations, I became increasingly aware of the structural life-span of such movements (I say structural as opposed to chronological, for a similar structure may be travelled in several months or a century). Indeed, this has been well documented: There is the early phase of dynamic innovation, often attributable to a few and even only one person's enthusiasm. This is followed, if development is to take place, by wider acceptance of the idea. In other words, the innovation must receive positive selection and support by a wider social group. Finally, the innovation reaches a point at which it becomes widespread and routinized (Dawson and Gettys, 1948; King, 1956; Smelser, 1962; Wilkinson, 1971). At this stage bureaucratic and systematic application supersedes innovation as the main goal; or, as Max Weber put it, this is the 'routinization of charisma' (Weber, 1948).

But this general pattern may take almost any length of time. What I would like to consider here are some of the processes which appear to affect the speed at which this structural life-span is travelled, how far and how quickly we would like to proceed, and the role of research in this. We have then three crucial points for consideration: initial innovation, wider selection and support, routinization and application. Various social and political processes can be identified in this life-span which affect the relevance and significance of research.

*Paper read at the Richmond Fellowship 2nd International Conference on 'the Politics of Therapeutic Communities', Washington, DC, August 1976.

Innovation

There has been considerable debate amongst sociologists and philosophers of science as to the nature of innovation (Kuhn, 1962; Medawar, 1969; Merton, 1968; Mulkay, 1972). Without referring to this debate in detail, we can illustrate how the way in which an idea is born can affect its ultimate fate. In this case we find that the therapeutic community was 'invented' simultaneously in two different places, unknown to each other, during the Second World War in Britain. (It is not disputed that considerable advances had been made earlier on ideas of milieu therapy in the USA (Myerson, 1939).)

On the one hand, it was invented by the Tavistock Clinic as a by-product of their investigations into group relations, personal selection, job placement, the promotion of health education and training, and even psychological warfare! (Dicks, 1970; Rees, 1945). In a sense it never 'stood out' as anything special in this collection of developments, and after the war seemed to become, in the hands of analytic Tavistock staff at the Cassel Hospital, subservient to Freudian analysis as the main therapeutic device. Tom Main led this development, becoming Director of the Cassel Hospital in 1946.

On the other hand Maxwell Jones, a research-trained, clinically oriented psychiatrist, also hit on this new approach, but without the aid (or perhaps distractions) of a social scientific 'Weltanschauung'. As a result he could concentrate on a method which his research training indicated worked most effectively without being side-tracked into generating other social psychological innovations. After the war Maxwell Jones did not slide back into a more trusted approach, but in an open-minded manner pressed ahead, and through not inconsiderable personal drive managed to push his idea through to stage two of our development structure, by getting wider institutional and, crucially, financial support at Belmont Hospital in 1947 (Jones, 1952).

In this first phase of innovation, we can see that both inventions occurred in the early part of the Second World War, and had attracted wider support within five to six years. Despite the caveat above about structural life-spans, this period would seem to be a typical lapse of time for a mental health innovation, after which without support it might well become forgotten. What were the roles of research and in particular the use of research as a political bargaining counter, at this time? It is clear from the literature (Bion, 1961; Kraupl Taylor, 1958; Jones, 1952) that research activity was a vital source of information about the effectiveness of this method — the primary function of research; but it is also clear that research results were an important source of legitimation and status for both of these independent innovations — a secondary function of research. For example, on the Tavistock side,

Bion's experimental intervention in Northfield Military Hospital from which later ideas developed was explicitly designed as research, and not as merely administrative change. More significantly both he (Bion and Rickman, 1943) and Tom Main (Main, 1946) published their findings at about this time, which increased support for their ideas.

Maxwell Jones also used research techniques. Although he invented the therapeutic community intuitively, he soon attempted to establish its efficacy, as he had been trained to do. And it is evident from his first book (Jones, 1952) that the results of his work were important for gaining wider institutional support: first at Dartford Hospital in 1945-6, and subsequently at Belmont Hospital (where, incidentally, its successor Henderson Hospital still thrives).

To summarize at this point: the structural movement from initial innovation to wider support, such as happened for the therapeutic community and must happen for any mental health innovation, is also likely to take a roughly standard length of time for this stage of development — five years. And the most crucial factor in this development is the demonstration through research that the method is effective. Hence research activity enters into this development in a vital way, to provide evidence and status that the new method works. But, of course, wider support in this case merely means financial and other resources being available to continue the work in one or two places. What sort of processes govern the development from this point to widespread routinization and application?

Wider support and routinization

If this new method were a drug, we would expect from studies of the diffusion of new drugs (Coleman *et al.*, 1957) that a demonstration of effectiveness would almost automatically result in widespread usage, subject to resource limitations. But for the therapeutic community these resources and other qualifications are more significant: application of therapeutic community techniques is not widespread even after thirty years. What are some of the factors which have limited the wider use of therapeutic community techniques?

First, therapeutic communities usually require above-average resources per patient or resident. They require: more staff; higher-quality staff; more space with suitable facilities for work activities and group meetings; etc. This immediately provokes the question 'what do we get for these additional resources?' And inevitably research is demanded to prove that resources pay off through better output.

Second, therapeutic communities, as are many new innovations, are weak in the face of powerful established positions. Initially they overcame this problem through having highly dynamic, charismatic leaders (and many still do). But this situation is unstable; leaders move on. The only way out is to gain status and therefore power by becoming professionally respectable; or to demonstrate in the language of the establishment (i.e. through research) that therapeutic communities deserve support because they are effective. Unfortunately, becoming professionally respectable is as unsatisfactory a solution as charismatic leadership, either because it distorts the therapeutic process (Manning, 1976b), or again because professionally acceptable personnel move on. A further alternative is to engage in collective action and fight a purely political battle for resources, as the Paddington Day Hospital did in London a few years ago. But this is not possible unless the therapeutic community is established in an organization which has resources available (like the British National Health Service), and may well be a tactic from which even radical therapists will shrink. The result of these difficulties is that once again research is looked to as the way out and forward in the struggle for recognition.

Third, we can turn to the culture of the therapeutic community as a hindrance to wider acceptance. As you know, Rapoport outlined the basic themes of democracy, permissiveness, and communality in which confrontation could flourish. I hardly need point out that these cultural themes contrast markedly with those of the conventional professional community, and thus have resulted in many professionals merely expressing sympathy with the ideas while politely declining to work in a therapeutic community. But if we look a little closer at the culture we find that self-examination and criticism are an essential ingredient. Indeed, as I have argued (Manning, 1976b), research was a central part of the early innovations, not just an activity grafted on to the side. And it is just this interest in research which can provide a cultural bridge to the more conventional professional establishment, who, like it or not, have an enormous influence over the distribution of resources, power and culture in this area of mental health.

Now, we can see where the argument is leading. On the one hand there is a much slower development from stage two (wider support) to stage three (widespread application), than from stages one to two (as I have argued at length elsewhere (Manning, 1976c)); and on the other hand research activity has played an important role in this differential rate of development. In the early stage it enabled the initial innovation to gain further support, but since then it has been less popular amongst therapeutic community practitioners — to their disadvantage; for each of the three areas of hindrance for expansion (resources, power and culture) could be helped through greater research activity.

Research in the therapeutic community

To understand this relative decline in the use of research we must look not only at the internal development of therapeutic communities, but also their relations with the outside world, especially the psychiatric arena in which many of them are embedded.

As far as the outside world is concerned, the therapeutic community has come under increasing pressure to change from an experiment to a conventional treatment alternative: that is to say, from 'innovation' to 'delivering the goods' in terms of patient treatment and improvement. This pressure is quite normal in that any new development is given a certain amount of licence to begin with, but after a while, in order to continue to attract interest and funds, and in general to remain viable, the innovation has to provide in some way a technically applicable product. Now, of course, this involves insidious invitations to forsake pressures for wide change which the therapeutic community implied, and to come under the wing of conventional psychiatry, as yet another specific treatment alternative. However, the point here is that experimental credit in a sense runs out.

Internally, the therapeutic community also developed away from research. Despite the early experimental approach, it was very tempting after a number of years to feel that the major idea was worked out. There was a tendency to move therefore from asking 'what ideas can we use here?' to proselytizing a finished set of ideas to those who had not yet heard the message. There was thus a move from innovation itself to the spreading of that innovation, already accomplished.

These changes, internally and externally, can be recognized clearly in the appointment in the late 1950s of a team of research workers from outside the therapeutic community to study what is now the Henderson Hospital. This arrangement epitomizes on the one hand the split between experimental and applied therapy demanded by the outside world (i.e., the unit no longer does research, it does therapy and therefore outside research workers must come in to do research); and on the other hand the internal change from asking 'How can we develop our ideas?', to asking 'We have our ideas and method already, how can we improve the application and wider use of these ideas?'

Given these changes, one may as well ask 'Well, this split is unfortunate, but has research in such a climate been useful?' One answer is to look at the impact of that research team's work, culminating in the book *Community as Doctor* by Rapoport (1960). Rapoport and I have been looking into this question, and have identified some of the social processes surrounding the reception of his book. By looking at book reviews and questioning relevant individuals, we have identified three major processes, and several more diffuse reactions.

291

The three major ones are rejection, implicit acceptance and reincorporation. These refer to Henderson Hospital's reactions. At first the book was rejected. Although this was partly due to the director, it fits in with the usual reaction to outside research reports. Implicit acceptance, however, was occurring simultaneously amongst more junior staff members. Thus, the second senior doctor used the book for the reason that its results were a very useful way of tackling some of the problems of translating ideals into practice in the hospital. Significantly, it was not until the director changed that full reincorporation could happen amongst a staff group less clearly associated with the original research period. The rejection process seems to have been a defence against anticipated threatening criticism, amplified by the deep commitment of staff, compounded for newer staff by the lack of personal contact with the research workers and therefore any confidence or support derived from this. Reincorporation on the other hand could occur only after a period of time had clearly elapsed, so that the book took on a more academic and less personal relationship with the hospital.

The lesson from this could be that one has always to wait for five years or so before research findings can be accepted. But this would be patently absurd, for the vitality of research work is surely bound up with its rapid feedback and use in developing further the practical work it has studied. There is, however, a more fundamental lesson to be learned. It is that the early splitting of the therapeutic community and research activity must be repaired. This split between practice and research activities, between systematic study from the outside and haphazard reflection on the inside, is, I suggest, the chief source of hostility towards research workers.

Thus Rapoport and I have summed up this issue in five maxims, which I will quote from our paper (Manning and Rapoport, 1976, p. 467):

1 The utilization and diffusion of social research are sensitive to different but interrelated processes.

2 The chances that there will be direct utilization by subjects of an applied research study will be enhanced if the research formulation is collaboratively arrived at, and the research results are fed back interactively.

3 If, for any reason, collaborative formulation and interactive feedback are incompletely achieved, a defensive *rejection phenomenon* may be expected.

4 Overt rejection does not preclude covert acceptance of many aspects of the research, particularly if there are mediating individuals in the action group.

5 Diffusion of the research on a broader basis may bring about a re-incorporation process within the action group at a later date, achieving a greater degree of ultimate utilization.

To summarize so far: many therapeutic communities have abandoned the research orientation which was a central part of their early development, and as a consequence have had less influence within the mental health field than they might have done, since research results appear to be one way of overcoming three important sources of hindrance to wider influence: shortage of resources, lack of power, and an unacceptable culture. The reason for abandoning research has been due both to external pressure to concentrate on providing a regular service, and to internal self-satisfaction that the basic idea had been sufficiently developed.

What is research?

But much of this discussion begs the question of quite what research is and can do, before it can be used as a political lever in the struggle for survival of therapeutic communities. It is quite apparent that therapeutic community practitioners have very ambivalent feelings about research. Those who perceive it as external to their 'real work', as I have suggested has become more common, tend to feel threatened, exposed; they often counter-attack by claiming that research is not sensitive enough, that it meets only the interests of research workers, and so on. There are also those who perceive research as the opposite: a kind of magic which if it can only be made to work will reveal clearly not only how to resolve chronic conflicts and problems, but also how to advance to greater heights. The image of the sorcerer's apprentice springs to mind: therapeutic community practitioners seeking to ease their work by recourse to the master's magic books.

But neither of these positions is fruitful. More useful are those who, like the earlier pioneers, saw themselves as engaged in a process of research about their community and its members (Jones, 1952; Lewis, 1952; Wiles, 1949), just as psychotherapy can be a joint process of research into the individual patient by both patient and therapist. From this point of view, research can become a joint participative exercise — sometimes with the aid of an expert, but not necessarily — whereby problems which the community wishes to resolve can be tackled, but without a naive faith that the solution, if it be found, will be easy.

Perhaps the most crucial step is the first: what is the question for which an answer is sought? For many people, both therapeutic community workers and interested outsiders, this question is 'Does it work?'

A simple enough request, one might think! But is this question being asked in the right way, so that it can be answered; and if it is appropriate what techniques can we use to find that answer?

Quite frankly, those of us who do research agree at least on one thing: that such a question cannot be answered in that form. The reason is simple. Therapeutic communities have more than one and often conflicting goals and activities: treatment versus rehabilitation, permissiveness versus democracy, insight versus adjustment, survival in the real world versus an ideal culture, professional intervention versus patients as therapists, psychotherapy versus sociotherapy, non-verbal versus verbal modes of therapy, etc. For this reason Paul has restated such a question more precisely as:

> *Which* treatment, by *whom*, is the most effective for *this* individual with *that* specific problem, under *which* set of circumstances? (Paul, 1967).

In other words, we must be much more precise about the questions which we wish research work to answer; and therefore such work will begin to take a more disjointed, bitty, messy style than a clean, clear-cut evaluation of the type: is drug X better than drug Y? (See Chapter 29 for an extended discussion.)

Perhaps it is worth while at this point to review the different types of research we could use. Cherns (1972) has suggested a fourfold typology:

1 Pure basic research (e.g. sociology of innovation).

2 Basic objective research (e.g. leadership and therapeutic communities).

3 Operational research ⎱ (e.g. the relative impact of specific groups
4 Action research ⎰ in a therapeutic community).

This ranges fairly obviously from research into problems determined purely by academic criteria, such as the sociology of innovation, to research into specific problems associated with ongoing practical work; for example, the therapeutic effectiveness of certain types of group activity within the weekly programme of a therapeutic community. We would choose our research according to the problems we wished to tackle, and neither pure nor basic research is more politically useful to a therapeutic community in itself, except in so far as the style of feeding back research results varies. Thus the first type uses academic journals; the second, professional journals; the third, administrators in the organization; and the fourth is a continuous feedback directly into the social situation under observation. Very broadly, the time taken for results to come back into a therapeutic community is longest for pure research, and shortest for action research. Thus, as far as the survival of a therapeutic community is concerned, the third and fourth types are most relevant, depending on the specific problem to hand.

But research personnel may often prefer to do 'purer' research, since this will enhance their academic and professional status and their personal careers. Thus, even though they tackle a problem seen as significant by both themselves and the therapeutic community, they may well approach it with a very different frame of reference, as Rapoport and I have noted in Henderson Hospital in the 1950s (Manning and Rapoport, 1976).

Having settled on an appropriate set of questions, the carrying out of research then becomes a more technical matter, which is pursued in Chapters 28 and 29. Rather we can skip here from this first crucial step to the last crucial step of using research results once we have them, particularly with regard to furthering the interests of a therapeutic community.

I must hasten to note that the real world is not always a totally rational one, and that research evidence will not necessarily smooth the path of political conflict. But in my experience the call for evidence of the effectiveness of therapeutic community activities is made time and time again by those to whom we have to turn for resources. For example, the Henderson Hospital in London has recently been threatened with closure unless it can produce positive evidence of its therapeutic success. This has arisen as a result of the 1974 National Health Service reorganization and the resulting emphasis on cost effectiveness, planning and review, and so on. Unfortunately the administrative authority has tended to pose the question in the simple form which I have just criticized. However, the important point is that, even with this most famous of therapeutic communities, evaluative research activity has been made a definite condition of continued financial support. Significantly, the emphasis has been more on doing the research than on what the results are; and this may be an important political use of research activity besides the use it may have in actually being applied to improve therapeutic results.

This is to reiterate an earlier point here, that research activity may enhance the status of a therapeutic community and hence be a vital ingredient in the battle for survival. Unfortunately, as is known only too well, it is dangerous to have to use outside professional personnel to enhance status, for they inevitably wish to impose their own styles, standards and techniques. But we are caught in yet another contradiction here, for to reject such help may mean you threaten the community's existence literally; yet to accept it may in the long run also threaten its existence in its present form. We must educate the research worker as much as he must help us to formulate questions which can be answered.

Having argued for the place of research in the survival of therapeutic communities in the first part of this chapter, and having all too briefly mentioned some of the issues surrounding the actual use of research in the second part (particularly the need for careful partnership between research activity and community activity — though preferably the two should not be split), I will conclude with an advertisement! It is that the Association of Therapeutic Communities in Britain has a research group, which meets regularly to discuss research issues and hear papers. For those who don't know this Association, it contains most major therapeutic communities in Britain. Contact can be made through the editors of this book.

28
Thinking about research in a therapeutic community

David Kennard

I am going to attempt to say something about what is involved in carrying out research, especially in thinking it out, and how this relates to questions which are relevant to therapeutic communities. In doing this I shall also be exploring these things for myself, for although I have been involved in research for some years I still find myself puzzling over these issues.

Therapeutic community staff, and for that matter patients, may have a variety of attitudes towards research. Three fairly common ones seem to be: (1) that it will eventually tell us whether therapeutic communities work or not; (2) that it cannot tell us anything helpful since there are far too many factors involved for anyone to understand properly; and (3) that it is ethically unacceptable, an impersonal, mechanical way of approaching people.

In answer to the last of these points, it is certainly true that any activity can become impersonal, whether research or therapy. However, research basically involves posing questions and trying to answer them, which we do all the time in our own lives, with other staff members and with patients. For example, when we try to get someone to adopt a realistic goal for themselves, we are trying to get them to ask questions which are capable of being answered, rather than dreaming of impossible goals or alternatively assuming that all the answers are foregone conclusions. Research similarly involves cutting questions down to size.

The problem with the other two attitudes is that a question like 'do therapeutic communities work?' is not capable of being answered as it stands; while the inclination to dismiss research completely as not being of practical use assumes that we are only interested in answers which reveal ultimate truths rather than piecemeal information. In our daily work we have to put up with much that is imperfect and unfortunately the same seems to be true of research. However, between them the two positions in fact define the limits within which any research must operate: balancing what is feasible to ask against what is important to ask.

When I said that the question 'Do therapeutic communities work?' was not answerable as it stood, this was because it assumes that we already know certain things, such as what is or is not a therapeutic community, which are in fact questions in themselves. It assumes that we know or agree what it means when we say something works. It also assumes more implicitly that whether a therapeutic community does work is unrelated to whom it is meant to be working for.

These three things – how we define our therapeutic community; how we define successful working; and how we describe the community's clientele – are all things which will vary in many ways and which will affect the answer to a question on the effectiveness of therapeutic communities. I shall try to list some of the actual possibilities that these three sources of variation introduce.

To begin with the patients: the question here basically is, does a therapeutic community work better for some patients than others? If we think the answer to this question is yes, or maybe, then we need to ask what characteristics are likely to be the most important ones. Is it the patient's age or sex, is it the type of illness or disorder that we consider him to be suffering from, is it his social class or the position he holds in his work or his family environment, is it something to do with his personality, his attitudes towards himself and his illness, or the attitudes that other people in his life have towards him? All of these things seem to be possible sources of influence when exploring the effectiveness of the therapeutic community approach for any individual patient or group of patients.

Moving on to the therapeutic community itself or the treatment environment, the basic question here seems to be: how we should define the treatment; how we should distinguish between different therapeutic communities and between a therapeutic community unit and any other kind of unit. The following variables seem to be important: (1) the size of the unit and the number of staff in it; (2) the range of treatments provided (for example, where therapeutic community techniques are the only ones employed as compared with units where these techniques are merged with other forms of treatment such as drugs or ECT); (3) the treatment ideology theoretically espoused by staff on the unit and the actual staff attitudes shown towards patients and treatment (for example, the extent to which decision-making is held to be a democratic process or the extent to which deviant behaviour is felt to be tolerable); and, last but not least (4), the length of time patients remain in the unit.

The final area of variation is perhaps the trickiest: what do we mean when we talk of success? What seems clear is that a simple criterion such as re-admission to hospital, as is often used as a measure of outcome, especially in large-scale studies, tells us little about the actual changes which have taken place in the patient or in his living situation.

From the therapeutic community point of view, if I can use that term, it seems that there are particular areas or dimensions of change which are seen as important: (1) the extent to which the patient is able to fulfil the social roles expected of him; (2) the extent to which he is able to reintegrate at an interpersonal level with the people in his immediate environment; and (3) his attitudes and feelings concerning himself. In addition, where the therapeutic community is situated within a National Health Service setting it is probably appropriate to include a measure of symptoms and of the continued need for social or medical support as relevant variables.

These lists present an already bewildering, although still partial, array of possible sources of variation. Each one presents the interesting question: does this one have anything to do with it? In the classic model of experimental research we would allow only one of these variables to vary at a time, keeping all the others (including all those not listed here) the same, so that we would be sure of the cause of any differences we found. Clearly this is not possible in practice. For a start, the researcher or community worker is seldom in a position to dictate either the type of treatment or the selection of patients in a particular setting. Second, although I have presented these variables separately, in practice they are likely to interact: for example, the type of patient being treated is likely to have an effect on the staff attitudes, while espoused treatment ideology is likely to have a strong influence on length of stay in the community. Third, the idea of keeping anything constant in the fluid, at times volatile, atmosphere of a therapeutic community is hardly on. Just as therapeutic communities defy orthodox notions about treatment, they also defy orthodox research methods. Yet no one can doubt that it is important to try to evaluate the place of therapeutic communities within the National Health Service, as Manning argues in Chapter 27.

A more practical approach seems to be to begin looking at which of these aspects do in fact vary in our own place of work and which of them are constant; i.e., things that we can't do anything to change. For example, the size of our community, the range of treatments provided, and the espoused ideology are all likely to be relatively stable. Certain patient characteristics may also be fairly uniform in some units; for example, the age, sex or social class of the patients, or the type of difficulties they come with. These things we can attempt to describe or measure, but must then leave as unknown sources of variation. Out of those things which do vary, we can select a number which seem to us to be both important and capable of being measured. This would depend to a large extent on the resources we have available, and it is at this stage that discussion and exchange of ideas will be most fruitful. Deciding what to leave out is often the most difficult and crucial aspect of any research project.

At this stage it may be helpful to describe briefly some of the research which we carried out recently at Littlemore Hospital, Oxford, in the Phoenix Unit.

We developed a number of rating scales and an interview protocol which required a lot of time not normally available to those employed in full-time clinical work. We also measured a number of variables which were relatively easy to measure and record, not least because they could be collected unobtrusively. These have subsequently provided some interesting insights into the factors influencing outcome in our particular community. It is these I shall describe. Full details of the research have been published elsewhere (Kennard *et al.*, 1977).

The **Phoenix** Unit acts as one of the acute admission units for the Oxford area. As such, a wide range of patients are admitted, providing a large number of sources of variation. Those which we decided to record were: the patient's age and sex, his diagnosis, whether he was admitted voluntarily or compulsorily, his social class, the position he or she held within the family (e.g., husband, wife, son, daughter), and his length of stay in the unit. The treatment situation was 'given' — we could attempt to describe it but not to vary it. In looking at outcome, one of the criteria we chose stemmed from the active day-patient policy of the unit, providing ex-patients with social support following their discharge. Since attendance as a day-patient was very much up to the patient, although influenced by staff attitudes, it was considered that this presented a reasonable indication of the patient's continuing dependence on the unit. I should point out that we are not saying that high dependence is necessarily bad or low dependence is good, but simply that it seems to be an important aspect of outcome. We measured this by taking the first three months following each patient's discharge, and counting up the number of days he was present in the Phoenix Unit and the number of weeks in which he attended at least once.

When we compared the patient variables with this particular measure of outcome, we found some rather interesting things. Whether the patient's diagnosis was one of schizophrenia, affective psychosis, or neurosis made no difference to the amount of contact he had with the unit after discharge. Neither did the age of the patient. Compulsory admission also seemed to have nothing to do with it. What did seem to matter, however, was the position the patient held in his or her family.

Wives who had one or more children at home had significantly less contact with the unit after discharge than all the other types of patient, while sons living at home had more contact than all other patients. Thus, the simple fact of the demands of the patient's role at home seemed to have a significant effect on the need for continued hospital support. This was further supported by our finding that patients who were both wives and mothers also spent a shorter time as in-patients than all other patients did.

This variable, length of stay, was also related to our measure of outcome. Patients who spent less time in hospital also spent less time attending the hospital as day-patients after they were discharged. This leads to the simple and perhaps well known equation that more treatment leads to more treatment.

The most significant finding, in statistical terms, was the relationship between social class and our measure of outcome. All our middle-class patients — about 30 per cent of our sample — had either no further contact with the hospital or at most only a few days. Working-class patients, on the other hand, tended to have considerably more day-patient contact; and all those patients re-admitted during the three months after discharge were also working class (i.e. Registrar General's Social Classes 3–5).

These results tell us that in a particular treatment setting two or three patient-attributes had a lot to do with patients' continued dependence on the treatment setting. They do not tell us whether this is a feature of the therapeutic community approach, hospitals in general, or just this unit. If we wanted to pursue this question, we could compare our unit with another run on different lines, or alternatively try to replicate the findings on similar units. In either case we would want to have as good an idea as possible of how the units differed from one another so as to narrow down the possible reasons for different findings, should we get them.

Another thing our findings do not tell us is how the aspect of outcome we measured relates to other aspects; for example, the presence of symptoms, emotional or behavioural problems, and the satisfaction of the patient or his relatives. In the full research project we did measure other outcome variables. The value of a piece of research, however, rests less on the number of measures of outcome it includes, than on their being aptly chosen. It is in the choice of what he intends to take notice of that the researcher takes his biggest decisions, and where most thought and consideration is needed. In our research we considered that the measures described here reflected both the patient's continued reliance on the therapeutic community and the converse, his speed of re-integration into his home environment. In the event we seemed to have picked on something which did relate to aspects of patients' social circumstances. We cannot know from these results whether a different outcome measure might have responded to different patient-attributes.

Having pointed out the limitations of our findings, what of their positive implications? They tell us that certain trends are occurring in this treatment setting, and this enables us to ask a few further questions. For example, is the unit providing follow-up support for patients who have the time for it, rather than those who might need it most? — in other words, for those whose social role commitments permit them to attend as day-patients. Or is the community operating within some more general Parkinson-type law: the patient's need for support/treatment expands to fill the time available? Also, are working-class patients more dependent than middle-class ones, or is there some aspect of the unit which makes it more attractive to working-class patients? And if so, is this felt to be satisfactory by the unit's staff? As you can see, the quite limited findings I have described raise some interesting questions and suggest possible lines of further enquiry or action.

What I have tried to get across is that research both is and is not a simple matter. It is not simple because it requires self-disciplined thinking, which we all try to avoid much of the time. It is as well to recognize this difficulty. Expecting even the simplest research to materialize of its own accord is uncomfortably akin to a patient's expecting to get better if he sits around the hospital long enough. On the other hand, it is, or can be, simple in that information is readily available on many things, and a rather straightforward enquiry into particular aspects of a therapeutic community may produce unexpected and thought-provoking results.

29
Evaluating the therapeutic community*

Nick Manning

One of a series of innovations emerging from the Second World War, the therapeutic community gained considerable status as a central concept in social psychiatry in the 1950s in Britain. It was based on the premise that just as a disordered personality may be produced by a pathological social environment, so a beneficial environment may remove such disorder. Evidence for this approach derived from theoretical advances in the social sciences, and detailed studies of the damaging effects of the repressive style of the large mental hospital.

But, just as the therapeutic community movement can only be understood fully by reference to the context in which it originated, changes in that context indicate some of the difficulties the therapeutic community has encountered in the last thirty years, and presage future developments. Politically and socially we now live in a very different Britain, in which the mental health services have virtually ceased to exist as a separate administrative entity. New principles of care and treatment, such as pharmacotherapy, community care, and the integration of hospital psychiatry into District General Hospitals, challenge the old institutional arrangements. The therapeutic community as an institutional alternative has itself been somewhat passed over by these innovations, although it has continued to appeal to social scientists as one of the few positive approaches to residential care, and as such has found new areas of application beyond psychiatry. But increasing pressure for unequivocal evidence of its effectiveness has mounted in recent years, and especially since the 1974 reorganization of the National Health Service.

*This paper was first read to the Research Group of the Association of Therapeutic Communities in 1974.

Evaluative research

Evaluative research has been traditionally associated with the medical field. Work within psychology and criminology has also developed, but often with the use of medical models, or modifications of them. The experimental drug-trial epitomizes this approach to evaluation. However, a growing body of literature in the late 1960s and 1970s has taken issue with many aspects of this model, as evidence accumulates to show its inadequacy when used to look at complex behavioural phenomena. This literature has appeared mainly in the fields of criminology, psychotherapy, and to a lesser extent social action programmes.

Much of the discussion revolves around the fact that previously accepted models and methods of research have not resulted in the answers sought in relation to the effect of a wide variety of change-induction techniques. This result has directed the discussion into two areas: (1) Is the question being asked in the right way, and indeed is it answerable at all? (2) If the question is appropriate, in what ways can the techniques be improved in seeking the answer?

These two questions reveal many contrasting approaches within this general area; and by means of a consideration of these, some problems of relevance to evaluating therapeutic communities will be tackled.

Outcome and process studies

Perhaps one of the most general concerns has been the question of the relationship between outcome studies (of the results of 'treatment') and studies of process (what happens in 'treatment'). Much earlier work can be classified as either one or the other. But Wilkins (1964), Clarke and Sinclair (1973), Clarke and Cornish (1972), Paul (1967), Bergin (1971), and Bottoms and McClintock (1973) have all pointed out that this opposition of outcome and process studies is misguided. Clarke and Cornish (1972) argued strongly against 'spot the winner' type studies, but found that on considering the processes that might affect outcome they were unable to isolate any clear causal factors. The dilemma is that unless the change-inducing techniques can be described in sufficient detail to reproduce them, then the knowledge that some unknown thing is effective is not very useful. On the other hand taking 'flight into process' (Zubin, 1964) will not answer the question of whether this technique works or not in the hands of a sample of therapists. Thus, Paul (1967) argues for a balance between process studies, and a complementary assessment of outcome, if real evaluation is to be achieved.

The dichotomy between outcome and process studies has arisen from the way in which questions of evaluation are posed. Wilkins (1964),

Clarke and Sinclair (1973), Paul (1967), and Bergin (1971) have stressed very forcibly that the single question 'Does X work?' is meaningless, unless divided into a series of smaller more specific questions which can be looked at in turn. Paul (1967) restates the question as: '*Which* treatment, by *whom*, is the most effective for *this* individual with *that* specific problem, under *which* set of circumstances?' Similarly, Bergin (1971) argues for specific interventions for specific problems with specific outcomes. Thus what may be improvement for one patient (relief from depression) may not be for another. In the same way, Wilkins (1964) prefers a step-by-step 'panzer' strategy to a 'mass attack'; and Clarke and Sinclair (1973) argue that for studying ongoing systems, small-scale studies are needed, focused on particular aspects, instead of 'monolithic' projects of the form 'Does treatment X work better than treatment Y?' They advise the avoidance of more formal evaluation designs.

Psychotherapy and criminological research

These two fields have flourishing traditions of evaluative research. The former has developed a whole battery of intra-psychic and behavioural measures of outcome over the years. The latter has advanced the technique of predictive analysis, and struggled with the problem of institutional evaluation. These fields have tended to favour psychology on the one hand, and sociology on the other. Neither has integrated these disciplines adequately, but rather:

> The current practice of sociologists is to standardize by matching persons on psychological factors, and of psychologists to standardize by matching on sociological factors, and thus try to avoid considering explanations of their observations which derive from the other's field of theory (Wilkins, 1964).

The therapeutic community falls between these two fields. Situated in the field of psychiatry, it uses both psychological and sociological ideas. Its psychotherapy is connected with institutional processes in common more with penal measures (such as approved schools or borstals) than with classic psychotherapy. On the other hand, it assumes, more explicitly than such penal measures, that the individual manifests some definitive pathological state which, if corrected, will lead to behavioural change. However, criminologists and psychotherapists would agree with Kurt Lewin that behaviour is a function of both personality and social environment. Indeed the split between the one dealing with personality disorders, and the other dealing with environmental disorders (such as sub-cultural or ecological theories) is rapidly giving way to the view on both sides that 'physical social life environments interact with socio-personal characteristics to produce behaviour' (Paul, 1967), and that pre-institutional behaviour and problems, attitudes and behaviour in the institution, and post-institutional conduct interact together and with the varying environment in complex ways (Bottoms and McClintock, 1973). This means that, for example, follow-up must entail a detailed study of the environment in which the subject is living, for this will affect the schizophrenic's chances of relapse (Leff, 1974), or the probationer's outcome (Davies, 1969).

Experimental and non-experimental designs

In all the fields discussed, both experimental and non-experimental designs have been used. However, not all experimental designs work out, as Clarke and Cornish (1972) found to their cost. Despite perfect conditions for randomization between a therapeutic community and a traditional house in an approved school, they found that the effects could have been explained by several factors other than the orientation to therapy. They argue that the controlled trial in institutional research is, therefore, not feasible. They have mistakenly considered a whole approach (the therapeutic community) as a single variable (Guttentag, 1971; Coleman, 1970). This is the real reason for their failure. A radical approach is not a unitary dimension, and hence 'spot the winner' research explains nothing. Thus Bergin (1971) showed, for example, how evidence now points to the fact that an increase in the variance, rather than the mean, of outcome scores is more common in psychotherapy, since some patients get very much better but also some, in fact, get worse.

Comparing whole institutions, then, is not very helpful when they are multi-dimensional. Rather each constituent dimension must be considered, and then experimental methods would be more useful. Until this degree of precision is possible, non-experimental designs can be used. In this case, systematic manipulation of independent variables is often not feasible. The only possibility is to exploit natural variations in the subject matter. Hence instead of experimentally comparing just two institutions, it is necessary to look at perhaps twenty or more and use their natural differences to explore relationships. Such a 'cross-institutional' design (Clarke and Sinclair, 1973) may involve the use of prediction methods to standardize the relative risks distributed in the populations of each institution, so that differences between predicted and observed outcomes will indicate the relative effectiveness of different institutions. Needless to say, such a design requires complementary process analysis to explain the possible causes of differential effectiveness.

Experimental designs are thus appropriate only when a single dimension can be isolated and manipulated. To the extent that multi-dimensional studies are undertaken (as with the therapeutic community), a cross-institutional approach must be used, together with a breaking down of the complexity of each case. Bergin (1971) dismisses the 'Bugaboo of complexity', whereby a process is claimed to be violated if reduced to its component parts, by pointing out that any understanding requires simplification, and then re-combination (as in the workings of a machine, for example).

Aims and criteria

Guttentag (1971) points out that evaluation research is qualitatively different from basic research: the subject matter is predefined; control over variables is small; a programme rather than a variable is studied; judgments of worthwhileness are involved; it is assumed that treatment effects overcome the cumulative effects of other variables; the relationship between inputs and effects is predefined; and inputs and outputs are fixed. In short, the researcher must accept the goals of the institution as his evaluative guide. These goals, derived from both stated and covert aims, will lead him to select the relevant criteria. For the therapeutic community, these goals are manifold, and hence alternative criteria are available. For example, it seems that staff dissatisfaction may be higher in the permissive atmosphere of a therapeutic community. There is also some agreement that therapeutic communities are exhausting for their leaders, and indeed have resulted in the breakdown of those in such positions. Should such criteria be used to evaluate such an institution? To the extent that a method is relatively new and one is trying to establish its validity, criteria most relevant will be those which set the method in a favourable light compared with other established techniques. Whether increased therapeutic gains are made at the expense of staff well-being and whether these two should be balanced are very different questions. The first may be fairly answered with research. The second depends on more political considerations.

Moreover, the ranking of aims may well vary over time. In the early 1950s Henderson Hospital (then the Belmont Social Rehabilitation Unit) was perhaps best known as an experimental therapeutic community unit (Wiles, 1949; Lewis, 1952; Jones, 1952; Freeman, 1952; Roscow, 1955). This goal was of sufficient importance to justify the unit's existence, whether great therapeutic gains were made or not. With the passage of time, the spread of new organizational concepts, and changing trends within the mental health services, the goal of experiment recedes in importance, while the need to prove that the hospital does produce therapeutic gains, and for types of patients not adequately dealt with elsewhere, becomes a more urgent objective.

Suchman (1967) has differentiated five areas in which evaluative data can be collected: effort, performance, adequacy, efficiency, profit. Obviously, a combination of the aims of the research and the programme determines which areas are examined. In general, studies have concerned themselves with the last factor of profit: is the outcome (of therapeutic gain) being attained? Therapeutic communities would certainly vary on these five areas. Many make considerable efforts, but the level of performance varies widely. The adequacy is also very variable. For example, Henderson Hospital deals with a very narrow range of patients, and is thus inadequate as a general source of treatment. Other units are more open. Finally, efficiency is often directly balanced against profit in the therapeutic community. A popular image is that where there is disorganization and inefficiency then sociotherapy can happen, but where there is quiet efficiency in a well-run unit, organizational goals have taken precedence over therapeutic goals and there will be little therapeutic profit, and may even be loss (e.g., institutional neurosis) (Barton, 1959).

To the extent that outcome is an essential goal to evaluate, appropriate criteria are hotly disputed. Bergin (1971) presents a useful list of outcome criteria available in psychotherapy. Generally measures may be divided into internal (intra-psychic) or external (behavioural). The latter are easier to measure (and favoured by criminologists), though the relative importance of each type is debatable. Paul (1967), for example, argues that ultimately we are interested in changing behaviour -- the way a patient relates to his social environment -- and that it is here that a therapeutic success or failure should be decided. Truax and Carkuff (1967), however, point out that the initial level of behavioural disturbance is generally negatively related to outcome, while the initial level of inner disturbance is generally positively related to outcome. This would seem to militate against the treatment of behavioural disturbance. On the other hand, Brooks (1972) has argued passionately against the idea of 'adjustment' as an objective. Although somewhat confused, he seems to feel that adjustment is a beneficial, though unintended, pay-off from helping delinquent boys to: develop their potential; become better-organized persons; find an authentic self; mature; gain insight; experience self-actualization; etc.

In a sense this debate is between those who look on the creative side of the human personality as a potential for growth, and those who are more concerned with adjusting behaviour that is unacceptable (to both the patient and his environment). In fact, many studies combine both aspects. Fairweather (1964), McCord and McCord (1956), Robins (1966), Clarke and Cornish (1972), Bergin (1971), and Bottoms and

McClintock (1973) have all used a combination of intra-psychic and behavioural measures. This combination is rather a blanket coverage of all possible indices. Clarke and Sinclair (1973) have, therefore, argued that intermediate criteria should be used so that outcome may be measured longitudinally during the career of the subject, rather than at one point in time, such as is usually done in follow-up studies. They mention two possible criteria which would give an indication of a subject's progress before it became swamped with post-treatment influences: absconding (drop-out from voluntary therapeutic communities); and 'treatment potential', a measure of popularity amongst both peers and staff, said to be related to outcome.

It seems then that studies of the careers of patients from pre-treatment, through treatment, to post-treatment, with sustained attention at each stage, may be essential to a better understanding of the place of treatment and the chance of effectiveness in such a career where other influences will be working before and after treatment (Fairweather, 1964; Hood and Sparks, 1970; Simon, 1971; Bottoms and McClintock, 1973; Sharp, 1975).

Randomization, matching and prediction

The choice between experimental and non-experimental designs discussed above often involves the practicalities of comparative methodologies. In the Clarke and Cornish (1972) study the opportunity for randomization of input was available, though not of input of staff, which Fairweather (1964) had achieved. This may be crucial in the light of Clarke and Cornish's finding that staff group variables may have been more powerful than treatment orientation effects.

When this is not the case, comparison requires some method of controlling for differential inputs to the treatment situation. Wilkins (1964) severely criticizes *ex post facto* matching, for without randomization any statistical inference is impossible. He prefers in this situation to use prediction or regression matching. Here the multiple correlations between independent (usually pre-treatment) and dependent variables (outcome criteria) enable the two groups to be matched by their regression weights. In other words, the pre-treatment distribution of risks of success or failure may be matched up, or differences compensated for. Then the relation of actual outcome to predicted outcome can indicate the differential effectiveness of various treatments. Unfortunately, correlation between pre-treatment variables and outcome can never be high, because the intermediate effects of the actual treatment experience and the post-treatment environment will have considerable power (Simon, 1971).

The derivation of prediction analysis has been comprehensively covered by Simon (1971). A crucial problem is to build the prediction equation for a specified population. It is impossible to transfer an equation built for one population (e.g., in treatment in a particular unit) to another, unless the populations are similar. If so, it is essential that it be re-validated on the new population. If this proves successful, then the equation may be used to match the two populations.

A further problem is obtaining sufficient information from the pre-treatment situation to devise a prediction of any useful power (Copas and Whiteley, 1976). This has in general been more problematic in the penal services than in psychiatry, where case notes contain more elaborate descriptions of the patients' background. Although, whereas it might be thought that intra-psychic factors would be more relevant in this latter situation, it is interesting that Ullman (1967) found marital status the best predictor of his 'early release criterion' of success (see also Kennard in the previous chapter). It is important that in general the prediction formula should include variables that affect the selection procedure in an ongoing system. If this is not the case the actual distribution of risk in a population may, for example, be better than shown by prediction, since in effect the selection procedure is acting as an undetected prediction device by choosing suitable cases which will do well subsequently. At Henderson Hospital, for example, where a selection committee of staff and patients votes for or against each applicant, the score obtained by counting positive votes may add strength to a prediction of the outcome of that applicant.

Whether one can randomize or not, comparison on more than one variable (as in the case of therapeutic communities) requires a rapidly increasing sample size of institutions for comparison. For example, if one wanted to compare the effects of treatment orientation, staff training, size, and patient-type on outcome (all factors which Clarke and Cornish (1972) felt could account for their results), using only dichotomized values, the number of therapeutic communities required would be vast in order to incorporate all the possible interactions. Path analysis (Hall, 1973) offers a solution to this problem, given a sufficiently large number of cases, but the measuring device would have to be easily applied and reliable, and hence rather coarse.

Therapeutic community evaluation

In the light of the above discussion, it can be seen that therapeutic communities present particular characteristics with respect to research methodology:

(1) They are multi-dimensional, and research is often designed to investigate single dimensions.

(2) They combine efforts at both intra-psychic and behavioural change.

(3) Up to now most studies have been descriptions and analysis of process, rather than outcome.

(4) They have multiple goals, of which outcome is but one. These goals have changed and will continue to change.

These factors militate very strongly against comparing, for example, the therapeutic community with the traditional institution, in a single-shot study. A more productive approach should be at four levels:

(1) Comparing a large number of therapeutic communities, in order to use natural variations to suggest relationships between constituent variables (such as size, staff training, leadership, environmental context, organizational arrangements, length of stay, etc.).

(2) Studying individual aspects which go to make up the therapeutic community; in other words, attempting to dissect the constituent parts to see how they work together, which are more effective, and why. For example, it would be very valuable to know how far the context of 'twenty-four-hour' treatment is important for small-group psychotherapy, or to what extent 'role-blurring' results in status competition amongst staff, or the way sub-grouping reflects treatment ideology and affects outcome (Sharp, 1975).

(3) Studying natural fluctuations within the community over time to ascertain relationships between, for example, levels of tension and the age-distribution of patients (Hall, 1973).

(4) Attempting to delineate more clearly the individual requirements of each patient (Bottoms and McClintock, 1973; Kiresuck, 1976), or at least of types of patient, so that on the one hand treatment can be more closely matched to needs, and also that 'improvement' may be more clearly defined for each case or category. Hood and Sparks (1970) argue for more basic typological research, in order to show empirically the relations, for example, between interpersonal maturity and role career, or self-image and rated 'amenability' (Sharp, 1975).

This approach will inevitably be messy, and will not appear to follow the single-shot orthodox experimental design. The overwhelming weight of opinion, however, rejects such classicism.

Bibliography

Official publications

Department of Health and Social Security, *Hospital Advisory Service Annual Report, 1972*, HMSO, London, 1973.

Department of Health and Social Security, *Better Services for the Mentally Ill*, HMSO, London, 1975, Cmnd 6233.

Department of Health and Social Security, *Priorities for Health and Personal Social Services in England*, HMSO, London, 1976.

Department of Health and Social Security, *The Way Forward*, HMSO, London, 1977.

Home Office, *Report of the Committee on Local Authority and Allied Personal Social Services*, HMSO, London, 1968, Cmnd 3703 (Seebohm Report).

Ministry of Health, *A National Health Service*, HMSO, London, 1944, Cmnd 6502.

Ministry of Health, *A Hospital Plan for England and Wales*, HMSO, London, 1962, Cmnd 1604.

Ministry of Labour, *2nd Report of the Standing Committee on the Rehabilitation and Resettlement of Disabled Persons* (Chairman, Sir H. Wiles). HMSO, London, 1949.

Books and articles

Algie, J. (1970), 'Management and Organisation in the Social Services', *Brit. Hospital Journal*, LXXX, p. 1245.

Allport, G. (1960), 'The Open System in Personality Theory', in *Personality and Social Encounter – Selected Essays*, Penguin, Harmondsworth.

Anastasi, A. (1968), *Psychological Testing*, Macmillan, London.

Apte, Z. (1971), 'Halfway Houses', *Occasional Papers in Social Administration*, Bell, London.

313

Argyris, C. (1970), *Intervention Theory and Method*, Addison-Wesley, Reading, Mass.

Association of Social Workers (1967), *New Thinking about Residential Care*, ASW.

Balbernie, R. (1972), *Residential Work with Children*, (rev. edn), Chaucer Publishing Co., London.

Barnes, E. (ed) (1968), *Psychosocial Nursing: Studies from the Cassel Hospital*, Tavistock Publications, London.

Barnes, J. A. (1972), *Social Networks, Addison-Wesley Modules No. 26*, Addison-Wesley, Reading, Mass.

Barton, R. (1959), *Institutional Neurosis*, Wright, Bristol.

Bazeley, E. T. (1928), *The Little Commonwealth*, Allen & Unwin, London.

Beedwell, C. (1971), *Residential Life with Children*, Routledge & Kegan Paul, London.

Benedict of Nursia (1943), in H. Beltenson (ed), *Documents of the Christian Church*, Oxford University Press, London.

Bergin, A. E. (1971), in A. E. Bergin and S. L. Garfield (eds), *Handbook of Psychotherapy and Behaviour Change*, Wiley, New York.

Berne, E. (1964), *Games People Play, the Psychology of Human Relationships*, Penguin, Harmondsworth.

Bick, E. (1968), 'The Experience of the Skin in Early Object-Relations', *Brit. J. Psycho-Anal.*, 49, p. 484.

Bierenbroodspot, P. (1972), 'Sharing or Delegation of Power: an important therapeutic decision in mental hospital development', *Third International Conference on Social Science and Medicine*, Elsinore.

Biestek, F. P. (1961), *The Casework Relationship*, Allen & Unwin, London.

Bion, W. R. (1946), 'The Leadership Group Project', *Bulletin of the Menninger Clinic*, 10, p. 77.

Bion, W. R. (1957), 'Differentiation of the psychotic from the non-psychotic personality', *Brit. J. Psycho-Anal.*, no. 38, p. 266.

Bion, W. R. (1961), *Experiences in Groups*, Heinemann, London.

Bion, W. R. (1962), 'A Theory of Thinking', *Brit. J. Psycho-Anal.*, 43, p. 306.

Bion, W. R. and Rickman, J. (1943), 'Intra-Group Tensions in Therapy', *Lancet*, ii, p. 678.

Bishop, J. and Foulsham, J. (1973), 'Use of Space in the Marlborough Day Hospital', *Architectural Psychology Working Paper No. 7*, Kingston Polytechnic.

Blake, R. (1974), 'Open Letter to Atkinson-Morley's Hospital', *Association of Therapeutic Communities Bulletin*, 14.

Blumberg, A. and Golembiewski, R. T. (1976), *Learning and Change in Groups*, Penguin, Harmondsworth.

Bott, E. (1957), *Family and Social Network*, Tavistock Publications, London (2nd edn 1971).

Bottoms, A. E. and McClintock, F. H. (1973), *Criminals Coming of Age*, Heinemann, London.

Bransby, E. R. (1973), 'Mental Illness and the Psychiatric Services', *Social Trends*, 4, HMSO, London.

Bridgeland, M. (1971), *Pioneer Work with Maladjusted Children*, Staples Press, London.

Briggs, D. (1972), 'Chino, California', in J. S. Whiteley, D. Briggs, and H. Turner (eds), *Dealing with Deviants*, Hogarth Press, London.

Brooks, R. (1972), *Bright Delinquents*, National Foundation for Educational Research, Slough.

Brown, G. (1972), 'The Mental Hospital as an Institution', paper read at 2nd Symposium on Psychiatric Epidemiology, Mannheim.

Brown, J. F. (1938), 'Freud v. Marx: Real and pseudo problems distinguished', *Psychiatry*, 1, p. 249.

Buckley, W. (1967), *Sociology and Modern Systems Theory*, Prentice-Hall, Englewood Cliffs.

Burn, M. (1956), *Mr Lyward's Answer*, Hamish Hamilton, London.

Caine, T. M. and Smail, D. J. (1966), 'Attitudes to Treatment of Medical Staff in a Therapeutic Community', *Brit. J. Med. Psychol.*, 39, p. 329.

Caine, T. M. and Smail, D. J. (1969), *The Treatment of Mental Illness*, University of London Press.

Caine, T. M. and Wijesinghe, B. (1976), 'Personality Expectancies and Group Psychotherapy', *Brit. J. Psychiat.*, 129, pp. 384–7.

Callwell, B. M. (1969), 'A New "Approach" to Behavioural Ecology', in J. P. Hill (ed), *Minnesota Symposia on Child Psychology, vol. 2*, University of Minnesota Press, Minneapolis.

Canizares, J. (1976), 'Nurses in the Making', *Proceedings of the International Conference on Adolescents* (Association for the Psychiatric Study of Adolescents).

Carpenter, M. (1851), *Reformatory Schools for the Children of the Perishing and Dangerous Classes, and for Juvenile Offenders*, Gilpin, London.

Caudill, W. A. (1958), *The Psychiatric Hospital as a Small Society*, Harvard University Press, Cambridge, Mass.

Central Council for Education and Training in Social Work, *Training for Residential Work, discussion document* (February 1973), CCETSW.

Cherns, A. B. (1972), 'Social Science and Policy', in A. B. Cherns, R. Sinclair, and W. I. Jenkins, *Social Science and Government*, Tavistock Publications, London.

Clark, A. (1970), 'Nursing Organisation in an Adolescent Unit', *Proceedings of the 5th Conference of the Association for the Psychiatric Study of Adolescents*.

Clark, A. W. (1967), 'Patient Participation and Improvement in a Therapeutic Community', *Human Relations*, 29, 3, p. 259.

Clark, A. W. and Yeomans, N. (1969), *Fraser House*, Springer, New York.

Clark, D. H. (1964), *Administrative Therapy*, Tavistock Publications, London.

Clark, D. H. (1965), 'The Therapeutic Community Concept, Practice and Future', *Brit. J. Psychiat.*, 111, pp. 947-54.

Clark, D. H. (1974), *Social Therapy in Psychiatry*, Penguin, Harmondsworth.

Clark, D. H. (1975), 'The Therapeutic Community in 1975', unpublished paper given at Richmond Fellowship Internat. Conference.

Clark, D. H. (1977), 'The Therapeutic Community' (review article), *Brit. J. Psychiat.*, 131, pp. 553-64.

Clark, D. H., Hooper, D. F., and Oram, E. G. (1962), 'Creating a Therapeutic Community in a Psychiatric Ward', *Human Relations*, 15, p. 123.

Clark, D. H. and Myers, K. (1970), 'Themes in a Therapeutic Community', *Brit. J. Psychiat.*, 117, pp. 389-95.

Clarke, R. V. G. and Cornish, D. B. (1972), *The Controlled Trial in Institutional Research*, HMSO, London.

Clarke, R. V. G. and Cornish, D. B. (1975), *Residential Treatment and its Effects on Delinquency*, HMSO, London.

Clarke, R. V. G. and Sinclair, I. (1973), *Towards More Effective Treatment Evaluation*, Council of Europe.

Coleman, A. (1971), *The Planned Environment in Psychiatric Treatment: A Manual for Ward Design*, Charles Thomas, Springfield, Illinois.

Coleman, J. (1970), 'Considering the Case against the Experimental Evaluation of Social Innovation', *Admin. Science Quart.*, 15, pp. 110-13.

Coleman, J., Katz, E., and Menzel, H. (1957), 'Diffusion of an Innovation Among Physicians', *Sociometry*, 20.

Cooper, D. (1967), *Psychiatry and Anti-Psychiatry*, Tavistock Publications, London.

Copas, J. B. and Whiteley, J. S. (1976), 'Predicting Success in the Treatment of Psychopaths', *Brit. J. Psychiat.*, 129, pp. 388-92.

Crabtree, L. and Cox, J. L. D. (1972), 'The Overthrow of a Therapeutic Community', *Int. J. Group Psychotherapy*, XXII, 1, p. 37.

Craft, M. (1965), *Ten Studies into Psychopathic Personality*, John Wright, Bristol.

Crocket, R. (1966a), 'Acting-Out as a Mode of Communication in the Psychotherapeutic Community', *Brit. J. Psychiat.*, 112, p. 383.

Crocket, R. (1966b), 'Authority and Permissiveness in the Psychotherapeutic Community: Theoretical Perspectives', *Amer. J. Psychotherapy*, XX, 4, pp. 669-76.

Crocket, R. (1967), 'Aspects of Communication in the Therapeutic Community Approach to Psychotherapy', *Proceedings of 3rd World Congress of Psychiatry*, Toronto.

Crocket, R. (1972), 'Initiation of the Therapeutic Community Approach to Treatment in a Neurosis Centre', *Int. J. Group Psychotherapy*, 12, pp. 180-93.

Crocket, R. (1975), '"Real" and "Abstracted" Network Relationships and Social Psychiatry', *Proceedings of the 9th Int. Congr. Psychother., Oslo, 1973; Psychother. Psychosom.*, 25, pp. 267-71.

Crozier, M. (1965), *The Bureaucratic Phenomenon*, Tavistock Publications, London.

Cumming, J. and Cumming, E. (1962), *Ego and Milieu*, Aldine, Chicago.

Davies, M. (1969), *Probationers in their Social Environment*, HMSO, London.

Davies, M. (1974), 'The Current Status of Social Work Research', *Brit. J. Social Work*, 4, 3.

Dawson, C. A. and Gettys, W. E. (1948), *An Introduction to Sociology*, Ronald Press, New York.

de Maré, P. B. (1972), *Perspectives in Group Psychotherapy – a theoretical background*, Allen & Unwin, London.

de Maré, P. B. (1975), 'The Politics of the Large Group', in L. Kreeger (ed), *The Large Group*, Constable, London.

de Maré, P. B. and Kreeger, L. (1974), *Introduction to Group Treatment in Psychiatry*, Butterworth, London.

Dicks, H. V. (1970), *50 Years of the Tavistock Clinic*, Routledge & Kegan Paul, London.

Dinnage, R. and Kellmer Pringle, M. L. (1967), *Residential Child Care – Facts and Fallacies*, Longman, Harlow.

Dockar-Drysdale, B. (1973), *Consultation in Child Care (Papers on residential work), vol. 4*, Longman, London.

Donnison, D. V. and Chapman, V. (1965), *Social Policy and Administration*, Allen & Unwin, London.

Edelson, M. (1970), *Psychotherapy and Sociotherapy*, University of Chicago Press.

Emery, F. E. (1969), *Systems Thinking*, Penguin, Harmondsworth.

Etzioni, A. (1960), 'Interpersonal and Structural Factors in the Study of Mental Hospitals', *Psychiatry*, 23, pp. 13-22.

Evans, J. (1970), 'Conflict, Crises and Tensions Within a Residential Unit', *Proceedings of 5th Conference of the Association for the Psychiatric Study of Adolescents*.

Evans, J. (1976), 'Development of Staff Training Programmes', *Proceedings of the International Conference on Adolescence* (Association for the Psychiatric Study of Adolescents).

Fairweather, G. (ed), (1964), *Social Psychology in Treating Mental Illness: An Experimental Approach*, Wiley, New York.

Festinger, L., Riecken, H. W., and Schachter, S. (1956), *When Prophecy Fails: a Social and Psychological Study of a modern group that predicted the destruction of the world*, Harper Row, New York.

Fishbein, M. (1967), 'A Behaviour Theory Approach to the relations between beliefs about an object and the attitude toward an object', in M. Fishbein (ed), *Readings in Attitude Theory*, Wiley, New York.

Fishbein, M. (1971), 'The Search for Attitudinal Behavioural Consistency', in J. Cohen (ed), *Behavioural Science Foundations of Consumer Behaviour*, Free Press, New York.

Forder, A. (ed) (1969), *Penelope Hall's Social Services of England and Wales*, Routledge & Kegan Paul, London.

Fortes, M. (1949), *The Web of Kinship*, Oxford University Press, London.

Foster, A. (1973), *Featherstone Lodge Project Annual Report*, 1972-3.

Foster, A. (1976), 'Helping Students through the Vac', *Community Care*, 129, p. 23.

Foster, A. and Christian, A. (1977), unpublished paper delivered to the Association of Therapeutic Communities, Supervisors' group.

Foulkes, S. F. and Anthony, E. W. (1957), *Group Psychotherapy*, Penguin, Harmondsworth.

Fraenkel, R. M. (1977), 'Community Development Goals and Citizen Participation', *Community Development Journal*, 12, 3.

Freeman, H. (1952), in M. Jones (ed), *Social Psychiatry*, Tavistock Publications, London.

Freud, S. (1912), 'The Dynamics of Transference', in J. Strachey (ed), *Complete Psychological Works*, vol. 12, standard edition (1953), Hogarth Press, London.

Fromm, E. (1960), *The Fear of Freedom*, Routledge & Kegan Paul, London.

Furedi, J., Szegedi, M., and K n, M. (1974), 'Methodological Problems of the Therapeutic Community's Large Groups', *Int. J. Group Psychotherapy*, 2, p. 190.

Goffman, E. (1961), *Asylums*, Doubleday, New York; and Penguin, Harmondsworth (1968).

Goslin, D. A. (ed) (1969), *Handbook of Socialisation Theory Research*, Rand McNally, Chicago.

Gouldner, A. (1954), *Patterns of Industrial Bureaucracy*, Free Press, New York.

Greenberg, I. (1974), *Psychodrama Theory and Practice*, Behavioural Publications, New York.

Greenblatt, M. (1972), 'Administrative Psychiatry', *Amer. J. Psychiatry*, 129, pp. 373-86.

Grunberg, S. R. and Hinshelwood, R. D. (1973), *The Therapeutic Community and its Politics*, ATC *Newsletter*, no. 7, February.

Guardian (1976), 'Hospital's methods "may do harm"' 25 June.

Guttentag, M. (1971), 'Models and Methods in Evaluating Research', *J. Theory in Social Behaviour*, 1, 1.

Hall, E. T. (1966), *The Hidden Dimension*, Doubleday, New York.

Hall, J. R. (1973), 'Structural Characteristics of a Psychiatric Patient Community and the Therapeutic Milieu', *Human Relations*, 26, 6.

Hampden-Turner, C. (1971), *Radical Man*, Duckworth, London.

Haring, N. G. and Phillips, E. L. (1962), *Educating Emotionally Disturbed Children*, McGraw-Hill, New York.

Hawkins, P. (1977), 'Between Scylla and Charybdis', *Association of Therapeutic Communities Bulletin*, 21 (February).

Heath, A. (1976), *Rational Choice and Social Exchange*, Cambridge University Press.

Higgin, G. and Bridger, M. (1965), *The Psychodynamics of an Intergroup Experience*, Tavistock Pamphlet no. 10, London.

Hinshelwood, R. D. (1972), 'A Treatment Model for a Community', *Association of Therapeutic Communities Newsletter*, 6.

Hinshelwood, R. D. and Foster, A. (1978), 'The Marlborough Experiment', in J. Abercrombie (ed), *Students in Need*, Guildford Society for Research into Higher Education.

Hobdell, R. A. (1972), 'Therapy in Groups', *New Society*, 11, May.

Hobson, R. F. (1959), 'An Approach to Group Analysis', *J. Analytical Psychology*, 9, 1.

Hobson, R. F. (1964), 'Group Dynamics and Analytical Psychology', *J. Analytical Psychology*, 9, 1.

Hobson, R. F. (1972), 'The Therapeutic Community Disease', unpublished Open Lecture, Institute of Psychiatry.

Hobson, R. F. (1974a), 'Loneliness', *J. Analytical Psychology*, 19, 1, pp. 71-89.

Hobson, R. F. (1974b), 'The Therapeutic Community Disease', in G. Adler (ed), *Success and Failure in Analysis*, Putnam's, New York.

Hobson, R. F. (1977), 'A Conversational Model of Psychotherapy', *Newsletter*, Association of University Teachers of Psychiatry.

Hobson, R. F. and Shapiro, D. A. (1970), 'The Personal Questionnaire as a Method of Assessing Change during Psychotherapy', *Brit. J. Psychiat.*, 117, p. 541.

Holden, H. (1972), 'On doing the Washing-up', Marlborough Day Hospital, privately circulated paper.

Hood, R. and Sparks, R. (1970), *Key Issues in Criminology*, Weidenfeld & Nicolson, London.

Hudson, P. (1971), 'Attention Structure in a Group of Pre-School Infants', *Architectural Psychology*, Kingston Polytechnic.

Huxley, J. (1964), 'The Emergence of Darwinism', in S. Tax (ed), *Evolution after Darwin*, University of Chicago Press (1960), reprinted in *Essays of a Humanist*, Chatto & Windus, London.

Illich, I. D. (1975), *Medical Nemesis: the Expropriation of Health*, Calder and Boyars, London.

Jaques, E. (1953), 'On the Dynamics of Social Structure', *Human Relations*, 6, p. 10.

Jaques, E. (1955), 'Social Systems as a Defence against Persecutory and Depressive Anxiety', in M. Klein (ed), *New Directions in Psychoanalysis*, Tavistock Publications, London.

Jaspers, K. (1963), *General Psychopathology*, Manchester University Press.

Jenkins, D. (1976), 'Some Assumptions about Learning and Training', unpublished manuscript quoted in A. Blumberg and R. T. Golembiewski, *Learning and Change in Groups*, Penguin, Harmondsworth.

Johnstone, T., Wilson, J., and Melling, J. M. (1969), 'A Brief Encounter with Psychotherapy', *Nursing Times* (3 July).

Jones, M. (1948), 'Physiological and Psychological Responses to Stress in Neurotic Patients', *J. Med. Sci.*, 94, p. 392.

Jones, M. (1952), *Social Psychiatry*, Tavistock Books, London.

Jones, M. (1953), *The Therapeutic Community: A new treatment method in Psychiatry*, Basic Books, New York.

Jones, M. (1956), 'The Concept of a Therapeutic Community', *Amer. J. Psychiatry*, 112.

Jones, M. (1962), *Social Psychiatry in the Community, in Hospitals and in Prisons*, Charles Thomas, Springfield, Illinois.

Jones, M. (1968a), *Beyond the Therapeutic Community*, Yale University Press, New Haven.

Jones, M. (1968b), *Social Psychiatry in Practice*, Penguin, Harmondsworth.

Jones, M. (1974), 'Psychiatry, Systems Theory, Education and Change', *Brit. J. Psychiat.*, 124, pp. 75-80.

Jones, M. (1976), *The Maturation of the Therapeutic Community*, Human Sciences Press, New York.

Jones, M., Pomryn, B. A., and Skellern, E. (1956), 'Work Therapy', *Lancet*, no. 7, p. 343.

Jourard, S. M. (1968), *Disclosing Man to Himself*, Nostrand, New York.

Kanter, R. M. (1972), *Commitment and Community: Communes and Utopias in Sociological perspective*, Harvard University Press, Cambridge, Mass.

Katz, D. and Kahn, R. L. (1969), 'Common Characteristics of Open Systems', in F. E. Emery (ed.), *Systems Thinking*, Penguin, Harmondsworth.

Kennard, D. and Clemmey, R. (1976), 'Psychiatric Patients as seen by self and others: an explanation of change in a therapeutic community setting', *Brit. J. Med. Psychol.*, 43, p. 35.

Kennard, D., Clemmey, R., and Mandelbrote, B. (1977), 'Aspects of Outcome in a Therapeutic Community Setting – how patients are seen by themselves and others', *Brit. J. Psychiat.*, 130, pp. 475-80.

Kesey, K. (1962), *One Flew Over the Cuckoo's Nest*, Viking Press, New York.

King, C. W. (1956), *Social Movements in the United States*, Random House, New York.

King, R. D., Raynes, N. V., and Tizard, J. (1971), *Patterns of Residential Care*, Routledge & Kegan Paul, London.

Kiresuck, P. J. (1976), 'Goal-attainment Scaling at a County Mental Health Service', in E. W. Makson and D. F. Allen (eds), *Trends in Mental Health Evaluation*, Lexington, New York.

Kirk, J. D. (1975), 'Towards a Theory of Residential Functioning', unpublished MSc thesis, Oxford University.

Klein, M. (1932), 'Early Stages of the Oedipus Conflict and of Superego Formation', in *The Writings of Melanie Klein*, vol. 2 (1975), Hogarth Press, London.

Klein, M. (1935), 'A Contribution to the Psychogenesis of Manic Depressive States', *The Writings of Melanie Klein*, vol. 1 (1975), Hogarth Press, London.

Klein, M. (1946), 'Notes on some Schizoid Mechanisms', *The Writings of Melanie Klein*, vol. 3 (1975), Hogarth Press, London.

Klein, M. (1952), 'The Origins of Transference', in M. Klein, *Envy and Gratitude and Other Works, 1946-1963* (1975), Hogarth Press, London.

Klir, G. J. and Valach, M. (1967), *Cybernetic Modeling*, London, Prague; printed in Czechoslovakia.

Kosin, J. and Sharaf, M. R. (1967), 'Intra-staff Controversy at a State Mental Hospital: an analysis of ideological issues', *Psychiatry*, 30, pp. 16-29.

Kraupl Taylor, F. (1958), 'A History of Group and Administrative Therapy in Great Britain', *Brit. J. Med. Psychol.*, 31.

Krausover, L. and Hemsley, D. R. (1976), 'Discharge from a therapeutic community', *Brit. J. Med. Psychol.*, 49, p. 199.

Kreeger, L. (ed) (1975), *The Large Group*, Constable, London.

Kuhn, T. (1962), *The Structure of Scientific Revolutions*, University of Chicago Press.

Leach, E. (1976), *Culture and Communications*, Cambridge University Press.

Leff, J. (1974), Personal communication, Institute of Psychiatry.

Letemendia, F. J., Harris, A. D., and Williams, P. J. (1967), 'The Clinical Effect on a population of chronic schizophrenic patients of administrative changes in hospital', *Brit. J. Psychiat.*, 113, pp. 959-71.

Lévi-Strauss, C. (1949), *Les Structures elementaires de la parente*, Presses Universitaires de France, Paris. English edition (1969), *The Elementary Structures of Kinship*, Eyre & Spottiswoode, London.

Lewin, K. (1951), *Field Theory in Social Science*, D. Cartwright (ed), Tavistock Publications, London.

Lewis, A. (1952), 'Introduction', in M. Jones, 1952, *Social Psychiatry*, Tavistock Publications, London.

Lewis, I. M. (1976), *Social Anthropology in Perspective*, Penguin, Harmondsworth.

Lewis, M. (1974), *Ecstatic Religions*, Penguin, Harmondsworth.

Lipman, A. (1968), 'Building Design and Social Interaction', *Architects Journal* (January).

Liss, J. (1974), *Free to Feel, Finding your way through new therapies*, Wildwood House, London.

McCord, W. and McCord, J. (1956), *Psychopathy and Delinquency*, Grune Stratton, New York.

McLoughlin, J. B. and Webster, J. (1970), 'Cybernetic and General System Approaches to urban and regional research: a review of the literature', *Environment and Planning*, 2, pp. 369-408.

Mahony, N. (1976), 'Hostel Project', *Association of Therapeutic Communities Bulletin*, 18.

Main, T. (1946), 'The Hospital as a Therapeutic Institution', *Bulletin of the Menninger Clinic*, 10, p. 66.

Main, T. (1975), 'Some Psychodynamics of Large Groups', in L. Kreeger (ed), *The Large Group*, Constable, London.

Main, T. (1976), 'Some Basic Concepts in Therapeutic Community Work', unpublished paper given at Richmond Fellowship International Conference, 1975.

Main, T. (1977), 'The Concept of the Therapeutic Community: variations and vicissitudes', *Group Analysis*, X, 2.

Mandelbrote, B. (1965), 'The Use of Psychodynamic and Sociodynamic Principles in the Treatment of Psychotics: A Change from Ward Unit Concepts to Groups and Communities', *Comprehensive Psychiatry*, vol. 6, p. 381.

Mandelbrote, B. and Gelder, M. G. (eds) (1972), *Psychiatric Aspects of Medical Practice*, Staples Press, London.

Mandelbrote, B. and Trick, K. L. K. (1970), 'Social and Clinical Factors in the Outcome of Schizophrenia', *Acta Psychiatrica Scandinavica*, 46, pp. 24-34.

Manning, N. P. (1975a), 'The Therapeutic Community Movement: a study in the innovation of social policy', unpublished MPhil thesis, University of York.

Manning, N. P. (1975b), 'Why bother with research?' in R. D. Hinshelwood and K. Seymour (eds), *The Changing Forms of Therapeutic Communities, Proceedings of MIND/ATC Residential Conference*, MIND (National Association for Mental Health, London).

Manning, N. P. (1976a), 'Innovation in Social Policy — the Case of the Therapeutic Community', *J. Social Policy*, 5, part 3, pp. 265-79.

Manning, N. P. (1976b), 'Values and Practice in the Therapeutic Community', *Human Relations*, 29, 2, pp. 125-28.

Manning, N. P. (1976c), 'What Happened to the Therapeutic Community?' in K. Jones and S. Baldwin (eds), *Year Book of Social Policy, 1975*, Routledge & Kegan Paul, London.

Manning, N. P. (1977), 'Social Psychiatry in the NHS — what happened to the therapeutic community?', unpublished paper delivered to the Heath Services Research Unit, University of Kent.

Manning, N. P. and Rapoport, R. N. (1976), 'Rejection and Reincorporation: A Case Study in Social Research Utilisation', *Social Science and Medicine*, 19, pp. 459-68.

Marcuse, H. (1955), *Eros and Civilisation*, Beacon Press, New York.

Martin, D. V. (1962), *Adventure in Psychiatry*, Cassirer, London.

Marx, K. (1889), Preface to 2nd Edition, Chapter XXXII, of 'Capital' in R. and F. de George, 1972, *The Structuralists from Marx to Lévi-Strauss*, Doubleday, New York.

Maynard, A. and Tingle, R. (1975), 'The Objectives and Performance of the mental health service in England and Wales in the 1960s', *J. Social Policy*, 4, 2.

Meares, R. A. and Hobson, R. F. (1977), 'The Persecutory Therapist', *Brit. J. Med. Psychol.*, 50, pp. 349-59.

Medawar, P. B. (1969), *Induction and Intuition in Scientific Thought*, Methuen, London.

Menzies, I. (1960), 'A Case Study in the Functioning of Social Systems as a Defence against Anxiety', *Human Relations*, 13, pp. 95-121.

Menzies, I. (1970), *The Functioning of Social Systems as a Defence against Anxiety*, Tavistock Institute of Human Relations, London.

Merton, R. K. (1968), *Social Theory and Social Structure*, Free Press, New York.

Meyer, R. (1969), 'Resistances to Occupational Therapy', *Brit. J. Occupational Therapy*, 32, pp. 39-42.

Midwinter, E. C. (1973), *Patterns of Community Education*, Ward Lock Educational, London.

Miles, A. (1969), 'Changes in the Attitudes to Authority of patients with behaviour disorders in a therapeutic community', *Brit. J. Psychiat.*, 11, p. 1049.

Miles, A. (1972), 'The Development of Interpersonal Relationships among long-stay patients in two mental hospital workshops', *Brit. J. Med. Psychol.*, 45, p. 105.

Miller, E. J. and Gwynne, G. V. (1972), *A Life Apart*, Tavistock Publications, London.

Miller, M. J. (1974), 'Residential Care: some thoughts and speculations on the literature', *Social Work Today*, 5, no. 9.

Mitchell, J. C. (ed.) (1970), *Social Networks in Urban Situations*, Manchester University Press.

Moos, R. M. (1974), *Evaluating Treatment Environments*, Wiley, New York.

Moreno, J. L. (1964), *Psychodrama*, vol. 1, Beacon House, New York.

Morrice, J. K. W. (1965), 'Permissiveness', *Brit. J. Med. Psychol.*, 38, p. 247.

Morrice, J. K. W. (1972), 'Myth and the Democratic Process', *Brit. J. Med. Psychol.*, 45, p. 237.

Morrice, J. K. W. (1973), 'A Day Hospital's Function in a Mental Health Service', *Brit. J. Psychiat.*, 122, p. 307.

Morrice, J. K. W. (1974), 'Crises, Social Diagnosis and Social Therapy', *Brit. J. Psychiat.*, 125, p. 411.

Morris, T. and Morris P. (1963), *Pentonville*, Routledge & Kegan Paul, London.

Mulkay, M. J. (1972), *The Social Process of Innovation*, Macmillan, London.

Myers, K. and Clark, D. H. (1972), 'Results in a Therapeutic Community', *Brit. J. Psychiat.*, 120, p. 51.

Myerson, A. (1939), 'Theory and Principles of the "Total Push" Method in the Treatment of Chronic Schizophrenia', *Amer. J. Psychiatry*, 95.

Nadel, S. F. (1959), *The Theory of Social Structure*, Cohen & West, London.

National Institute for Social Work Training (1967), *Caring for People: Staffing Residential Homes (the Williams Report)*, NISWT, 11.

Neill, A. S. (1968), *Summerhill*, Penguin, Harmondsworth.

Newman, O. (1973), *Defensible Space*, Architectural Press, London.

Nokes, P. (1960), 'Purpose and Efficiency in Humane Social Institutions', *Human Relations*, 13, 2, pp. 141–51.

Osgood, C. E. (1957), *The Measurement of Meaning*, University of Illinois Press, Urbana.

Palmer, B. W. M. (1973), 'Thinking about Thought', *Human Relations*, 26, p. 127.

Parker, T. (1971), *The Frying Pan: A Prison and its Prisoners*, Panther, London.

Parsons, T. (1957), 'The Mental Hospital as a Type of Organisation', in M. Greenblatt, D. Levinson and R. Williams (eds), *The Patient and the Mental Hospital*, Free Press, New York.

Pattison, M. E. (1976), *The Experience of Dying*, Prentice-Hall, Englewood Cliffs.

Paul, G. L. (1967), 'Strategy of Outcome Research in Psychotherapy', *J. Consulting Psychology*, 31, 2.

Perls, F., Hefferline, R. F., and Goodman, P. (1973), *Gestalt Therapy*, Penguin, Harmondsworth.

Perrow, C. (1965), 'Hospitals: Technology, Structure, Goals', in J. G. March (ed), *Handbook of Organisations*, Rand McNally, Chicago.

Pines, M. (1975), 'Overview', in L. Kreeger (ed), *The Large Group*, Constable, London.

Pines, M. (1976), 'Doctor–Patient Relationship', in S. Krauss (ed), *Encyclopaedic Handbook of Medical Psychology*, Butterworth, London.

Polyani, M. (1958), *Personal Knowledge*, Routledge & Kegan Paul, London.

Polsky, H. (1962), *Cottage Six*, Russell Sage Foundation, New York.

Punch, M. (1974), 'The Sociology of the Anti-Institution', *Brit. J. Sociol.*, 25, p. 312.

Punch, M. (1977), *Progressive Retreat*, Cambridge University Press.

Radcliffe-Brown, A. R. (1952), *Structure and Function in Primitive Society*, Cohen West, London.

Rapoport, R. N. (1960), *Community as Doctor*, Tavistock Publications, London.

Rees, J. R. (1945), *The Shaping of Psychiatry by War*, Chapman & Hall, London.

Rice, A. K. (1963), *The Enterprise and its Environment*, Tavistock Publications, London.

Richardson, E. (1973), *The Teacher, the School and the Task of Management*, Heinemann Educational, London.

Robins, C. N. (1966), *Deviant Children Grown Up*, Williams & Wilkins, Baltimore.

Roethlisberger, F. L. and Dickson, W. J. (1939), *Management and the Worker*, Harvard University Press, Cambridge, Mass.

Rogers, C. (1961), *On Becoming a Person*, Houghton Mifflin, Boston.

Rosenbaum, M. (1973), *Drug Abuse and Drug Addiction*, Gordon & Breach Science Publisher, Inc., New York.

Rosenberg, P. (1970), 'Hospital Culture as a Collective Defence', *Psychiatry*, 33, pp. 21–38.

Roscow, I. (1955), 'Research Memorandum: Patterns of patient referral to the Belmont Social Rehabilitation Unit', unpublished manuscript.

Rowan, J. (1976), *Ordinary Ecstasy*, Routledge & Kegan Paul, London.

Ruitenbeck, H. M. (1970), *The New Group Therapies*, Avon Book, New York.

Russell, B. A. W. R. (1967), *The Autobiography of Bertrand Russell*, Allen & Unwin, London.

Sanders, R., Smith, R., and Weinmann, B. (1967), *Chronic Psychoses and Recovery: An Experiment in Socio-Environmental Treatment*, Jossey-Bass, San Francisco.

Schiff, S. B. and Glassman, S. M. (1969), 'Large and Small Group Therapy in a State Mental Health Center', *Int. J. Group Psychotherapy*, XIX, 2, p. 150.

Schoenberg, E. (1972), *A Hospital Looks at Itself*, Cassirer, London.

Schon, D. (1970), 'The Stable State: Reith Lectures', *Listener*, 84, p. 2173.

Schutz, W. C. (1973), *Elements of Encounter*, Joy Press, Big Sur, California.

Seager, C. P. (1973), 'Psychiatry and Architecture: Brief for an Architect', Society for Clinical Psychiatrists.

Sharp, G. A. (1964), 'A Perspective on the Function of the Psychiatric Halfway House', *Mental Hygiene*, 48, p. 552.

Sharp, V. (1975), *Social Control in the Therapeutic Community*, Saxon House, Farnborough.

Simon, F. H. (1971), *Prediction Methods in Criminology*, HMSO, London.

Simon, H. A. (1948), *Administrative Behaviour*, Macmillan, New York.

Sinclair, I. (1971), *Home Office Research Studies: 6 hostels for probationers*, HMSO, London.

Skynner, A. C. R. (1974), 'An Experiment in Group Consultation with the staff of a comprehensive school', *Group Process*, 6, p. 99.

Smelser, N. J. (1962), *Theory of Collective Behaviour*, Routledge & Kegan Paul, London.

Sommer, R. (1969), *Personal Space – A Behavioural Basis for Design*, Prentice-Hall, Englewood Cliffs.

Sommerhoff, G. (1969), 'Abstract Characteristics of Living Systems', in F. E. Emergy (ed), *Systems Thinking*, Penguin, Harmondsworth.

Springman, R. (1976), 'Fragmentation as a Defence in Large Groups', *Contemporary Psychoanalysis*, vol. 12, p. 203.

Stanton, A. and Schwartz, M. (1954), *The Mental Hospital*, Basic Books, New York.

Stotland, E. and Kobler, A. C. (1965), *The Life and Death of a Mental Hospital*, University of Washington Press, Seattle.

Strauss, A., Schatzman, L., Erlich, D., Bucher, R., and Sabshin, M. (1963), 'The Hospital and its Negotiated Order', in E. Freidson (ed), *The Hospital in Modern Society*, Free Press, New York.

Street, D., Vinter, R. D., and Perrow, C. (1966), *Organisation for Treatment*, Collier-Macmillan, London.

Suchman, E. A. (1967), *Evaluative Research*, Russell Sage, New York.

Sugarman, B. (1968), 'The Phoenix Unit – an alliance against illness'. *New Society*, vol. 11, pp. 830-3, 6 June.

Suttie, I. (1935), *Origins of Love and Hate*, Routledge & Kegan Paul, London.

Syz, H. (1961), 'A Summary note on the works of Trigant Barrow', *Int. J. Soc. Psychol.*, VII, 4, p. 283.

Szasz, T. (1970), *Ideology and Insanity*, Doubleday, New York.

Szasz, T. (1974), *Ideology and Insanity: Essays on the Psychiatric Dehumanisation of Man*, Penguin, Harmondsworth.

Szasz, T. and Hollander, M. (1956), 'A Contribution to the Philosophy of Medicine: The Basic Models of Doctor-Patient Relationship', *A.M.A. Arch. Int. Med.*, 97.

Talbot, E. and Miller, S. C. (1966), 'The Struggle to Create a Sane Society in the Psychiatric Hospital', *Psychiatry*, 29, p. 365.

Titmuss, R. M. (1968), *Commitment to Welfare*, Allen & Unwin, London.

Tooth, G. C. and Brooke, E. M. (1961), 'Trends in the Mental Hospital Population and their effect on future planning', *Lancet*, 1, pp. 710-13.

Townsend, P. (1962), *The Last Refuge*, Routledge & Kegan Paul, London.

Trist, E., Higgin, G. W., Murray, H., and Pollack, A. B. (1963), *Organizational Choice: capabilities of groups at the coal face under changing technologies*, Tavistock Publications, London.

Truax, C. B. and Carkuff, R. R. (1967), *Toward Effective Counselling and Psychotherapy*, Aldine, Chicago.

Turner, V. (1969), *The Ritual Process*, Routledge & Kegan Paul, London.

Ullman, L. P. (1967), *Institution and Outcome*, Pergamon, Oxford.

Vickery, A. (1974), 'A Systems Approach to Social Work Intervention, its uses for work with individuals and families', *Brit. J. Social Work*, 4, No. 4, pp. 389-404.

Walk, A. (1976), 'Medico-Psychologists, Maudsley and The Maudsley', *Brit. J. Psychiat.*, 128, p. 19.

Walton, H. J. (1970), Introduction to *The Management of Alcoholism*, B. Ritson and C. Hassall (eds), Livingstone, Edinburgh and London.

Walton, H. J. (ed) (1971), *Small Group Psychotherapy*, Penguin, Harmondsworth.

Weber, M. (1947), *The Theory of Social and Economic Organization*, Oxford University Press, New York.

Weber, M. (1948), 'Bureaucracy', in H. Gerth and C. Wright Mills (eds), *From Max Weber*, Routledge & Kegan Paul, London.

Wepman, J. M. and Heine, R. W. (1964), *Concept of Personality*, Methuen, London.

White, W. F. (1967), 'Models for Building and Changing Organisations', *Human Organisation*, 26, 1/2, p. 22.

Whiteley, J. S. (1970), 'The Response of Psychopaths to a Therapeutic Community', *Brit. J. Psychiat.*, 116, p. 517.

Whiteley, J. S. (1978), 'Dilemma of Leadership in the Therapeutic Community, *Group Analysis*, vol. 11, pp. 40-7, 1 April.

Whiteley, J. S., Briggs, D., and Turner, M. (1972), *Dealing with Deviants*, Hogarth Press, London.

Wilensky, H. and Hertz, M. (1966), 'Problem Area in the Development of a Therapeutic Community', *Int. J. Soc. Psychol.*, XII, 4, p. 299.

Wiles, H. (1949) (Chairman), *Second Report of the Standing Committee on the Rehabilitation and Resettlement of Disabled Persons*, HMSO, London.

Wilkins, L. T. (1964), *Social Policy, Action and Research*, Tavistock Publications, London.

Wilkinson, P. (1971), *Social Movements*, Pall Mall Press, London.

Wills, D. W. (1941), *The Hawkspur Experiment*, Allen & Unwin, London.

Wills, D. W. (1971), *Spare the Child*, Penguin, Harmondsworth.

Wittgenstein, L. (1968), *Philosophical Investigations*, translated by G. E. M. Anscombe, Blackwell, Oxford.

Wootton, A. J. (1977), 'Sharing: Some notes on the organisation of talk in a therapeutic community', *Sociology*, 11, pp. 333-50.

World Health Organization (1953), *Report of Expert Committee on Mental Health*, WHO, Geneva.

Yablonsky, L. (1965), *The Tunnel Back*, Macmillan, New York.

Zeigenfuss, J. T. (1976), 'The Therapeutic Community from 1970 to 1975: A review and comment', unpublished thesis, *Dauphin County Commission for Treatment and Programme Developments*, Harrisburg, Penn.

Zeitlyn, B. (1967), 'The Therapeutic Community — fact or fantasy', *Brit. J. Psychiat.*, 113, p. 1083.

Zubin, J. (1964), in H. H. Hoch and J. Zubin (eds), *The Evaluation of Psychiatric Treatment*, Grune & Stratton, New York.

Index of therapeutic communities and support institutions

General Index